BABY CATCHER

 Chronicles of a Modern Midwife

PEGGY VINCENT

Scribner

NEW YORK   LONDON   TORONTO   SYDNEY

SCRIBNER
1230 Avenue of the Americas
New York, NY 10020

First Scribner trade paperback edition 2003

SCRIBNER and design are trademarks of
Macmillan Library Reference USA, Inc., used under license
by Simon & Schuster, the publisher of this work.

For information about special discounts for bulk purchases,
please contact Simon & Schuster Special Sales:
1-800-456-6798 or business@simonandschuster.com

Designed by Kyoko Watanabe
Text set in Bembo

Manufactured in the United States of America

10

The Library of Congress has cataloged the Scribner edition as follows:
Vincent, Peggy, date.
Baby catcher : chronicles of a modern midwife / Peggy Vincent.
p. cm.
1. Midwives. 2. Midwives-Anecdotes. I. Title.
RG950.V563 2002
618.2'0233-dc21
2001054988

ISBN-13: 978-0-7432-1933-4
ISBN-10: 0-7432-1933-3
ISBN-13: 978-0-7432-1934-1 (Pbk)
ISBN-10: 0-7432-1934-1 (Pbk)

The author has changed the name of some individuals and
the details of some births in this book.

Baby Catcher is dedicated to
all the midwives everywhere.

Acknowledgments

During my fifteen years as a midwife, many babies timed their arrivals to coincide with the night of our family's annual Christmas party, my children's birthdays, school pageants, family gatherings, and the hours between midnight and four A.M. Every midwife should be blessed with a partner like Rog, my husband of thirty-six years. He unfailingly appeared at my side, ready to carry my equipment to my VW bug as I headed out for yet another inconvenient birth. With patience and versatility, he filled in whenever I was absent, doing everything except fold laundry.

Eternal love and gratitude to our three children, Colin, Jill, and Skylar. They could have resented the little souls that took me away from them, but they never made me feel guilty, not even when I missed Christmas morning two years in a row.

But even before my husband and children, there were my parents, Mary and Bill MacRobert, who always believed I could do whatever I set out to do. They still do.

For years, many people urged me to write this book, but none were as persistently obnoxious as Sally Gambrill, my friend from college days. Nag, nag, nag. Like a puppy with a sock, she just wouldn't quit, promising to line edit for free if I'd just write it. So I did, and she kept her promise, eventually reading these chapters so many times she knows them by heart. All she wants in return are California Meyer lemons, but even if I dedicate a whole tree to her, I'll still be in her debt.

A serendipitous chain of events resulted in my contract with Scribner. It all began with a class at Book Passage in Corte Madera that led to Dorothy Wall, a Berkeley writing consultant. She helped me hammer my book proposal into shape and then pointed me toward an agent, Felicia Eth. A week later, Felicia and I agreed to our partnership before we'd even finished our lattés.

Felicia smiled at my neophyte enthusiasm, patted my sweaty hand, and mailed my proposal off to several New York publishing houses. Two weeks later, I had a contract with Scribner, where Jane Rosenman nurtured me through the first edit. When Jane left to spend more time with her children, Jake Morrissey assumed the role of doula and helped me deliver *Baby Catcher* on its due date.

Thanks to *San Francisco Chronicle* columnist Adair Lara, my first writing teacher, for teaching me how to "show, don't tell"; for scrawling "death to adverbs" all over my first efforts; and for hooking me up with Marie, Lyssa, Bibby, and Holly, my first writing partners.

I would happily sit forever at the feet of Philip Lopate, who assured me I'd be published and then added, "I'd be honored to write a blurb for your book."

I can't say enough about the nonfiction group of The Internet Writing Workshop. Ann Hutchins, Barbara Mullins, and many others provided invaluable critiques, but I'm especially grateful for the relentless nit-picking of Dawn Goldsmith, who hacked at these chapters till her keyboard bled.

Humble thanks to Dr. Bill Stallone, who first backed my practice and seemed to enjoy swinging from the branches as much as I did. Jim Jackson, Joe Weick, and his partners Hank Streitfeld and Betsy Kanwit, and Lisa Keller followed. I know they faced resistance from their peers, and I'm grateful for their faith in me and for their support of women who wanted home births.

Thanks to Carole Hagin, the gifted midwife who nurtured me through my first ten home births and allowed me to ride her coattails for a year before cutting me loose to dance on my own.

Heartfelt thanks to Sandi MacKenzie. She served not only as my first home birth assistant but also presided over the home birth of Skylar, my youngest child. In addition, she gave permission for me to share her caramel recipe (see Appendix VI).

After Sandi left for midwifery school, Kathy Heilig, Margaret Love, and Bonnie Bruce assisted me. My thanks for their speedy response, enthusiasm, and skilled help at hundreds of home births.

Many thanks to the nurses at Alta Bates Hospital who welcomed my patients and gave them special attention. I especially thank Ann Beckes, Cherie Campbell, Cheryl Jacques, Cindy Speltz, Doris Burleson, Holly Wagner, Irene Terestman, JoAnne Koury, Lois Carelli, Lori Prescher, Lynn Polon, Maggie Halliday, Marion Johnson, Marybeth Abarbanel, Mijo Horwich, Rita LaBarge, Robin Calo, and Wencke Roed. Many of them honored me further by asking me to deliver their babies.

I appreciate the women who have attended my strength training class at the Oakland Hills Club. They laughed at my stories, advised me what to wear when I met my agent, and took me to lunch at Oakland's Garibaldi's restaurant to celebrate the sale of *Baby Catcher*. The hamster Beanie Baby they gave me sits on my computer and is my muse.

Perhaps most of all, I thank the Berkeley couples who trusted me to deliver their babies. I see them all the time at places like Cody's Books or Safeway. At Peet's Coffee or the Cheese Board I'm likely to spot someone with a six year old that I caught. While waiting at my son's orthodontist's office, I recognized another mom, and she pointed out her teenager whom I'd delivered.

I'm profoundly thankful for my years as a baby catcher. I've had a good run.

Contents

PART VII

PART I

As it was in the beginning

"As it was in the beginning, is now,
and ever shall be, World without end."

Gloria Patri
The Declaration of Absolution
Book of Common Prayer, 1928 version

~ *You Have to Lie Down*

Please lie down," I begged Zelda. "Please."

Wearing nothing but a shiny coat of sweat, the young black woman stood upright on her hospital bed, stomping from the lumpy pillow to the foot rail and then back again. For the past fifteen minutes she'd been running laps on top of her bed, towering four feet above me as I raced along the floor with my arms outstretched in the futile hope that I might catch her if she fell.

"It's against the rules to do that," I whined, aware of how prissy and juvenile I sounded, but I was just a student nurse, and I'd be in trouble if I couldn't control this crazy pregnant woman. I tried another line of reasoning. "You might hurt yourself, not to mention your baby." Yeah, that sounded better. But she wasn't buying it.

Moaning, she sped to the head of the bed, tromped on the pillow with her callused feet, and grimaced as another labor pain began. Shaking her head from side to side, she banged on the wall with her thin hands. I watched the line of her vertebrae sway like beach grass in the wind while she dealt with the pain.

"Lordy, lordy, sweet Jeeeesus, help me, Lord. Yes, Lord, stay with me and guiiiiide me. Mmm-hmm, yes, yes, sweet baaaaaby Jesus. Umm-hmmm . . ." As the contraction wound down, she murmured, "Thank you, thank you."

She was twenty-two, in labor with her third child, and so skinny I could see the tendons in her arms and the sharp angles of bones in her face. Even with her belly sticking out in front, her hipbones jutting beneath the brown skin were easily visible. I saw the baby's knobby heels and elbows moving just below the surface of Zelda's taut abdomen. It was the only part of her that was big. It looked as though the child in her womb had drained all the nutrition out of her body and into its own, like sand in an hourglass moving from one chamber to another.

Short of tackling her, I didn't think I could convince her to lie down, so I pulled up the safety rail but saw the low barrier would contribute nothing toward preventing a fall. I lowered it, shaking my head in confusion and wondering what Mrs. Purdue, my instructor, might say. But then I figured rules are rules, especially when you're a student nurse, so I hauled it up again. I saw Zelda's half-smile as she watched me from the head of the bed. Blushing, I could just imagine what she was thinking: up, down, up, down, what is this crazy white girl gonna do next?

Then Zelda turned again and headed toward the foot of the bed, lurching and reeling above me, and I thought, Lord, she'll just trip over the bar and land on her head. So I lowered the rail and this time I left it down. Besides, it gave me better access to her. I thought maybe I could rebound her onto the bed like a basketball if she fell.

Zelda mostly ignored me, and I knew I looked as ridiculous as I felt. Earlier that morning as I snapped up my denim-colored uniform, I had no hint I'd be assigned to an uncooperative woman who refused to follow the rules. A year on the medical and surgical floors where so many of the patients seemed to be suffering from rare or lethal diseases had left me wondering if perhaps I should transfer into elementary education. Maybe I wasn't cut out for nursing.

But just the week before, I had discovered a passion for obstetrics. All it had taken was seeing my first delivery, and I knew I'd found a reason to stay in nursing school. Everything changed the day that little baby unfolded into the doctor's arm, threw his hands overhead, and screamed. It was more astonishing than any magician's stunt. Seeing a white dove fly free from a wizard's cupped hands paled in comparison to watching a glistening baby with pink fingernails and wet eyelashes appear from inside a woman's body. It wasn't magic. It was real. In that moment I knew I wanted to spend my life caring for women having babies.

But now as I stared at Zelda, I thought, Maybe I should become a teacher after all.

Hints about some Frenchman named Lamaze and a fad called Natural Childbirth bounced about in obstetrical circles, but doctors still believed the worst kinds of pain people experience are childbirth and kidney stones. Consequently, the few women whom I had seen give birth received narcotics during labor and breathed gas while pushing.

But Zelda was different. Zelda refused pain medication. And Zelda was making my life miserable.

"Just lemme outta this bed, girl. I need to walk these pains off, umm-hmm, you know what I'm talking about?" She slung one foot over the edge.

I planted myself in front of her with my arms out. "Zelda, we can't have labor patients walking all around the department. Really, I can't let you out of the bed. Are you absolutely sure you don't want some pain medicine?"

"Uh-uh, no needles for me. No, ma'am."

"But it seems like it hurts a lot."

"It wouldn't hurt so much if y'all would just lemme up. You had any kids?"

Oooh, I wanted to lie. I wanted to say, 'Sure I've had kids, two of them, and I was a good patient who stayed in the hospital bed. I kept my skimpy hospital gown on the whole time, tied right up the back. And I was quiet,' but I didn't think she'd believe me. Although I'd just turned nineteen, I looked about fourteen. On top of the blue uniform I wore a pinafore, and the hospital laundry used so much starch that the skirt never moved, even when I bent my hips or knees. With my blond hair confined behind my neck, the effect was more Alice in Wonderland than mother-of-two.

"No," I admitted, "I don't have any children. I'm not married yet."

"Oh, well, shoot, honey, neither am I, but I've had me two babies. They was delivered by my granny down in Tennessee, and I can tell you, I'm going back to Granny Vida if I have another one. Mmm-hmm, I'm sure not comin' back to Mr. Duke's hospital. Mmm-mmm, no. Granny let me walk, see, yes, she let me walk and sing and dance my pains away. Ooooh, here come another one. Ohhhhh, Lordy, oh, sweet Jesus, umm-hmm, come to me and help me, mmm-hmm, yes, guide me and bring me up out of these troubled waters, up and into your arms. Ahhhhh, yeoooow, oh Baby Jeeeeeesus! Yes, yes, yes, yes . . . and I thank you."

Wow, I thought, shaking my head, this woman sure read a different rule-book from all the other women I'd seen give birth. I'd just never even heard of anyone behaving like Zelda.

I glanced for the umpteenth time at the doorway. Any minute Mrs. Purdue would swoop around the corner again. The instructors didn't leave us alone for more than half an hour in obstetrics, a service where conditions often change with dramatic suddenness.

"Why you keep lookin' out that door, huh? Ain't nobody out there having a baby, is there?" She stood still and craned her neck to see past the bedside curtain.

"No, it's just that my instructor'll be here soon . . . umm . . . and I don't think she's gonna, you know . . ."

"What, girl? What you tryin' to say?" With one hand on her cocked hip, she peered at me with narrowed eyes. Staring straight ahead at her knobby knees, I knew that to her I was just a foolish white girl who'd never had a baby and wouldn't let her get up.

"Zelda, I wish you'd lie down. I've never heard of anybody walking on the bed before."

"Oh, I see. She gonna get mad at you for what I'm doin'. That it?"

"Well . . ."

"Tell you what. You ain't gonna let me outta this bed, right?" and I nodded so vigorously my cap slid toward my eyebrows and I had to pin it back in place. "I'm fine, honey, and trust me, I ain't gonna fall. So you just stand where you can see when she's acomin' and then you give me a sign, and I'll lay me down in this here bed quick as a face-slap upside the head. Ohlordlordlord, here comes another one and it's a *biiiiiig* one. Oooooooh, yes, Jesus, Jesus, Jeeeeeeesus, oh Lord, raise me up unto the highest mountain where thy mercy shiiiiines the brightest. Yes, oh yes, my Saaaavior. Ummm-hmmm, oh my Lord. Lordy me . . . Whew, that'n' made me sweat some, girl, sure did."

So that's what we did. When Mrs. Purdue's white uniform rustled toward us, Zelda slumped to the bed, and I yanked the sheet over her angular nakedness. She grabbed my fingers, and I stroked her forehead. When Mrs. Purdue bustled through the doorway with every teased poof of hair in place, Zelda and I presented a perfect picture of cooperation and competent nursing care. As soon as my instructor left, Zelda leapt to her feet and continued her pacing, pausing now and then to hum a churchy tune and drum her fingertips on the overhead light.

Then Zelda winked at me, and as she flashed her smile full of crooked teeth I knew we were in it together, conspirators at a birth. An hour passed this way, and I smiled and nodded my head in rhythm to her Gospel chanting. And she was right. She didn't fall. I was the one who did the falling as I fell under her spell. It was as though I'd stumbled into a piney woods revival tent and been transported by the spirit of a new religion. She made the process look like so much fun, I almost wanted to dance with her.

Then her dance changed. She turned her back to me and leaned her elbows against the dingy wall. In a slight crouch she stuck her bony bottom way out behind her and rotated it like a hula dancer. All the while she crooned to herself and beat on the wall with her fists. "Oh, Vida, Vida, Granny Vida. Help me, help me, oh, my Lord and Saaaaavior. I will lift up mine eyes unto the hills from . . . whence . . . cometh myyyyyyy help!!! Yeowy, ummm-hmmm, oh yes. Oh, my soul. Lord, now baby, don't you be takin' much longer, y'hear?"

She glanced down and said, "Is it okay me making some noise, honey? Do they allow that around here in Mr. Duke's fancy hospital? I mean, havin' babies takes some *talking,* girl, you know?"

I giggled and said, "Well, so far you're getting away with it, Zelda."

"Thank you, sweetheart, thank you. I'll keep singin', but I'll try keepin' it soft, for your sake. Don't wanna get you in no trouble, no ma'am, 'cause you bein' real good to me. You gonna make a fine nurse, you know that?"

About half an hour later her sounds changed again as she began to grunt and moan. A feral smell invaded the room. Puzzled, I watched while she squatted lower, pressing her hands on her thighs as sweat dripped from her chin and ran in glistening trickles down her back. She became very quiet, and now and then she gasped and held her breath. Bright shreds of bloody mucus dripped from her body, leaving scarlet smears on her legs and the sheet beneath her.

Suddenly it occurred to me what she was doing. She was pushing her baby out, still standing on top of her bed.

I grabbed her knees, trying to pull her down as I shrieked, "Zelda, you can't stay like that! Lie down! You have to lie down! What if the baby falls out?"

She pushed at my hands, and her eyes locked onto mine. Between teeth clenched in a grimace, she said, "What if the baby falls out? What if . . . it . . . falls . . . out, is that what you said? Well, darlin' *that's the whole point,* ain't it?"

I stared at her for a moment with my mouth hanging open as her words sank in.

The whole point. Of course.

But when she squatted lower and pushed harder, I jerked back to reality. "Oh, my God, I need to get the doctor," I muttered, turning away.

Zelda's claw-like fingers stopped me. Radiating heat from the sweat and passion of birth, she pushed her face close to mine and rasped, "No. Nonononono, just leave it be. You can do it. Just you. You and me, girl."

The blood left my face. My hands went numb as a cold stone of fear landed in my stomach. An instant one-way ticket right out of the university loomed before my eyes.

But the next moment an army of nurses and doctors pushed past the curtain, propelling a stretcher ahead of them. Zelda's cries and grunts had been heard, and within half a minute they wrestled her onto the stretcher and whisked her toward the delivery room. She screamed and kicked and begged them to leave her alone, but there were too many of them. I followed behind, staring at her hand grabbing for me like a lifeline, a way out, a piece of floating debris on a stormy ocean.

They rolled her from the gurney to the delivery table, tied her legs high in stirrups, strapped her hands at her sides with thick leather cuffs, and put a mask over her face. Zelda fought them at every turn. Like an octopus, she grew what seemed to be eight arms and legs and the nurses struggled to restrain her, throwing their full weight against her as she fought with the unholy strength of panic and despair.

"She doesn't want drugs or gas," I whispered. "She just wants to do it her way."

"What? Did you say something to me?" muttered the doctor with the gas mask, battling to keep it over Zelda's face while she slammed her head from side to side.

"She doesn't want gas. She told me." I blushed beneath his stare. Student nurses didn't talk to doctors. Not ever.

"Oh, Christ. She's a crazy woman, totally out of control. She's gotta have the gas or she'll do herself harm, and her baby, too. Wacko, goddam bitch."

Zelda somehow wiggled one hand from the leather restraint. She tore the mask from her face, and it separated from the plastic tubing. Finding the hated mask free in her hand, Zelda threw it across the room where it crashed into the metal door of the sterile supply cabinet. Then she spit at the doctor and reached across to undo the strap that held her other hand down. Two nurses rushed forward, and I watched them yank both cuffs to their tightest link around her thin wrists.

"Jesus Christ, why do we let these women breed?" growled the doctor standing between her legs. A quarter-sized patch of baby's hair shone in the glare of the overhead spotlight. Another push or two would do it.

Zelda rolled her head toward me and looked into my soul.

Tears clouded my eyes, and I bit my trembling lips. She mouthed the words, *help me,* as the anesthesiologist pulled another mask from the cabinet. Zelda took a huge gulp of air just before the mask descended. I saw the doctor crank the mixture higher, hoping to put her under before she attacked him again. But Zelda wasn't breathing.

Slowly, slowly, the baby's head slipped free of her body, and then the rest of the little boy flip-flopped head over heels into the doctor's lap. I smiled down at Zelda. Her eyes bulged above the mask. She looked like she was about to explode.

She knew the baby was out. So did the doctor. Why didn't he take the mask off her face? "It's born," I said to him, stating the obvious. "The baby's out."

"I know, I know," and he pushed the dial even higher.

Zelda realized he was determined to knock her out, no matter what, and she went wild again, tossing her head and making strangled sounds from beneath the cushioned mask. She kicked and bucked with every ounce of her strength but succeeded only in rattling the delivery table till I feared the bolts would shake loose.

She couldn't keep it up forever, but her face turned deep purple before she finally sucked in a tremendous mouthful of the gas. Her fists and spine relaxed, and her head rolled to the side as she slumped into unconsciousness. When the doctor lifted the mask, dribbles of spit hung out the side of her slack mouth before dripping to the pillow.

"Jeezis, I'm glad this one's over," growled the doctor.

Invisible in my student uniform, I stood beside her as they untied her arms and legs and moved her onto the gurney. A tall nurse carried the bundled baby out the door, and I thought, Zelda doesn't even know it's a boy. I slipped my fingers into her loosely curled hand and held it as I watched another nurse jam a white sanitary pad between her dark and bloody thighs. When they stretched her legs out flat, her belly wrinkled like a deflated brown balloon and slumped between her angular hipbones.

I stared at her a moment, and then I grabbed a sheet from the linen shelf and covered her nakedness, wanting to do more.

So much more.

~ *Babies, Babies, Babies*

I f I'd been born ten years later, I'd have probably become a doctor or lawyer. But when I wrestled with college and career choices in 1958, midway through my junior year of high school, good little girls could be secretaries, nurses, or schoolteachers, and that was it.

"Be a nurse. You'll always be able to get a job," Mother said. She looked forward to returning to nursing as soon as my little sister began kindergarten.

"Be a nurse," my father echoed. "It's the best preparation for being a good wife and mother." Dad always felt motherhood represented a woman's highest calling.

Even then, I sensed something wrong with his line of thinking, but as a docile child of the fifties, I followed their advice and embarked on Duke University's four-year path to a Bachelor of Science in nursing. I could study the Reformation, the Revolutionary War, and Rimbaud while completing my nursing studies at a top-ranked medical center. Besides, Duke was a thousand miles from my parents' Michigan home—an extra ace in the deck of life for any seventeen year old.

Along with Duke's hundreds of other madras-shirted, starry-eyed freshmen, all 110 first-year nursing students shouldered a typical load of six liberal arts classes. But the next year the nursing school began piling science courses onto our bouffant heads: anatomy, biology, physiology, chemistry. Nearly a third of our class abandoned ship, but I hung on.

Day one of sophomore year, our corseted nursing arts instructor taught us that properly made beds have mitered corners and a pan of reeking vomit is called an emesis basin. All the patients who crossed my path had come to Duke because of its research facilities, and they all had terrible, terminal, or disfiguring diseases. Not my cup of tea at all, at all, as my Irish grandmother would've said. My brain screamed, "Honey, you've made a big mistake. Run home, find a nice secretarial school, and learn shorthand."

But just before I threw up my hands in surrender or threw up my lunch into an emesis basin, my obstetrical rotation began. The first time I saw a baby born, the mother lay moaning on the stark delivery table as her enormous belly heaved with each contraction. "Push harder!" shouted the nurse, and then a squirming, squalling baby lay in the doctor's hands. A big baby. I blinked and, struggling with sudden tears that blurred my vision, thought I must have missed some important piece in the mystery. How did that happen? I looked between the mother's legs. The umbilical cord led up through a small, bloody opening into a dark and unknown world. How could that huge baby have come out of that little hole?

I was hooked. I thought if I saw lots more babies born, perhaps I'd discover that missing bit of information, the secret of that enchanted moment when one person suddenly becomes two people. But even now as I look back on the thousands of babies I've watched enter the world, I still don't understand it. I kneel between a woman's legs with an eight-pound baby in my hands, and I glance at the vaginal opening—and something from the scientific left side of my brain wants to scream in disbelief. Impossible, I say. It's all mirrors. It simply can't have happened.

Then came Zelda. After her delivery, I knew I'd make it through med-surg, psychiatry, and public health. I knew my passion for obstetrics would last a lifetime.

Passions other than my own stirred in the South during the sixties. Although no students of color attended Duke at that time, geography alone should have given us front row seats. But we listened and watched from a distance declared safe by the dorm mothers, middle-aged women whose permanent waves curled as tightly as the cramped restrictions under which we lived. It was as though we'd bought SRO tickets and peeped over the heads of others, craning our necks for a view of the social drama. Voting drives and school desegregation. Governor Wallace with his dogs. Joan Baez and Bob Dylan singing songs of protest. Conflict spread from Detroit to Los Angeles, from Selma to Washington, D.C. Battles raged everywhere, but they didn't penetrate Duke's hallowed Gothic campus. Our honeysuckle world remained serene, protected, and oh so white.

As the sun set at the end of those long, hot afternoons, frogs croaked in the woods, magnolia blossoms drifted to the grass, and the Westinghouse fans whirred in our windows. We sat on the cool linoleum floor in white cotton underwear, and between bridge hands we shared snippets of our day. Some of my classmates told of bizarre behavior on the locked psych unit. Others talked about children with cystic fibrosis or toddlers maimed by drinking lye. Diseases we'd never heard of a year earlier now spiced our dinner table conversations: lupus, scleroderma, Huntington's chorea.

My stories all revolved around babies. Black and white babies. Big and little babies. Breeches, twins, preemies, and stillborn babies. Childbirth provided the drama I craved, the thrill of peeking over the primal edge of creation, the rush of the unexpected. Textbooks taught me the science of obstetrics, but I learned the art of birth from babies and their mothers.

Every time a baby unfolded like a butterfly from the cocoon of its mother's body was a moment I suspended rational thinking and accepted a miracle. I watched one day as a woman lay straining on the delivery table, and slowly her baby's head emerged. Beneath the pale green drapes covering the mother from chin to toes, I rested my hand on her belly. When the baby's shoulders came out, I felt something that made me gasp. The baby's tiny bum rose up against my hand, and I felt him curling into a tuck. A moment later, he thrust his legs out straight and flutter-kicked like a dainty swimmer as he left his watery environment and made his way into our world.

I blinked and held my breath, trying to memorize the moment. I figured maybe another piece to the puzzle had dropped into place. I didn't realize that no matter how many times I felt the baby leave the womb with my hand as I saw it enter the world with my eyes, still I would not have the answer. How can this be?

But not all my stories ended with happily ever after.

There was Princess Ann, a thirteen-year-old who brought a stuffed bunny to the hospital with her. Like many young teenagers, she progressed quickly. When she became noisy, I gave her a shot, and she dozed through the next couple of hours. Suddenly Princess Ann sat bolt upright, staring at me in stony silence as she grimaced. Her smooth brown face darkened to deep blue, and she pushed only twice. I delivered her baby's head before the doctor arrived to catch the rest of the skinny little boy, a baby with high cheekbones and close-set eyes. Mostly ignoring the real live baby in the crib beside her, she slept with the dusty bunny tucked under her chin.

Princess Ann had five sisters under eighteen, and three of them had also given birth in the past year. A month later, I took a bus to her tarpaper, shantytown shack across the tracks to examine her infant. John Kennedy's photograph torn from a recent issue of *Life* magazine gazed from the wall opposite the front door. A bedroom door hung ajar, and in the dim light beyond I saw a tangle of arms and legs. On any other day, the grunting and thrashing in the sheets would have riveted my attention, but just to my left lay Princess Ann's baby. Lying on an overstuffed chair, he cried, kicking his little frog legs four inches below a sputtering electric skillet teetering on the broad armrest.

I picked up the damp baby and navigated an obstacle course among a mass of squirmy babies and toddlers with gray diapers hanging half off their bottoms. A striking sameness to their high cheekbones and close-set eyes made me think they were siblings, but they were too close in age for that to be possible.

One sister, Margaret Rose, caught my eye and turned proudly in profile, posing. She didn't move until she saw that for sure I'd noticed. About five months along, I guessed.

Then a blade-jawed, ebony man swaggered from the dark bedroom and leaned against the doorjamb while he buckled his belt. I met his eyes and stared into his insolent face, a face with eyes set much too close together atop those now familiar high cheekbones. A girl of about sixteen came from the darkness behind him and leaned against his hip, trailing her fingers across his bare chest. She wore only a thin slip, and the soiled strap hung off her shoulder.

With sweat beading my brow, I looked away first, blushing as I wiped my clammy hands on my slacks. He saw and laughed, a harsh barking sound. Then he lit a cigarette and turned back into the bedroom, yanking the girl-child along behind him.

"That my momma's boyfriend," said Princess Ann.

I licked my dry lips, checked the baby, and fled back to the safe predictability of the campus. That evening I told my friends about Princess Ann, my fingers trembling as I rolled my hair on curlers the size of juice cans.

"Well, you can't save the world," they said. But I didn't sleep that night.

Another sultry evening I shuffled the cards, sipped Budweiser from a cardboard milkshake container—we called them chocolate Buds—and talked about babies born to the wives of university professors, doctors, and tobacco barons, pretty women schooled in the southern art of "making nice."

There were women like Melinda Bascomb, who curled her hair and applied fresh makeup before coming to the hospital. Thanks to twilight sleep, a combination of a narcotic and an amnesia agent, she didn't give a hoot what she looked like by the time she delivered. Anyway, the next day she wouldn't remember anything. She wouldn't remember climbing over the side rails and squatting above the wastebasket. She wouldn't recall throwing the water pitcher at me or using cusswords she'd probably never before said aloud. She kicked and scratched and pulled out her IV, but she wouldn't remember.

Melinda finally delivered her baby, sleepy and blue-tinged from drugs. She smiled a goofy smile and thanked the doctor for a wonderful birth as I shook my head and thought, If you only knew.

A few weeks later I told my roommate, Marcia, about Mrs. Richardson, a forty-five-year-old woman who'd just delivered her eleventh child. Blind from congenital cataracts, she'd passed her affliction to half her children. Her wiry, seventy-six-year-old husband sprinted up two flights of stairs to the family planning clinic and zoomed back down with handfuls of free condoms, leaving the tired young residents open-mouthed in awe.

Because Mrs. Richardson didn't pee every time she coughed, the doctors refused her request for a tubal ligation. Incontinence and imbecility were the only valid grounds for sterilization. It's the law, they said. The laws changed before I graduated, however, and sterilization became available on demand. Doctors holding clipboards jogged a two-step alongside the gurneys of groggy welfare moms who'd given birth twenty minutes earlier, catching them while memories of the pain were still fresh.

"How many babies you got, momma?" the doctor asked.

"Four, sir, yassuh, I got me four babies, mmm-hmm," came the tired response.

"How was that labor for you? That sure looked like it hurt some."

"Lordy, yes, that hurt me somethin' awful," and I knew what would come next.

"You wanna be doin' this again next year, momma?"

"Uh-uh, no sir. May sweet Jesus be my witness, I don't wanna go through that pain no more."

"Sign right here," purred the doctor. The next morning the same woman lay in the recovery room after her tubal ligation, not exactly sure what had been done to her.

More often, though, I told happier stories. As we sat around a circular cafeteria table wolfing down eggs and grits, I told my friend Nancy about Marianna, the schoolteacher wife of Jerry, a third-year medical student. As she neared the end of labor, we rolled her onto a gurney, and Jerry went to the waiting room at the far end of the hall.

We wheeled Marianna through two sets of heavy double doors and into the enormous delivery theater, a room with a set of bleachers at one end, five rows deep and twelve feet wide. When an unusual delivery absorbed everyone's attention, those bleachers would be packed. It could be a baby coming feet first that caused a crowd to gather, or a forceps rotation of a baby facing the wrong way. Perhaps twins or triplets made the medical students come running, or the consummate skill required by a difficult mid- or high-forceps delivery. Today all those babies would greet the world through a cesarean incision.

But Marianna's delivery was routine, so no audience gathered. I stood by her side, watching her grip the mask of Trilene anesthetic to her face. As her baby's head filled the vaginal opening, she gasped once and then shrieked in a high, soaring tone that made me flinch. The reverberations still hung in the air when we heard another sound.

Bang! went the first set of double doors.

Bangity-bang-bang went the second set.

Then, *Wham!* The delivery room door slammed against the tiled wall, and Jerry skittered into the room.

Jerry's blue jeans, Kingston Trio T-shirt, and scruffy, high-top basketball shoes constituted a serious break in sterile technique, and I waited for the doctor to send Jerry out the door with his tail between his legs. But Dr. Hammond, one of the more relaxed physicians, just snorted with laughter as Jerry glanced around, pinned to the spot by his own embarrassment. Almost any other doctor would have yelled at him to go put on a scrub suit, mask, and shoe covers, and Jerry would have done it. But he'd have missed the delivery, because the baby was so close its bald head looked like a tennis ball about to be ejected from a sock.

Jerry laid his head on his wife's shoulder, wrapping her in his arms as he stared over the mound of her diminishing belly. I pressed my hand to my lips, and my eyes glittered with unshed tears. The nurse saw me and smiled like a fond auntie. I saw her catch Dr. Hammond's eye and nod in my direction. He looked at me and then back at the nurse, and the two of them knew they'd just seen a student nurse hit by a sentimental sucker punch. I'd never before seen a father present at his child's birth. As I stared at Jerry and Marianna, their tears mingling on each other's cheeks, I knew I'd want it like that when I birthed my own babies.

Fortunately, those same swinging doors ushered other women like Marianna and Zelda into the delivery room. They came in huffing and puffing, and I gravitated toward them like steel to a magnet—women who knew what they wanted and didn't want anyone messing with them. Such women were the stuff and substance of the best stories I brought back to my indulgent, bridge-playing friends, stories that made my heart sing in the retelling.

I lived for these occasional women, the ones who were different, who thrived on the challenge and the passion. The women who wanted to sigh and moan and deep-breathe through their labors, to move around in the bed, to squeeze my hands and look into my eyes. They pressed their sweaty foreheads against mine as they hissed in and out between clenched teeth—and I hissed along with them, pulling the curtains to keep the world away. I shut the doors and tried to keep them quiet, to shield them until it was too late for intervention. Too late for anyone to steal their births from them.

These were the ones who touched my heart and fed my fire.

~ Mrs. Purdue

John F. Kennedy was killed two days after I turned twenty-one. One day, Camelot; the next, chaos. Although graduation hovered six months away, nothing seemed certain any more. For hours, my friends and I did nothing but stare at the TV in the third floor lounge, transfixed.

I dragged myself to work at the hospital the next afternoon. Hushed conversations and shocked expressions replaced the usual hubbub in the delivery room. Nurses in white stockings and doctors in blue scrub suits stood hugging their elbows, shaking their heads, wiping tears from their cheeks.

I didn't think anything could overshadow the mind-numbing national events, but I received an assignment intimidating enough to take my mind off JFK, at least for a little while. Because of short staffing, the head nurse put me in charge of all the uncomplicated laboring women. There was only one. Mrs. Purdue, my obstetrical instructor from last year, would be my patient.

"But-but-but," I sputtered.

"Can't be helped, dear. You'll do fine," said the head nurse as she swished into the room of a woman in premature labor.

Mrs. Purdue, I thought. She was nice enough, but she was my teacher, for heaven's sake. I couldn't believe it. I sighed and walked into the large labor room.

Mrs. Purdue lay in the far-left bed. My shoes squeaked. A curtain on an overhead pole hid her from my view. I strained my ears. Not a sound. Should I knock? How do you knock on a curtain? What if I found her on a bedpan expelling her enema? Oh, Jesus, Mary, and Joseph, help me get through this shift. Let her not deliver till I'm off duty. Let me get back to Dallas and Jacqueline Kennedy's bloodstained pink suit. Even listening to LBJ's swearing in on

Air Force One appealed to me more than pulling back the curtain and saying hello to Mrs. Purdue.

But that's exactly what I did, knocking my cap askew as I pushed back the swinging folds of pale yellow cotton. I blushed and muttered, "Hello, Mrs. Purdue." Covering my embarrassment, I ducked my head and pinned my cap back in place.

She looked up from the pillow, her sprayed bouffant hairdo an exact duplicate of Jacqueline Kennedy's, except Jackie had dark brown hair and Mrs. Purdue was a bleached blond. And Mrs. Purdue wasn't wearing a pink suit. She wore a hospital gown with a blue-gray print that looked like my grandfather's pajamas.

"Peggy? No, they wouldn't do that."

I knew what she was about to say, and I didn't want to hear it. "Actually, Mrs. Purdue, they would. They did. I can't believe it myself. I just don't . . ."

She reached out her hand and placed it on my arm.

I froze. "What?" I said, wondering what I'd done wrong so soon.

But she smiled, a big, sincere smile, and her eyes went all soft like she saw not an uncomfortable senior nursing student, but a cuddly puppy. "Oh, you poor thing!" she crooned. "You must be so nervous."

"Nervous? Me? Why would I be nervous, Mrs. Purdue?" I babbled. "I'm not nervous. But I know you were expecting the head nurse to care for you." I took a breath and blathered on. "But we're short-staffed, and there's a woman with toxemia and another in premature labor and one who's bleeding, and, well, I'm the only one left."

"Shh, here it comes."

Startled, I looked over my shoulder, thinking she meant someone might overhear us, but that didn't make sense. I took another look at her and realized she meant a contraction had started. She pressed her hands to the mattress, rocking back and forth and humming deep in her chest like a cat purring.

Should I touch her? I wondered. What did she expect? As the contraction ended, I put my hand on her shoulder and said, "Uh, good job. How close are they?"

"Oh, not closer than four or five minutes, but they're starting to get a little stronger." She sat up and swung her legs over the side of the bed to face me.

"Can I lean against you?" she asked.

"Sure, sure," I gushed, grateful to be told what to do.

Half an hour passed, and with each contraction I touched her with more confidence. I rested my hands on her shoulders between pains, retied her gown so it wouldn't slip off, and draped a wet washcloth across the back of her neck.

Soon I began to hum with her, and before long I almost forgot who she was. This felt like familiar territory. She stared into my eyes, and I met her gaze, nodding my head in time with her steady breathing. I heard myself talking softly to her, unaware of the actual words I spoke, just fitting them into the pattern of her humming. I rocked with her swaying body and allowed her to slump against me toward the end.

And often she smiled and patted my hand. She still made me feel like a waggle-tailed puppy, but I kind of liked it. She relaxed and took a deep breath. So did I.

"We'll do fine together. And we'll have fun, you'll see," she whispered.

Fun? Well, I wasn't too sure about that. The fun part, I mean. I'd never heard a woman say that labor held the promise of fun. That possibility stretched my imagination a little too far. And although I began to feel better about relating to her as just another woman in labor, in between the contractions she was still my teacher.

"Mrs. Purdue, would you like . . ."

"Peggy, you're going to have to stop calling me that."

"What?"

"Mrs. Purdue. Just call me Kay. In hard labor I won't respond to 'Mrs. Purdue,' so you might as well start saying 'Kay' right now."

"Okay . . . Kay. Sure."

I wondered if she'd like her husband to come for the birth. It would be unusual, of course, but they'd begun making exceptions for bigwigs and doctors' wives, and I thought they'd probably extend the privilege to Mrs. Purdue.

"Mrs. Pur . . . Kay, shall I see if I can get the doctors to let your husband be with you? I think it'd be possible."

"Oh, I've already cleared it with Dr. Hammond, but I don't want John here till the end. He's taking care of our little boy, and Timmy's not too keen on being left with our neighbor."

"But Dr. Hammond's not on call. It's Dr. Atkinson."

"Chuck—Dr. Hammond—agreed to come in and deliver me, even though it's his night off. We've been working on hypnosis for pain control."

"Whoa, hypnosis! That's great. Did you use it with your first child?"

"Oh no, I had Timmy in a military hospital. What a nightmare. Those memories haunted me when I got pregnant again, so Dr. Hammond offered to try hypnosis. I figure it's got to be better than what happened before."

As she talked, I learned her first birth hadn't been complicated or danger-ous, just frightening. She'd been drugged, neglected, and left alone for hours at a stretch. Mrs. Purdue wanted more control this time.

We watched the sun set, and by six P.M. her pains crowded close together. She sat upright at the bedside with her legs apart. I stood between her knees with my hands on her shoulders, and she rocked me back and forth, follow-ing some internal rhythm I could only imagine. In between, she rested her head on my chest while I massaged her shoulders, waiting for the next one.

She even dozed, something I'd always associated with women sedated with drugs in labor. But here was Mrs. Purdue sleeping between the contractions, and I found I could tell when one started even before she could. She became restless, her spine tensed, and her breathing quickened. Then she jerked awake and began deep breathing, swaying just as Zelda had. Also like Zelda, Mrs. Pur-due began talking to herself. Different lyrics, but the tune sounded so familiar.

"Oh, yes, open, open, open wide, no tension, no fear, no pain. Just open-ness and acceptance. Mmm-hmm, I can do this. Yes . . . I can do this."

Swaying and chanting. Zelda and Mrs. Purdue. I couldn't help noticing the similarities in their behavior. Perhaps it was a common response of women laboring without drugs, without fear. And with support.

Mrs. Purdue shifted to let me rub her lower back. As she lifted her thigh, I saw bright blood on the cotton pad beneath her. She saw it, too. "Maybe you should check me," she suggested, using her damp gown to blot the sweat from her cheeks. Her eyes looked even greener than usual, green as dragonfly wings in the middle of twin smudges of mascara. Some of her lipstick had smeared onto the bib of my uniform.

"I'll get someone, um, yeah . . ." I hedged, edging away.

"Peggy. This is your job. Check me."

"Oh, sure, no problem," I muttered, feeling the heat of my blush. God, I could not *believe* I was going to do this.

I put on the exam glove without looking at her. When I turned around, she lay on her back with her knees bent and her thighs spread, completely exposed. With her grandfather-print gown tucked under her armpits, Mrs. Purdue lay naked from her breasts to her toes. I looked at the ceiling as I felt between her legs, groping for anatomical landmarks. I finally found the hills and valleys that told me I was in the right county.

Oh, wow, eight centimeters! And a big bag of water bulging pretty low. No wonder she had all that bloody discharge. If her water broke, she'd hop onto a speedy, one-way street toward delivery. Time for her husband and Dr. Hammond to be on the scene. Any later would be too late.

I hollered down the hall, telling the clerk to make the necessary phone calls.

In my desire to protect her modesty, I'd waited too long to call the doctor. Mrs. Purdue's labor shifted into high gear, and for the next thirty minutes I worried I'd blown it.

Mrs. Purdue struggled with tension, too, and the closer she got to delivery, the more she sounded and acted like Zelda. She perspired heavily and began to tremble. "Mmm-mmm-mmm, yes, uh-huh, I can, I can, I can. Open wide, oh, wider still! Relaaaaax, softly, now. Soft. Soft. Soft. Ahhhh."

She sat up again, legs dangling a foot above the floor. She banged her heels into the bed frame, rocking and moaning. Her voice strained toward a new high as she gripped my shoulders and pulled me back and forth till I felt like a sapling in a hurricane. It was a birth dance of sorts, but she'd definitely taken the lead. I could only let her use me any way she saw fit. I hummed when she hummed. I crooned when she crooned. I swayed when she swayed. When she squeezed me, I squeezed back.

At the end of each contraction, Mrs. Purdue smiled at me. I smoothed back her damp hair, rubbed her tight shoulders, fanned her with the empty glove wrapper, gave her ice chips—and smiled back.

Finally, after about twenty years, Dr. Hammond and Mrs. Purdue's husband arrived. Their broad shoulders collided in the doorway—one in blue hospital scrubs, the other in blue madras plaid. Mrs. Purdue stretched her arms and cried, "John!" as another contraction began. I stepped back.

She tried doing with John what she'd been doing with me, pulling, swaying, rocking, but he had just walked in, uninitiated to her style.

"Come on, Kay. Hold still. Relax," he urged, trying to take charge.

"Open, open WIDE. Aagh, move with me, John!" She shook him, trying to force him to dance the dance, but he gripped her shoulders. "Shh, Kay, Relax. Be quiet."

"Yeeeeeoooowww."

Dr. Hammond intervened. "Look into my eyes, Kay, and blink slowly . . ."

"It's too late for that shit!"

I stared at her. Swearing? Screaming? Until the two men arrived, we'd just been two women doing a pas-de-deux. Something had shifted.

"I'll get someone to give her a shot," the doctor said.

"No! Nonononono! Don't want drugs, dammit. Just gimme her!" She grabbed the starched bib of my uniform, yanking me toward her with enough force to risk whiplash.

Zelda, young, poor, black, on welfare, a nobody in the eyes of the establishment, had had no support for her desires. But Mrs. Purdue? A white woman with private insurance, a nursing instructor with the university, a professor husband, and a favorite patient of the chief resident? She had an ample power base from which to make demands.

The two men froze at her imperious tone. They watched as once again she and I melded. Once again I hummed and swayed and crooned. Once again she rocked, pulling me with her as if I were in a rocking chair, rhythmically, on and on, until the endless contraction faded away.

And once again I smoothed her hair and fanned her. And smiled at her. She squeezed my shoulders and flopped her head on my chest. I felt her spine relax. She fell asleep.

Dr. Hammond laughed and said, "I think we're going to be having a baby real soon, and it's gonna be on her terms."

Again I thought of Zelda. Her terms. Her terms that had not been honored.

Suddenly Mrs. Purdue reared back and looked straight into my eyes. She didn't say a word, but her face turned purple, and her fingernails dug into my shoulders. I knew how a mouse must feel when an owl swoops from the sky on soundless wings and snatches him from the meadow. I flinched, but she just dug in deeper as if she feared I'd try to escape.

Dr. Hammond ran to the doorway and yelled down the hall, fast, garbled words ending with " . . . and she's *pushing!*"

People in blue and white rushed in and jockeyed a gurney to the bedside. Dr. Hammond fumbled between Mrs. Purdue's legs. John clenched his hands under his chin and backed up till I thought he'd disappear into the wall. With her sharp nails imprisoning me, Mrs. Purdue pulled my face into her chest. I smelled her sweat. Her chin dug into the top of my head as she curled into another silent, Olympian push.

An orderly wrestled her shoulders toward the gurney, but Dr. Hammond shoved him aside and shouted, "Jesus, leave her alone. The baby's right here."

A flustered nurse hollered, "Get a precip pack!"

Mrs. Purdue yelped as the bag of water broke with a gush that drenched Dr. Hammond's arms from the elbows down. He jerked back momentarily and then lunged forward, pressing his whole palm over her crotch. From my vantage point on her chest with my nose about ten inches from the action, I saw the doctor cup his spreading fingers over a growing mound of dark hair as if he were palming a fuzzy tennis ball.

"John, you can't see from back there," said Dr. Hammond, sounding surprisingly calm. "Come over here."

"I'm okay. Right here is fine." John didn't sound nearly as calm as Dr. Hammond. I couldn't see him because Mrs. Purdue had wrapped both of her arms around my head, hugging it as if she were trying to deflate a beach ball.

As she started to push again, Dr. Hammond said, "Hey, Kay, Kay, listen to me, woman. Slow down a little, will you? Just blow or yell or something, but don't push so hard. Christ, it doesn't *need* to come any faster."

So she screamed. She screamed right into my ear. She screamed with a high, soaring, House of Horrors sound that reverberated inside my head and then faded away as another sound filled the room, the soft, uncertain wail of a newborn trying out her lungs for the first time.

Suddenly Mrs. Purdue let go of my head.

I stood up very slowly. I rotated my head and shrugged my shoulders a few times. I moved my jaw this way and that. When I stretched my back with my arms over my head, something popped. Dr. Hammond glanced at me and smiled as he clamped the umbilical cord. John moved a few steps closer and took a peek. Mrs. Purdue pushed herself onto her elbows and stared at her flailing daughter, crying now with more self-confidence.

The smell of birth hung heavy in the room. The sharp odor of sweat, the cloying sweet scent of blood, the faint bleachy smell of the amniotic fluid. The astringent tang of the Betadine poured into a basin that suddenly appeared at Dr. Hammond's elbow.

I backed into the cluster of professionals standing around with smiles on their faces. John reached one fingertip toward the baby, and Mrs. Purdue grabbed his other hand, pulling it to her lips. A nurse lifted the baby, dried her off, and wrapped her in a huge bundle of thick blankets till she looked like a big-eyed Eskimo baby lost in the depths of a parka. The nurse started to whisk her away to the nursery, but Mrs. Purdue's strangled, keening "Nooooooooo . . ." stopped her.

The nurse stood still and looked at Dr. Hammond. If conscious, new mothers usually had a quick glimpse of their newborns before an obligatory four-hour observation period in the nursery. Most of the mothers were too drugged to care.

Dr. Hammond looked from Mrs. Purdue to the nurse and back again. Then he said, "Let her have the baby, okay?"

"But, Doctor, what if she drops it?" said the thin-lipped nurse, pulling herself up to her full height.

"I don't think that's very likely. I'll take full responsibility."

I could see the nurse wrestling with The Rules, but she returned to the bedside and placed the baby into Mrs. Purdue's outstretched arms. Then she grabbed my elbow and jerked me closer. "Stand here, missy, and be useful. Be sure she doesn't drop that little baby, y'hear?" I nodded. She adjusted her cap and marched out of the room.

Mrs. Purdue tore her gaze from her baby's big searching eyes and looked into mine. She said, "Well, that certainly wasn't how I planned it, but I have no complaints. None at all. And I never could have managed it without you. Thank you so much."

"Oh, you're welcome, Mrs. Purdue," I gushed, and if I'd had a tail, I'd have wagged it. "I loved it, and you were right. It was fun!"

"Please, call me Kay. To you, I'm Kay. Forever."

"Sure, Kay."

When I climbed the stairs to my dorm room that night, I avoided the end parlor where the bluish light of the television illuminated hushed and somber faces. I couldn't deal with them, with the assassination, the sadness and broken dreams, the national heartache. I needed to stay with that birth a little longer, with Kay and me swaying and humming together, with the sight of the baby emerging just inches from my eyes, with Dr. Hammond's kindness. With the smells and sights and sounds of a special birth.

I'd just witnessed a birth unlike any of the others I'd seen. One in which the woman herself made the decisions. In six months I would graduate into a world in which Lyndon Johnson sat in the White House as Vietnam sucked young men into early graves. Jim Ayton, my high school prom date, flew jets over the Mekong Delta; he never came home. Neither did Bill Heep, a gentle boy I had a crush on at fifteen. Nor Sean, the freckled redhead who sat beside me in a Duke history class. Civil rights marches, student demonstrations, Kent State, and hippies. Haight Ashbury, Patty Hearst, and little girls in white dresses in a church in Birmingham.

The country trembled in transition, everything changing.

Including obstetrics. I wanted to be part of that change. I wanted to help create some of the changes. I wanted more women to have births they could look back on and say, "That was fun."

~ *The Hippie Effect*

How did a nice Midwestern girl like me end up in Berkeley, California, in 1970, with twenty-two scruffy hippies crowded into her living room? It was love, of course. I live surrounded by extremes of lifestyle because I love a man with an aversion to extremes of temperature. Roger Vincent, the boy who would become my husband, chose a university in the South because he hated Boston's winters, and he planned to live in California because he hated Boston's summers.

While we were at Duke together, he taught me to double-clutch his 1931 Model A Ford down the meandering, dogwood-lined roads between Durham and Chapel Hill, and we became engaged in Duke's Rose Garden. In June 1965, as the shadows lengthened on the lawn of an ivy-covered Episcopal church in Michigan, we strolled arm-in-arm down the aisle, then headed for a honeymoon in Bermuda in a pastel cottage that bore a striking resemblance to our wedding cake.

On our return, we loaded wedding presents in the trunk of our new blue Buick Skylark, stashed luggage and snacks in the back seat, and drove straight west toward the Pacific Ocean. Oncoming cars flashed their headlights, signaling for us to turn down our high beams. We blinked back to show we didn't have them on. Those beleaguered other drivers had no way of knowing our trunk was weighted with so much wedding booty that it tilted down in the back like a jet as its front wheels leave the runway, almost airborne.

It all feels normal now, but back when my wedding ring gleamed like a newly minted coin, Berkeley took some getting used to: foggy summers cold enough to demand goose down, autumns warm enough to be summer, rainy winters so short I barely noticed, and springs erupting in February with freesias and poppies, lupine and wild iris.

"Everybody here eats foods beginning with A," I wrote home. I learned the art of eating an artichoke and the joy of scooping the pulp from an avocado cupped in my palm. I devoured arugula salads, abalone with lemon and capers, and my first fresh asparagus.

I worked as a public health nurse in a Mexican barrio for the first four years of my marriage, years during which the country struggled under the influence of anti-Vietnam War demonstrations and the resulting peace movement. Public health nursing hadn't been an interest of mine at Duke, but I succumbed to the lure of regular hours, a sweet benefits package, and a pay rate 25 percent higher than hospital nursing offered.

I visited elderly TB patients in their homes, ran a prenatal clinic, immunized hundreds of dark-haired, large-eyed babies against polio and diphtheria, and taught a birth control class, the first one ever offered in the local Mexican community. Many bureaucrats swore none of the neighborhood women would dare attend a clinic offering birth control pills and IUDs, but within a week the lines of patient women snaked down the tiled hallway and stretched across the lobby.

"Well, I'm Catholic, but not *that* Catholic," said one shy matron when I routinely asked, "Religion?" while recording her intake history. She left the clinic that day with three months' worth of contraceptive pills.

Thanks to twice-weekly Berlitz classes, I augmented my high school Spanish with enough additional medical terms, verb tenses, and a sprinkling of new nouns and adjectives to permit me to get by without a translator. I also used my Spanish to order lunch from the noisy neighborhood mom-and-pop restaurants. I ate *albóndigas* (another "A" word!), *quesadillas, menudo,* and *flautas,* listening to loud mariachi music interspersed with Jimi Hendrix, Janis Joplin, Bob Dylan, and the Beatles.

Although I enjoyed the work, grew to love my little eight-block neighborhood, and really liked having weekends free and no night shifts, I began to miss the excitement of the delivery room and wondered what I was doing in a public health uniform. I wanted to share again the intensity of those moments surrounding birth, that instantaneous transition from great pain to great joy that transforms women's faces as they push babies into the world. In the spirit of those serendipitous years, I quit my cushy day job and took a position in labor and delivery at Berkeley's Alta Bates Hospital.

Everyone living in the Bay Area has heard of Alta Bates. Known as one of the best hospitals in California, it was still privately owned when I began working there in 1970. Alice Minor Bates, a diminutive, single-minded woman of uncommon compassion and drive, founded the hospital in 1905, and in the next twenty years, the eight-bed facility expanded to a 112-bed hospital. A full-service medical center with 555 patient beds and more than 900 physicians on staff now stands on the original site. From its inception, Alta Bates Hospital was known as *the* place to give birth in the East Bay, and it still proudly carries that distinction.

Three hours into my first day of orientation, a frantic ER orderly shoved a stretcher into my hands, hollered, "She's pushing," and fled. The purple-faced patient dug her fingernails into my wrists as I spun the gurney into the nearest empty labor room. Twisting free of her grip, I wiggled her maternity pants down and, as the next contraction began, I caught her flailing, wailing baby with my bare hands. Slippery amniotic fluid trickled from my elbows, and I knew I'd come home, home to the place where a tight pair of maternity pants might be the only barrier to birth; where the rhythm of the day can change with the suddenness of a handclap. It was desire for that unpredictable and fast-changing rhythm that had brought me back.

Along with the back-to-the-earth, bread-baking, and tie-dying philosophies of the hippie era came the belief that nothing could be more natural than having babies. "Lamaze" became as common a word as "layette." On that issue, at least, I seemed finally to be in sync with the counterculture population. I became a certified Lamaze teacher and offered a six-week series of evening classes in my home.

I actually believed that, if you followed the method, childbirth oughtn't to hurt—at least, not much. I realized Zelda had tried to show me something important, but I figured she probably wouldn't have needed to do all that pacing and chanting if she'd been trained in Lamaze.

Those eleven hippie couples in my living room that night didn't know I was three months pregnant with my own first baby. When I'd cared for Zelda eight years earlier, I'd been tempted to lie and say I had a couple of kids, just to provide validation for my daring to presume to tell her how to act. I still felt embarrassed by my childlessness. Who did I think I was to teach women how to handle labor? Why should they believe me, a childbirth virgin? But they did. I'd been teaching for nearly a year already, and those trusting couples soaked up every word I said. I kept thinking one day someone would expose me as a charlatan. I'd feel a lot more qualified to teach these classes once I'd finally been through the experience myself.

I looked around again at this new group of credulous faces. The men, mostly bearded, wore overalls or bell-bottoms. The women, mostly long-haired, wore long skirts and no bras. They each clutched two pillows, and they all had the same goal: to learn the Lamaze method so the women would be awake and aware when they gave birth. And their men would be there, too, coaching them through each contraction, wiping their brows, and sharing the exciting moments around the actual delivery.

The women sneaked looks at each other, probably checking out who looked like she'd gained the most weight. The men knew they were revolutionaries on more than just political frontiers. After centuries of society's viewing childbirth as strictly women's work, these men aimed to be labor coaches and had faithfully followed their pregnant wives into the Lamaze arena. Persuaded into spending one night a week talking about heartburn, leg cramps, hemorrhoids, backaches, leaking breasts, cervical dilation, and all things vaginal, a few of them still had a trapped look in their eyes. They stared at the ceiling, their fingernails, their tattered sandals, anywhere other than the fecund bellies surrounding them. Yep, just a standard group, I figured.

I began by asking them some questions. Turning to one fellow, I checked his name tag and said, "Steve, what do you want to learn most of all?"

The only guy in the room with short hair and no beard, Steve wore overalls that looked cleaner than most, and his shirt might even have been ironed. Probably a recent transplant from Iowa, I mused.

He folded his hands in his lap and said, "I want to learn to deliver a baby."

"That's not really the focus of these classes, Steve," I said. "It's not likely you'll ever need it."

"Well, I needed it. Outside. In the rain. So I really want to be prepared this time."

Dead silence. Everyone stared at him, especially the guys.

Steve smiled like a second-grader in the front row, waiting for class to begin.

"I think you're going to have to elaborate just a teeny bit, Steve."

"Yeah, man," said a scrawny guy in patched overalls. "I mean, like, *what?*"

"Oh," Steve said, looking surprised at the sudden attention. "Well, we were watching TV, and Polly here," and he put his arm around the wispy Mia Farrow look-alike at his side, "... well, she was kinda antsy, right? Squirmy. She got up to go to the bathroom, but before she'd taken four steps she dropped to the floor and screamed the baby was coming. She was pulling at her pants, these really tight capris with elastic sewn across the top of the open zipper. They were all wet and bloody, and she was screaming and rolling around on the floor. So I picked her up and carried her to the car."

His blond wife piped up, "We lived in an apartment on the third floor with outside stairs."

"Yeah, and then I delivered our baby, Jason. I'd just like to know how to handle things better if it happens again."

He looked at me calmly, thinking he was finished.

"That's it? That's all you're going to tell us?" said a burly guy with fluffy hair and a Jerry Garcia beard. "Uh-uh, no way, brother, we need details!"

"I don't want to take up too much class time . . ."

I laughed. "Steve, trust me, you've got our total attention. No one's gonna listen to me till you fill in the facts."

"Well, so I picked her up and ran out of the apartment. It was rainin' like hell, and I had my slippers on, I remember. I got almost down to the first landing when she wiggled out of my arms like a wet tuna and kinda flopped around on the steps."

He paused and gave his young wife another hug while she twirled the wedding ring on her finger. "Then she started futzing with that elastic again," he continued. "And she's screaming and thrashing all over the place. And pushing. Yeah, I could see that she was pushing. I hollered at her, 'Jeez, don't push!' but she just keeps screaming, 'My pants! Get my pants off!'"

Polly peeked from her curtain of straight hair and said, "He wouldn't help. He just picked me up again and threw me over his shoulder like a fireman would've."

"I did not," Steve insisted with disgust in his voice. "I carried you in my arms as if you were Miss Scarlett O'Hara."

"Uh-uh, Stevie. You threw me over your shoulder. I remember looking down and seeing your butt crack."

Tension eased for a moment as couples exchanged looks and laughed.

Steve shrugged and looked sheepish. "Anyhow, I got down to the bottom with her kicking and screaming the whole way, but then she grabbed the wrought iron railing and damn near jerked me off my feet. And she's outta my arms again and down in the marigolds beside the walkway, diggin' her heels in the mud and tuggin' at those goddamn pants. And oh man, was it raining!"

I looked around the room. The men sat with their hands clenched between their knees and their jaws hanging down. The pregnant women stole quick glances at Polly and then at each other, praying, I was sure, that such a thing wouldn't happen to them.

"I could hardly see for the rain in my eyes," continued Steve, "but I ran to our VW bug by the curb and pulled the passenger seat forward. In those few seconds Polly shifted her slacks down to her hips."

"He just wouldn't help me get them off," repeated Polly in her little-girl voice.

"Well, damn, I'm thinking those pants were 'bout the only thing keeping that baby *in,* and that seemed like a fine plan in my mind, you know what I mean?"

Vigorous nodding from all the men.

"But it *hurt!*" insisted Polly.

Vigorous nodding from all the women.

"So anyhow," he continued, with an impatient glance at his wife, "I put her in the back seat of the bug . . ."

"Headfirst, on my back, and only halfway. Most of me was still in the rain."

"Well, yeah, that's true. I still wonder why I did it that way. I mean, on her back? No wonder I couldn't get her all the way inside." He shook his head at the memory. "Then she lifted her hips and worked the pants below her butt, and Jason's head came out right into the crotch of those capris."

"What?" shouted the Jerry Garcia guy. *"Judas priest!"* He turned and pointed to his wife. "Don't you even *think* of doing that!" She shook her head, wide-eyed.

"With those pants still around her thighs holding her legs together, there was no room for me to wiggle the rest of the baby out, so I hauled 'em down a little more. Then Polly screamed once, really loud, and she pushed the whole baby out. And I caught him."

He paused and glanced around the room. Ten speechless couples, hanging on his every word. Me, too.

"So I'm standing there in the rain, holding this screamin' baby. And I'm thinkin', what next? And then the afterbirth comes shooting out and drops right into the street. I stomped on it to keep it from floating away and dragging on the baby's 'umbiblical,' you know? I mean it was still attached. So there I am. Soaked. With a naked baby in my hands and my slipper on a bloody placenta in the gutter. And Polly with her legs wrapped around my knees and falling half outta the car. And the rain comin' down like it's the Great Flood, and it's cold, Christ, so cold. I didn't know what to do."

A young woman whispered, "So what *did* you do?"

"I did what any of you guys would have done, I guess. I just started screaming 'Help' over and over at the top of my lungs. And this nice couple came outside with an umbrella and a flashlight. The lady took care of Polly, pushed her the rest of the way into the back seat, and wrapped the baby in her jacket. That woman was so cool. She folded some newspaper around the placenta and tucked it right in beside the baby. She said it was okay about the cord and stuff."

"But don't you hafta cut it right away or something?" asked a woman in a long patchwork skirt.

Everyone looked at me, and I explained that there's no rush with cord cutting, and that the Good Samaritan woman had been correct. "Circulation through the cord stops quickly after the baby's born. It was wise for them to wait till they got to the hospital to cut it, though, so it could be done with sterile scissors."

"Yeah, that's what she said," agreed Steve, and all eyes turned back to him. "And she put her raincoat around me. Her husband called an ambulance, then came back with blankets and some brandy. And it all turned out okay. I mean, Jason's three now, and he's great. But I really don't want to do it like that again, see?"

Dead silence. I cleared my throat, and their faces spun my way as if I'd blown a whistle.

"Well, then. Yes, indeed. How 'bout if we begin this first class with emergency childbirth procedures? Anybody have a problem with that?"

Twenty-two heads shook. As I went over the nuts and bolts of supporting the perineum, crowning, delivering the shoulders, the basics of CPR, and what to do with the cord and the placenta, not one man stared at his sandals or inspected his fingernails.

Not one.

Five classes still remained. Plenty of time for me to teach them the Lamaze method of painless childbirth. And plenty of time for me to wonder what my own labor would be like.

PART II

The meditation of my heart

"Let the words of my mouth and the meditation of my heart be always acceptable in thy sight, O Lord, my strength and my redeemer."

PSALMS 19:14
THE HOLY BIBLE, KING JAMES VERSION, 1611

Painless Childbirth?

In 1971, pregnant with our first child, I expected labor to be a cakewalk. I'd been teaching natural childbirth classes for two years. I'd seen hundreds of deliveries. Although many of those women had taken Lamaze classes, most of them asked for drugs. I figured they must not have practiced enough. Surely I'd have no trouble at all. Who could be better prepared?

Talk about a setup. An hour after labor started, I realized I didn't know diddly.

My bag of water broke at midnight. Immediately, the contractions slammed into me every three minutes. I whimpered like a lonesome puppy in a big, dark backyard. The three kinds of Lamaze breathing didn't work. I didn't know if there were too many to choose from or not enough. I arched my back and groaned as I watched a possum prowl back and forth on the fence outside our open window. She peered at me as I gasped, "Uff-hee, uff-hee, uff-hee."

The Lamaze books advised, "Don't waken your partner until necessary." I grabbed the pamphlet from my cluttered bookshelf, just to be sure. "Let him sleep as much as possible," I read, "so he can be helpful to you later, when the going gets rougher." Rougher? I didn't want to think about rougher.

I resembled the composed woman in the booklet about as much as a toad resembles a prince. Clawing at my belly, I squirmed on the wrinkled sheets. She, the woman in that piece of Lamaze propaganda, reclined against pillows and rested delicate fingertips on her belly—and she was smiling.

I'll bet she wasn't really in labor when they took that photo.

My eyes fell on another line: "They'll feel like strong menstrual cramps."

Uh-uh. They didn't feel like that at all. It felt as though a meat grinder was doing unspeakable things to my lower abdomen. I silently apologized to the many women to whom I'd said, "Breathe quietly. Relax. Slow down."

My labor quickly became a global experience. My toenails curled backwards. The roots of my hair hurt. My fingers cramped up. Every muscle of my body felt connected to my uterus, and my five-foot-eight-inch self contracted into a concentrated knot of pain the size of a softball. I imploded into a black hole of efficient, uncaring pain and . . . disappeared. It wasn't even me anymore. I became Labor.

Time warped. I stared at the mocking minute hand, but, like a Dali clock melting over the edge of a table, it made no sense. I tried recording the start of each pain in a spiral notebook, but my desperate, scrawled numerals slanted and ran off the paper.

I never gave the baby a thought. This was epic, far bigger than one single baby. I was birthing a galaxy, a supernova. Lost in a void, my thoughts scattered like pinpoints of light from a Fourth of July firecracker.

"A deep pulling from within," the book had said. No, mine felt close to the surface, and I scratched my belly, trying desperately to touch the pain. I was outside, frantically digging toward the source of my pain. But I was also within, in and of the pain itself. Trying to rip free.

My contractions had no buildup, no "ah-another-one's-starting" phase. Unlike the "sounding brass or tinkling cymbal" mantra that repeated in my brain, my cymbals crashed offstage, without warning—exclamation points in a heroic symphony. Each contraction pounded me, just *there,* full force.

Between pains, I collapsed into a space of tense and empty silence. Empty for never more than a minute of waiting, waiting. Then, crash, lost again. The bang and battle of labor annihilated all that used to be Me.

I know from experience that earthquakes are loud. The roar of the shifting earth drowns out all thought. That's how my contractions felt, as though the pain transposed into the discordant screech and clamor of Mother Earth's sliding tectonic plates, my shifting pelvic bones, the whole world moving aside. I could hear them all—and nothing else.

Around three A.M., I hunkered on the bathroom floor and examined myself. Four centimeters. Still too soon to go to the hospital, I told myself, nearly sobbing.

Around five A.M., I clawed at my husband's back. He rolled over and stared at me. "What's wrong?" he whispered.

"Water broke. Labor. Hospital. Now."

We arrived at the hospital half an hour later. I gritted my teeth, denying my intense desire for drugs until the morning shift arrived and my favorite nurse came on duty. She examined me and said, "Seven centimeters."

I grabbed her hand and begged, "Drugs. Half dose."

With her, I didn't feel shamed by my weakness. She'd never had children, and I knew she believed that labor hurt like hell. She'd often said she couldn't understand why women would want to do it without drugs.

She laughed, patted my hand, and went to the narcotic cabinet.

The narcotic made me groggy and thick-tongued, but I no longer had an urge to leap from bed and pound the doorframe. An hour passed in that hazy space, and then my eyes flew open as a steamroller chugged down my belly. Without warning, I pushed.

That little blue book of lies had said, "Pushing is a relief. Finally you can work with your body." I'd believed it. I'd said it myself to rooms full of unsuspecting, pregnant women. "Pushing will feel wonderful. You'll love it."

Bullshit. Pushing hurt worst of all.

I screamed. Rog recoiled. Nurses rushed in. The doctor arrived in a swirl of white, examined me, looked over the tops of his dark-framed glasses and said, "Your tailbone's fused." The tailbone should operate like a swinging door; mine was latched.

He slipped forceps like salad tongs with extra-long handles inside me, and I had visions of the Inquisition, men in hoods with their faces covered, screams from other hidden chambers, clanking chains, and dripping water. The forceps handles locked, and when the doctor pulled on them, I howled. It felt like he was turning me inside out.

"Push!" everyone hollered.

Somehow I pushed, and with a crack that sounded like a grenade had exploded inside my pith helmet, my tailbone broke. Then . . . my son lay in my arms.

"It's Colin!" I gushed. "Oh, he's beautiful!"

No one agreed. No wonder. Mostly bright red, my baby had several large navy splotches on his face where it looked like he'd been pelted with ripe plums. His head went straight up, then slanted to the right where two huge hematomas bulged like lopsided Mickey Mouse ears. His whole face tilted asymmetrically, and a bloody gouge marred the corner of his left eye.

"Forceps trauma," someone explained. "It won't leave a scar." But it did— just a little crater, like a memento from chicken pox.

As I nursed my son during the following weeks, I brooded. Yes, my son's birth was a little unusual. A slam-bam-thank-you-ma'am labor and a fused tailbone aren't common, but I still felt humiliated that I'd asked for drugs. I thought of Zelda. I'd wanted to do the same things she had done. I'd wanted to get out of bed, to moan, to rock. To dance and writhe and boogie into the pain. I thought she'd needed her chanting and her rhythmic movements because she hadn't learned the Lamaze Method of Painless Childbirth. Now I wondered.

Painless childbirth? I don't think so.

Furious at the line I'd been sold, I wondered about this conspiracy to avoid the word "pain." My labor had hurt like hell, and I knew I'd never teach a straight, formulaic approach to childbirth preparation again.

During the following two years, I developed an eclectic kind of birth class.

"Every birth is different," I told the women. "Since you have no idea what kind of labor you'll have, how can you realistically train for it? Give yourself permission to experiment, to see what works best for you."

In each series, I spent a full hour acting like a woman in labor. I asked the guys to support me, two at a time, so they would get a sense of how it really feels to be with someone about to have a baby. I swore a little, hollered, twisted their belt loops, pressed my forehead to theirs, and made them rock with me in a dance that probably had origins in primitive Africa. I demonstrated a whole smorgasbord of options. I wanted the women to feel that anything that occurred to them, if it helped, was acceptable. I said, "Each woman needs to find her own path through the labyrinth of labor."

This role-playing proved to be the most popular part of my classes. Other childbirth teachers came to observe and incorporated the technique into their own classes.

One father, after his wife delivered, told me, "It was easy being with Rachel when she was in labor. She acted just like you did, so I felt like I'd been through it before."

While I was doing my little labor act on one occasion, I saw a look of real fear pass across one woman's face. Worried I'd overdone it, I called her after her birth to ask how it had gone. I laughed when she said, "Oh, it was perfectly normal, and by the way, I handled myself much better than you did."

When I found myself pregnant with my second child in 1973, I vowed I would listen to my body's wisdom. But once again, labor tricked me.

Three weeks before my due date, I awoke with a feeling of something expanding inside me. No contraction and certainly no pain, but throughout the morning, the expansions came every twelve to fifteen minutes. I did some laundry, nibbled cinnamon toast, helped Colin with a puzzle, and every time one of those surges began, I stood and rocked.

"Do they hurt?" Rog asked, watching me hum and sway through another one.

"Not a bit. It just feels better like this."

"Are they contractions?"

"No, more like expansions."

When I squatted, he raised his eyebrows.

"Pressure," I said, "like someone's inflating a beach ball inside me."

It dragged on all morning. Wondering if it might be the start of the real thing, I crouched in the bathroom with a sterile glove but couldn't find my cervix. Too difficult, I figured, in the weird yoga position I had to assume to reach over my belly and into my own vagina.

So I called Linda, a nurse friend, to come check me. She arrived with a big smile, but her face froze when she examined me. "You're complete."

"Bull. Can't be. They don't hurt a bit, and they're so far apart."

She checked again and pulled her hand out even faster, "Oh my yes, you're definitely complete. You need to get to the hospital. Now."

Rog deposited Colin in the arms of our neighbor, bundled me into his ancient VW van, and pulled away from the curb. My contractions became closer during the one-mile ride to the hospital, and the pressure localized down low, about as low as it could get without something coming out. In fact, I couldn't tolerate sitting on top of that pressure. I slid onto my knees on the floor of the car and gripped the handle above the glove compartment, the one we always called the chicken-shit bar.

At 1:10 P.M., I walked into the hospital, navigating the hallways as if I walked a tightrope. Spreading my hands to each side, I warned everyone away. It felt as though I was wired with dynamite. At the slightest touch, I'd explode.

I was so close to delivery that the nurse grabbed the first available doctor in the department. He hustled in and broke my bag of water. Until that moment, I'd felt suspended in a bubble of control, tense with the nearly heroic effort of staying calm and still in the core of my being. But as the amniotic fluid gushed out in an arc that soaked the doctor's chest, once again I heard the earthquake roar of labor.

I shrieked, then my mind left my body. Only the fact that the labor room had a high ceiling kept me from going into orbit. Looking down from my vantage point beside the overhead light, I felt like a celestial observer watching a total stranger give birth. At 1:20 P.M. my daughter flew out. The doctor had only one glove on and bobbled her twice in midair before crouching and snagging her in his lap.

"It's Jill!" I shouted. "Wow, it's a girl!"

"No, honey, it's another boy," said my dazed husband, who only moments earlier had been preparing for many long hours of labor. "But that's okay. We'll still love him."

Amazed, I looked at him. Then I glanced back at the baby and understood Rog's confusion. The umbilical cord snaked around her hips and looped up beside her puffy labia, swollen like the genitals of all newborns. Yeah, I figured, I could sorta see how he might think she was a boy.

"It's a girl," I repeated, but he shook his head.

I sat up and grabbed the baby's feet. Spreading her legs beneath the doctor's astonished eyes, I said, "That's a girl. Trust me. I know what girls look like."

We went home the next morning. Joy flooded my whole being, and right behind it came pride. I felt so smug. Smug that I'd figured out how to labor painlessly. Smug that the thought of drugs never entered my mind. Smug that I had a boy and a girl. Smug at how terrific I felt, like Miss America with a tiara, cape, and bouquet of long-stemmed roses.

During the following weeks, I cuddled Colin with one arm while holding my nursing baby girl with the other—and I pondered. Why had I felt almost no pain? Why, when I thought it was just false labor, did I allow myself to rock and chant and sway instead of doing fancy breathing? I'd given myself permission to do things I'd denied myself during my first birth. How might Colin's birth have been different if I'd behaved differently? I couldn't believe it had taken me so long to internalize the lessons that Zelda and Mrs. Purdue had tried to teach me ten years earlier.

A month later I sat at our kitchen table nursing Jill while Rog stood at the counter cutting spiny tops from artichokes. "Wouldn't it have been something if my bag of water had broken at home?" I said.

"Lord, Peggy, we'd never have made it to the hospital."

"Yeah, we'd have had her at home. Probably right there," I said, pointing to a spot in the middle of the kitchen floor, "and you'd have delivered her."

He stared at me, knife motionless. "Oh, my God."

"It would have been fun."

"Fun?" His voice rose with disbelief.

"Yeah. Let's think about having the next one at home with a midwife."

He laid the knife down and faced me. "Midwife? At home? The . . . next one?"

I smiled at him.

~ *To Be or Not to Be*

I'd never paid much attention to the local lay (unlicensed) midwives. They'd always been a shadowy presence lurking on the fringe of organized medicine. But as I realized how close I'd come to an unattended home delivery with Jill's birth, I began watching for these mystery women. They were hard to spot.

They never showed up at all, of course, if their planned home deliveries went off without a glitch. We saw them only when a complication made it necessary for the laboring mom to come to the hospital. Some of the midwives disappeared at the door of the emergency room, but a few stayed with their patients, trying to act like a sister or friend. Usually they ducked into the bathroom or hid behind a pillar at the approach of any doctor or nurse. None of them had a license or hospital privileges, and very few had a friendly backup doctor.

I began to realize their furtive behavior didn't reflect a lack of confidence. They simply feared exposure. When her patient's labor stalled or problems developed, the lay midwife had two choices: abandon the woman, or stay and risk prosecution for practicing medicine without a license. No wonder they were elusive.

Then in 1974, a labor dispute at Alta Bates left us so short-staffed that doctors mopped the dirty delivery rooms and we had to divert many patients to other hospitals. That's how I met Carole Hagin. The chief of obstetrics asked her to come sit with the laboring moms to relieve the nurses of some of their tasks. At last I had an opportunity to watch the most respected of the local lay midwives in action.

Carole had had seven children before becoming a childbirth teacher. She attended many births as a labor coach, a person we now call a *doula,* and soon she was catching babies on her own. I'd heard people say she'd been born with her midwifery skill, that it was in her DNA.

Remembering those words, I watched her. She cradled and rocked the women in her arms, and I wondered if she crooned magic spells into their ears. The women stared into her eyes, did whatever she told them, and sang her praises forever after. When I asked her later what she was doing, she laughed and said, "Just using verbal anesthesia, talking them through labor."

I wondered what it would be like to be cared for in that calm, nurturing way by such a wise woman. And then I had another thought: how wonderful to actually BE that wise woman myself. For the first time, I considered becoming a midwife.

A revolution erupted in the field of women's health during the early and mid-seventies, The hippie ethos of the late sixties expanded to encompass feminist politics. Many women turned to herbalists and acupuncturists for health care. Copies of *Our Bodies, Ourselves* appeared on bookshelves, and women used plastic disposable speculums to examine their own cervixes. They performed Pap smears on each other, some learned simple abortion procedures, and they attended each other's births. They wanted more than permission to use Lamaze or Bradley techniques. They wanted a full menu of birth options. During those years, my style of teaching birth classes dovetailed perfectly with what many Berkeley women wanted.

The medical establishment swayed and then buckled to the wishes of the pregnant population. The first local alternative birth center, staffed entirely by the midwifery service, opened in 1975 at San Francisco General Hospital. In 1976, San Francisco's Mt. Zion Hospital also started a birth center, decorating a room with ferns swinging from macramé hangers, a brass queen-size bed, a round oak table, and no hospital equipment in sight. Just for the thrill of being on the cutting edge of the whole birth center phenomenon, I drove across the Bay Bridge several times a month to moonlight at Mt. Zion.

Back in the East Bay, Alta Bates was one of two hospitals fighting for the obstetrical dollar. In Berkeley, in 1977, it seemed common sense to suppose that any hospital boasting a birth center with liberal policies would pull in the money. Applying their collective influence, two nursing administrators and a female obstetrician obtained the go-ahead from the necessary committees. The birth center proceeded from idea to reality with astonishing swiftness, and suddenly they realized they needed a nursing coordinator. Since I'd had six months of hands-on experience at Mt. Zion, they asked me.

"Only if I can write policy," I bargained, and they agreed. Adapting boiler-plate sets of procedures and protocols from other birth centers to the unique situation of Alta Bates, a hospital with no in-house resident obstetrical staff, I typed practically around the clock and hammered out the guidelines in just over a week.

I expected a major tussle around some of the policies—freedom from the confines of routine IVs and fetal monitors, limited access to narcotics, and no epidurals. When the protocols passed through the OB committee almost unchallenged, I realized the doctors did not understand what was about to hit them.

During the next two weeks, workmen gutted a postpartum room and trucked in a queen-size bed, foldout couches, brass lamps, and enough potted plants to rival a rain forest. With carpeting, paint, and furniture in shades of sage, terracotta, and teal, decorators transformed the chrome-and-linoleum room into something resembling an upscale southwestern motel, and we opened for business.

The physicians' planning committee estimated that six to eight women might sign up in the first month. Forty came to the introductory meeting, twenty of them due within the next few weeks.

In the early years of the birth center revolution, most doctors seemed confused about the whole concept. They'd never learned the pain-relieving techniques used for centuries by wise women, witches, and midwives. Some doctors lacked the ability to assess labor without relying on machines. Because they'd lost sight of what normal labor looks like and how unmedicated women really behave when artificial barriers are removed, they didn't understand what made birth center deliveries so different.

We nurses, on the other hand, basked in our newfound power. We volunteered extra hours of work for the satisfaction of choreographing very special births for women who hoped to experience the births of their babies as potentially transforming events.

Julie, a delivery nurse who used the birth center for both of her drug-free deliveries, later said, "It hurt a lot, but it was *my* pain, and it wasn't something I wanted anyone to take away from me."

Julie's attitude, common among the women, was foreign to many of the doctors; they just didn't know what to make of it all. One evening during the beginning months, Dr. Clark looked anxious as he stood beside me in the hallway. He glanced into the birth center where his patient labored in the queen-size bed, her seven or eight invited guests snacking on Brie and sipping Chardonnay. "What am I supposed to do in there?" he asked.

I smiled. "Nothing. She's doing fine. Just catch the baby."

"The hell with that. I didn't go to medical school to do nothing at a birth."

"But if the birth is normal, then what's there to do?"

"Normal birth is a retrospective diagnosis," he said. "No birth is normal until after the fact. All births are complicated until proven otherwise." Straightening his shoulders, he walked into the room.

Dumbfounded, I stood in the corridor staring at his back. I realized that he had just provided me with the definition of the difference between doctors and midwives. Midwives believe birth is normal till proven otherwise. Doctors don't.

For a couple of years I'd considered applying to midwifery school, but the enormity of the decision paralyzed me. I'd be giving up a lot: steady income, job security, day shift hours, five weeks of annual paid vacation, and health care for myself and my family. Although Rog thought midwifery school was the inevitable next step in my career, I stalled, knowing better than he how much impact it might have on our lives.

But Dr. Clark's statement resolved my dilemma. How could I continue following the orders of physicians who believed that normal childbirth is a retrospective diagnosis? My entire belief system rebelled at the very idea.

Given the freedom offered by the birth centers that popped up everywhere, nurses, midwives, and the pregnant women themselves rediscovered a wisdom more valid than any method we tried to superimpose on the natural process. Women's bodies have near-perfect knowledge of childbirth; it's when their brains get involved that things can go wrong. When we force external rules on laboring women's behavior, their births may veer off track. The intrinsic intelligence of women's bodies can be sabotaged when they're put into clinical settings, surrounded by strangers, and attached to machines that limit their freedom to move. They then risk falling victim to the powerful forces of fear, loneliness, doubt, and distrust, all of which increase pain. Their hopes for a normal birth disappear as quickly as the fluid in an IV bottle.

Given a normal labor and supportive, permissive surroundings, women are capable of finding their own unique ways of dealing with labor. They need only a guide, a calm and experienced woman who can help the struggling mother-to-be along the rocky paths of Laborland, as we frequently called it.

In Alta Bates's birth center, I saw deliveries where mothers had carte blanche to behave however their bodies dictated. No one vested in a particular method shouted at them to breathe shallowly, breathe deeply, blow, hold your breath when you push, exhale as you push, do abdominal breathing, do chest breathing, take short fast breaths or long slow breaths, keep your eyes open, close your eyes. No one, in short, telling them they were doing it all wrong.

I saw women dance to Grateful Dead music. Some sang golden oldies, moaned like the wind coming down a chimney, stared at flickering candles, showered for hours, clapped their hands, rocked while holding onto door-knobs, swayed while gripping their husbands' belt loops, trudged up and down stairs, howled toward the ceiling, crawled from bed to bathroom, tossed their heads like circus ponies, or just grabbed the nearest warm body and hung on for dear life.

Some used mental tricks like reciting multiplication tables or repeatedly subtracting a random number from one hundred. One woman quoted Wordsworth. Another chose Shakespeare. A Jewish woman, to her husband's amazement, asked me to recite the Hail Mary over and over while she floated in a warm tub.

Many women reacted to labor musically, and it was fun trying to identify the primal origins of their songs. Gregorian? Byzantine? Native American? Did she sound like a Jewish cantor? Or like the muezzin in a Marrakesh minaret calling the faithful to prayer? A few produced high, bell-like tones, but most gravitated toward the deeper pitch of Tibetan monks.

A cellist surrounded herself with four musician friends from the San Francisco Symphony, requesting they each take a different instrument's part of Beethoven's "Ode to Joy" and hum to her while she labored. She carried the main melody, and her friends wove in and out in counterpoint, louder as the contraction peaked and fading to a whisper as it died away. With tears in his eyes, her awed husband knelt at her side and watched her wave her hand in the air as she conducted her labor opus.

With memories of those pure voices still humming "Ode to Joy" in my head, I went home, stuck a stamp on an envelope, and mailed my application to midwifery school.

Only If You Can Be There

Pregnant women flocked to Alta Bates's birth center, bringing along bean-bag chairs, flowers, champagne, incense, musical instruments, excited kids, and bemused grandparents. We quickly added two additional birthing rooms to cope with the demand.

Most of the OB nurses wholeheartedly supported the idea of natural birth with freedom from hospital-imposed rules. One organized a sibling preparation program, and another suggested a workshop to inform grandparents of changes in obstetrics and baby care. My friend Sandi, a nurse whose fourth baby was due any day, offered to have photos taken of her birth for use in the orientation classes.

The doctors, however, were divided over the very existence of the alternative birth center. A handful thought it was the best idea in obstetrics since the banishment of chloroform from delivery rooms. Another group acted as if their professional competence had been challenged. The majority drifted in the middle ground of confusion, probably hoping this latest Berkeley fad would disappear along with acupressure for the treatment of anemia, hair analysis for diagnosis of dietary deficiencies, Chinese moxabustion for converting babies from breech to headfirst, and macrobiotic diets for everything else.

Dr. Rider belonged to the offended group, and his negative comments went beyond birth centers to include physician's assistants, midwives, and nurse practitioners.

"Did I hear right?" he asked, stomping into the birth center where I was caring for his patient. "You're going to midwifery school?"

"Yes, but not for another year."

"Well, I certainly hope you're not going to do home deliveries. Pizzas should be delivered at home, not babies. Pretty soon, people will want to die at home."

I didn't reply, but Erica, his patient, frowned and said, "Well, I'd sure rather die at home than in a sterile hospital. What's wrong with that?"

"Birth and death belong in hospitals, and that's that." Dr. Rider examined her and left without another word.

Erica stared after him, turned to her husband, and said, "He didn't even look at my face."

I'd never liked Dr. Rider much, and I could see from Erica's expression that she was having some doubts of her own. A tense man with deep creases at the corners of his mouth and rabbity eyes that darted everywhere, Dr. Rider never expected that any woman in his practice would use the birth center. He liked control, preferring his patients mildly sedated, on their backs, draped from chin to toes in blue cotton sheets—and quiet. Above all quiet, asking no questions—certainly none about the birth center.

Somehow Erica, a feisty woman with long black hair and a lush, statuesque body, had slipped into his practice and signed up for the birth center without even discussing it with him. His first clue came when he arrived in labor and delivery and couldn't find her.

"She's in the birth center," one of the nurses said pointing down the hall.

He was not pleased, and Erica could tell. "He'll just have to cope," she said after he'd left. "I'm getting into the shower now, and I'm going to stay there," she told me. "I'll let you know when I feel like pushing."

"Fine with me," I said. "Just let me check the baby now and then, and I'll need time to get Dr. Rider here for your delivery."

Her husband, Jordan, said, "Did Erica tell you she plans to give birth on the floor, on her hands and knees?"

I whooped with amusement. "Oh brother, Dr. Rider's gonna freak right out."

Erica raised an eyebrow and said, "Well, he'll just have to freak right back in, won't he?" With a sassy toss of her head, she disappeared into the shower.

An hour later, she peered around the sliding glass door. With hair streaming in her face, she hollered, "I'm feeling pushy!"

I checked her dilation while she stood in the shower, the water running over both of us. Then I made a quick call to Dr. Rider.

He swept into the birth center and, just as I'd predicted, freaked out. He took one look at Erica crouched naked on a blanket in the middle of the floor and dragged me into the hallway.

"She's on the floor," he sputtered. "What the hell am I supposed to do with her?"

"Just catch the baby," I replied. "She's doing great, isn't she?"

"She's on the floor!"

"Yeah, she likes it there."

"She's on her hands and knees!"

"Mmm-hmm."

He snorted and fumed and then decided to wait in the call room till she was truly crowning, clearly wanting to spend as little time as possible in "that baby center or birthing place . . . whatever you call it."

With about three contractions to spare, I phoned him again. He gowned and gloved as if preparing for open-heart surgery, lowered himself awkwardly to one knee, and caught the baby. Other than to say "Push . . . now stop pushing," he didn't speak. As soon as the placenta slid into the stainless steel basin, he shook hands with Jordan and stalked away with rigid shoulders.

I looked at Erica. She looked at me. We started laughing. "Did he say you're going to midwifery school?" she asked, when we'd tamed our giggles.

"Yes, next December."

"Well, I'm having my next baby at home—but only if you can be there."

"I'll look forward to it," I assured her.

The very next day I was restocking the birth center's supply cupboards when Sandi called to say she'd started labor, and I admitted her at noon. A Tinkerbell of a woman, she donned a pink T-shirt that just covered her bottom and ambled around the room to speed up her labor. Her husband, Steve, moved to her side with each contraction.

Sandi and Steve's two oldest children, aged ten and eleven, glanced over their shoulders at regular intervals but devoted most of their attention to a picnic hamper Sandi had packed. It was laden with Evian water, Camembert, Belgian chocolate, fresh raspberries, baguettes, and paté—not your usual kid-fare, but Sandi's children had sophisticated palates; the contents of that basket represented their version of peanut butter and jelly.

They spread runny cheese on hunks of bread and then turned back to an ongoing game of Monopoly. I suspected that they were trying hard to appear more worldly than Seth, their little brother.

Looking like a cherub in a Raphael painting, five-year-old Seth clutched a teddy bear to his chest and stared at his mother. Seth's light brown hair tumbled into soft curls above his serious blue eyes. While his brother and sister feigned indifference to the drama unfolding just ten feet away, he locked onto his mother's face. Her every change of expression showed in his eyes.

Seth buried his nose in the teddy bear's head and peered at his mother from between the bear's furry ears. A little wrinkle creased his brow each time Sandi paused, one foot twisting behind the other, to lean against Steve or to hold onto the back of a chair. A second wrinkle joined the first one when Sandi began to moan.

Just as my replacement nurse arrived at three P.M., Sandi reached six centimeters of dilation, and her labor intensified. I'd planned to stay for her delivery, but Sandi's next words changed everything.

"Peggy, do you want to get your kids and bring them back for the birth? It's fine with me. Is it okay with you, Steve? Kids?"

Steve and the children shrugged their assent, and off I went like the wind, hoping I'd make it back in time. Colin and Jill had lobbied long and hard for permission to see a baby born, and now it was about to happen. I pulled in our driveway, ran into the house and said, "Hey, guys, you wanna come see Sandi have her baby?"

"Yeah? When? Now?" They scrambled to their feet, and we slammed the door behind us, leaving Scooby-Doo blaring on the TV.

On the way back to Alta Bates, however, I began wondering what I was doing. There'd been no time to prepare seven-year-old Colin and five-year-old Jill for the nitty-gritty, get-down-and-funky event they would be witnessing. The birth center's sibling program readied children for the sights, sounds, and smells of birth, but here I was about to introduce my own totally unprepared children to childbirth. Unprepared, that is, except by a lifetime of exposure to mealtime conversations that often focused on bags of water breaking, bloody discharge, timing of contractions, and the effects of intercourse on the onset of labor—issues other families might consider unmentionable under any circumstances, let alone at the dinner table.

So as I led my children through the electronic doors and up the elevator, my only thought was, What have I done? The kids raced ahead of me and dashed into the birth center. I breathed a silent prayer, crossed my fingers, and followed.

"We made it," Jill whispered as I came through the door. I hugged her and nodded, looking around the room, crowded now with five children, a photographer, two adult friends to supervise the kids, two nurses, Sandi and Steve—and me.

Colin stood in the background holding onto his elbows with his arms crossed in front of his thin chest. He looked like he'd figured out how to strike just the right attitude of not appearing *too* interested while indulging his bug-eyed curiosity. The slanted afternoon light caught the tiny scar at the corner of his eye, and I thought of his own birth, the bloody forceps mark they'd said would disappear. It hadn't, but he racked up lots of mileage telling classmates, "It's just a superficial wound I got while fighting off a mugger."

Jill, on the other hand, wiggled her way to the foot of the bed. She rested her elbows on the mattress between Sandi's feet and propped her chin in her cupped hands. Occasionally she looked into Sandi's grimacing face, but mostly she kept her gaze fixed on the dark, slick, slightly bloody spot between Sandi's thighs where a baby's head would soon appear. It looked as if she wanted to crawl between Sandi's knees.

But Seth. A third wrinkle had appeared on his lightly freckled forehead, and nothing short of his mother's finishing this relentless process would relieve his anxiety. I smiled and said, "It's hard work, Seth, but your mom's doing fine. It'll be over soon."

He nodded and tried a little smile, but he didn't take his eyes off Sandi. He hugged the teddy bear tighter as he took a deep, shuddering breath.

Dr. Bill Stallone, a tall Italian with a hawk-like profile, came through the door. He didn't even blink at the room full of children, cheese, chocolate, and Chardonnay. His gentle eyes smiled, and he spoke quietly to Jill and Seth. One of the few doctors who wholeheartedly supported the birth center, he helped himself to a piece of chocolate, smiled at Sandi as he smoothed her hair back from her forehead, and settled himself beside my daughter at the foot of the bed.

Just then, right in front of Jill's face, Sandi's bag of water broke. My daughter jerked back a foot or two, but even that watery surprise didn't persuade her to abandon her ringside seat. As soon as we mopped up the water, Jill moved back into place.

Seth had jumped, too, when the water splashed. Sandi rolled her head to the side and smiled at him. "It's okay, Seth. I'm fine." Seth's eyes grew even bigger with the magnifying effect of unshed tears. Steve pulled him into an embrace and kissed his head. Seth swallowed and rested his chin on his dad's chest, the little bear dangling at his side.

Sandi's first push produced a spontaneous bellow that riveted everyone's attention. Dr. Stallone pulled a stool to the foot of the bed behind Jill. He sat down, opened a small equipment tray, and smiled at the children crowding at his elbow. Monopoly money and chocolate bars lay forgotten on the cluttered table.

With Sandi's second push, the oval opening became rounder and a little bit of a bald head showed. Sandi's older boy peered at it and said, "Is that the baby's brain?"

The doctor and I laughed, and I explained, "I know what you mean. It does look like photographs of a brain. Kind of like a walnut, right?" He nodded, and I continued, "It's the skin of the baby's head all smooshed together from the pressure. It'll look totally different as soon as it comes out."

"Cool!"

"Whoa, here she goes again," hollered my son as Sandi roared with another push. The baby slid way down. Another push or two would do it.

Seth covered his ears and shut his eyes at the sound of his mother's cry, but as far as Jill was concerned, Sandi might have been crooning a lullaby. That incredible, powerful roar never even registered on my daughter. Spellbound, she inched closer and, like Adam reaching his finger toward God's, she stretched her hand to the little head that almost filled the opening between Sandi's legs.

"Jill . . ." I cautioned, and she jerked back.

"Do you want to touch it?" asked the doctor, and Jill's head bobbed up and down like a parakeet in front of a mirror.

He took her hand and guided it forward. With the tips of two fingers, she gently stroked the shiny head, and a smile spread over her face.

"It's warm—and so slippery," she said softly.

Except for Seth, who hid his face in his dad's armpit, the other children crept closer to watch.

Jill inched between Sandi's knees, blocking the doctor's view. "Jill, could you give me a little room here?" he requested. She backed up and sat on his knee. Before I could remove her, the baby's head emerged. With my daughter still sitting in his lap, a laughing Dr. Stallone delivered Sandi's baby.

The infant, petite at only five-and-a-half pounds, tumbled into the doctor's hands on a second, even bigger wave of fluid. She threw her arms above her head like a child saying "Soooo big!" and added her own voice to the already noisy room as everyone erupted in cheers. The doctor laid the baby in Sandi's outstretched arms, and one of the nurses covered her loosely with a warm blanket.

Seth dropped his bear and climbed onto the big bed to crouch behind Sandi's head. His brow smoothed and his curls dangled over his forehead as he bent forward to gaze into his baby sister's face.

Jill leaped off Dr. Stallone's lap and crawled up to Sandi's shoulder. She gazed at the baby's flailing arms and captured a frantic hand in her grasp. The baby latched onto Jill's finger with the characteristic monkey grip of all newborns.

Jill said, "Her head's ticking," as she saw the pulsing soft spot, and then she squealed, "Look out, she's peeing."

Thirty minutes later I peeled my daughter away from the baby, dragged my son away from the Belgian chocolate, and steered them both out the door. They bounced and jumped and skipped at my side, bubbling with excitement. As the elevator opened to the lobby, I pulled Colin close and said, "How did that make you feel, seeing Sandi have the baby?"

"It was really cool, Mom. It was like a stunt in a sci-fi movie, you know? I mean a person coming out of a person is creepy, in a way. But it was fun. And I'm really glad I'm a boy and won't ever have to do that myself!"

Jill stopped and looked at her brother with a strange expression. She looked back at me and then at Colin again. As wheelchairs and visitors streamed past us in both directions, she stood lost in thought. I could almost see the little wheels turning as she realized—probably for the first time—that it's only women who do this thing called "having a baby."

"How about you, honey?" I whispered, kneeling and looking into her blue, blue eyes. "What did you think of that?"

She put her arms around my neck before answering, and I felt her shoulders lift as she heaved a sigh fit for Broadway. "Oh, Mom, I'm going to have twenty-five babies."

"Twenty-five?" I asked. "Are you sure?"

"Oh, yes. But only if you can be there. Okay?"

Fog

I jerked upright in bed as the phone rang beside me. Grabbing blindly, I knocked it to the floor. "Damn," I muttered, hauling it up by the cord and looking at the clock. 12:07. "Hello?" I finally whispered.

A soft voice said, "Peggy, it's Maria. Were you asleep?"

"Maria! Oh wow, are you in labor?"

Then I realized Rog had leaped up when the phone rang. He'd put on his bathrobe and now stood blank-faced at the edge of the bed, hands dangling at his sides.

"Rog, what are you doing?" I asked.

"The alarm clock," he mumbled.

"No, honey, it was the phone. It's midnight. Go back to sleep."

He crawled obediently back under the covers, and I suspected he'd awaken in the morning wondering why he had his bathrobe on.

"Okay, Maria, what's up?"

"It's started. I've been having contractions for about an hour. Could you come check me to see if it's time to call Carole yet?"

"No problem," I replied, all business now. "I'll be right there."

A home birth. I was going to my first home birth. As an obstetrical nurse for more than a decade, I'd seen thousands of babies born. I'd seen births in delivery rooms, labor rooms, alternative birth centers, operating rooms, emergency rooms, on gurneys in hallways, even in an elevator a couple of times. But I'd never seen a baby born in someone's home.

In two weeks I would be starting midwifery school with eleven other women. Unlike me, many of them were coming from a lay midwifery background with hundreds of home births already behind them. Lay midwives practiced their calling on the extreme edge of acceptance by the medical community. They acquired their training by apprenticing themselves to another lay midwife. Their approach to childbirth and midwifery was usually experiential and holistic, often employing techniques from various alternative medicines. While some of them were nurses, most were not. When they decided they "wanted to get legal," they first had to complete nursing school, then put in time working in a hospital delivery room. Only then were they eligible to apply to midwifery school.

That's what Carole Hagin had done. Since that first time I had met her at Alta Bates in 1974, five years earlier, she'd completed nursing school, worked briefly at a hospital near her Martinez home, and graduated from San Francisco General's midwifery school, the same program I would begin in just two weeks.

I, however, was approaching midwifery school from the opposite direction. Standard, allopathic, Western medical philosophy stuffed every hemisphere of my brain, and I hungered for some breathing space. I wanted to poke holes in my rigid education and let the fresh air of new (to me) ideas fill the empty spaces. Acupressure, herbal preparations, Native American chants, reflexology, homeopathy—I knew nothing of them.

So when my friend Maria, an obstetrical nurse herself, asked me to help at the home birth of her third baby, I eagerly agreed. And now her labor had started. I'd finally have a chance to see Carole Hagin practice her sorcery right through to the actual delivery of the baby.

I peeled off my nightgown and groped for warm clothing, shivering in the kind of deadly, silent cold that tourists refuse to believe ever happens in California. Amazed at how much louder the squeaky armoire door sounded in the dark, I finally found sweatpants, a loose T-shirt, and a long-sleeved sweatshirt, then dragged my shoes from among the dust kittens beneath the bed. I picked up a stethoscope and some sterile gloves, grabbed my down jacket, and eased the door shut behind me. It had taken almost fifteen minutes to get going. At least I was wide-awake.

As soon as I turned to walk down the steps, I saw my future. Fog as thick as a winter whiteout blanketed my world, and I realized that, as a midwife, I'd have to face weather like this regularly. Alone. In the middle of the night.

As my car rolled through the quiet streets, I squinted into the miasma as if sheer willpower could give me better vision. Once, fearing I was lost, I left my car at an intersection and walked to the curb. Holding the slick metal pole of the street sign, I peered into the mist to read the street names.

Twenty-five minutes passed before I knocked on Maria's front door. Her husband, Steve, answered right away and then stared at the fog. "Gee," he breathed, eyes wide.

I accepted a cup of coffee with gratitude and curled my cold hands around the warm mug. Maria was crouched on a futon in front of the fireplace. With glossy black hair falling in loose waves halfway down her back, she had the wide smile and dramatic, flashing brown eyes of many women from her native Argentina. But now a quiet and dreamy Maria knelt before me, her body rocking to a universal rhythm as if governed by the gentle surge of the tides. She came forward onto all fours with a deep sigh as another contraction began. She swung her head from side to side, letting her long curls ripple onto the futon.

I knelt beside her, checked her baby's heartbeat, and felt the strength of the next contraction with my fingertips as she breathed through the pain. Strong, and just three minutes apart. I called Carole. Maria wasn't in heavy labor yet, but this was her third baby, and I knew her midwife faced a difficult drive.

"Hello, this is Carole Hagin." She spoke in a normal tone of voice without a trace of sleep in her speech. Would I ever learn to do that? I wondered.

"Hey, Carole, it's Peggy, and I'm at Maria's. I hope I didn't wake your husband."

"Wake Bob? You kidding? A phone ringing in the middle of the night hasn't bothered him for fifteen years. Can't you hear him snoring? You havin' a good time? It's your first time at a home birth, huh?"

I started to answer, but she kept on talking.

"I remember how excited I was at the first home birth I attended, especially as it happened right in my own house. A pregnant friend stopped here on her way to the hospital because the fog was so bad, and I delivered her about twenty minutes later. All my kids were . . ." and she went on and on.

How could her husband sleep through this? The next time she paused, I jumped in. "There's bad fog tonight, too. Maria's getting active, and I think you should start now."

"Sure, I'll be out the door in three minutes. I always . . ." and she talked on.

I wondered if she was going to talk till the fog cleared, but finally she said, "So if it's as bad as you say, I'd better get going. See ya in about an hour."

The hour passed. Maria labored so quietly. If she stayed this composed, I knew her two children sleeping in a bedroom just five steps down the hall wouldn't hear a thing. She looked cozy in her crocheted, long-sleeved sweater, colorful Peruvian knee socks, and Garfield bedroom slippers.

After waltzing around the room with Steve for a while, she wandered into the bathroom, saying, "I think I'll try the shower." Steve followed. I poured another cup of coffee, listened to the splash of the shower, and thought about what the coming year would be like as I juggled midwifery school, a job, marriage, and two young children.

Every five minutes I pulled the front curtains aside to look for Carole.

Then Steve called, "Peggy? Can you come in here?" With one last desperate glance out the window, I jumped up and headed toward the bathroom.

The steam in the tiny room was as thick as the fog outdoors, but much warmer. Maria sat on the toilet, naked and soaking wet. Rivulets of water ran down the mirror. I couldn't see Steve's eyes behind the misty lenses of his glasses, and he swiped uselessly at them with the heel of his hand. In the heat and humidity, he'd stripped down to just his Levis.

God, it was hot. I took off my sweatshirt and hung it on the doorknob, glad I had a T-shirt underneath.

"She won't talk, and she's making grunting sounds. I think she's starting to push."

"Do you feel like you want to push, Maria?"

No answer. It didn't surprise me. I'd seen that dazed look on many women's faces. Maria drifted in her own world, far beyond our reach. She sagged to one side, letting her head droop against Steve's chest.

"Steve, does she have any hospital equipment? Clamps, scissors, anything? Carole should be here any minute, but . . ."

"There's an emergency kit somewhere, but I don't know where she put it."

Maria righted herself and curled forward, placing just the fingertips of both hands on top of her round belly. As I saw her lean into a push, instinct and experience guided my bare hand between her thighs.

I gasped at what I felt. The bag of water bulged from the opening like a Florida grapefruit, and I suspected the baby's head floated right behind it.

"Maria, do you have any birth stuff around here? Clamps? Maria?"

Not a word.

A little desperate, I looked at Steve again, kneeling at the side of the toilet. I stared at his glasses, wondering if he could see anything at all. I still had my hand on the taut water sac as I glanced into Maria's face. She looked remote, so serene and confident. I didn't feel quite so confident. Where the devil was Carole? Every nerve in my body strained, listening.

The next contraction began. Maria gasped once as the bag of water burst with the suddenness of a handclap at dawn. The water exploded onto my palm with such force that it flowed uphill, up the full length of my arm and through the sleeve of my T-shirt. I yelped as it splashed into my armpit and cascaded down my body, soaking my entire right side with hot water. Then the baby's whole head landed in my palm.

I blinked fast and said, "Well, now."

I had two choices: panic and deliver the baby, or stay calm and deliver the baby.

I knew how to do it, of course. For more than fifteen years I'd worked with women having babies. I'd even delivered about fifty of them myself when the doctors hadn't arrived in time, but in this foggy bathroom I had no support system, no equipment, no helpers, no paraphernalia to handle problems. Nothing. Just a half-naked man who probably couldn't even see me and a laboring mom who wouldn't talk to me. And she was on the toilet.

Maria's eyes opened wide and stared straight into mine. With a silent grimace she gripped her knees and gave a quick push that thrust the entire baby into my hand. Trying to balance the wiggling, upside-down baby as I struggled to get my other hand between Maria's thighs, I felt the slippery little body get away from me. Holding the baby's head above water, I heard the rest of him splash into the toilet. He screamed in shock and began paddling his fat legs in the cold water, every muscle devoted to an escape effort.

Maria snapped out of her trance, and her mouth opened in a big grin. Laughing together, we hauled the baby from the toilet and dried him off.

Steve removed his glasses and squinted at us, trying to make sense of all the commotion. "Whoa, that was fast," he said.

The baby needed nothing except gentle handling to recover from his dramatic delivery. We wrapped him in a clean towel, and he played finger-dancing games with his mother while we waited for the placenta.

Not wanting to fish the placenta, too, out of the toilet, I spied a small blue bucket on the far side of the tub, a bathtub toy. I grabbed it just as Maria moaned, "Ooooh, I think it's ready."

"Here, just let me get this little bucket in there," I muttered. As I crammed it over the toilet seat, she gave a soft push, and the bucket instantly filled with the afterbirth.

We needed to leave the bathroom, but I was really, really wet. I asked to borrow dry clothing, and Steve took a long nightgown off the back of the bathroom door. It wasn't quite what I had in mind, but I stepped into the bathtub, pulled the shower curtain closed, peeled off my wet clothing, and put on the flowered flannel nightie. Then we formed a little parade and marched into the living room.

First came Steve, bare to the waist, backing out the door and steadying Maria by her shoulders. Then came Maria, naked, carrying the baby with one hand and clutching the front end of a towel between her legs. I brought up the rear in a flannel nightie, holding the other end of her towel and carrying the placenta bucket aloft like a bowl of salsa. The cord looped between bucket and baby, swinging with each step.

We settled Maria in front of the fire, and Steve found some scissors. I chuckled. He'd brought me a delicate pair of thread snippers shaped like a stork. After boiling the scissors in a saucepan, I tied the cord with dental floss, and Steve cut it.

I looked at the three of them and took a deep breath. I'd just done my first home birth—all alone. All of a sudden, I felt shaky. Steadying myself with a hand on the wall, I walked into the kitchen and gripped the edge of the counter for support. I took a deep breath.

For years and years, I'd followed doctors' orders. Sure, I'd caught a bunch of babies, but help had always been nearby, and usually the tardy doctor arrived seconds later. This midwifery stuff was very different, I'd just discovered. No doctor's orders, no nursery staff down the hall, no cabinets full of sterile equipment, no obstetrician bursting through the doorway. And where the hell was Carole, anyway?

Comfort food, that's what I needed. When I was sick as a child, my mother always brought me breakfast in bed. Sweet tea, a sliced orange, a soft-boiled egg, and cinnamon toast. Well, eggs and oranges seemed a bit much, but cinnamon toast I could manage. Cinnamon? Right there on the spice shelf. Sugar? In the bowl on the table. Butter, bread, toaster. In ten minutes I made enough toast for a troop of starving Boy Scouts.

More than two hours had passed since my call to Carole, and I was seriously worried. As I stacked the tower of buttery toast on a plate, I stared out the kitchen window where the fog swirled thick as ever. Where was she?

Then we heard a knock, and Steve opened the door. Carole came in talking, as if we had interrupted a conversation she'd been having with herself on the front porch. "Can you feature this fog? And it's even worse in Martinez, so close to the river . . ."

Boxes and bags of birth equipment hung off both sides of her body. From the edges of a brown knitted cap, her graying curls sparkled with dewy condensation, like a halo. Her face radiated confidence and humor as she walked into the living room.

"I got out of my car three times before I reached the end of my driveway," she continued, "just to see if I was still . . . Oh." She stopped briefly but missed only a single beat when she saw the baby at Maria's breast. "Well, I thought the baby might get here before me. Did Maria have a birth kit? Did you come in your nightgown, Peggy? Why didn't you take time to change? God, weren't you cold? What time was the baby born?"

Overwhelmed, I didn't know which question to answer first. But that last one grabbed me. I hadn't given the time of birth a thought. "I have no idea," I said, looking at Steve, who shrugged.

"Are you into astrology?" Carole asked him. He shook his head, puzzled. She smiled and turned toward the cinnamon toast. "Well, then, it doesn't matter, does it? Pick whatever time you like."

What a concept. In the hospital where everything is so regimented, it had always seemed critical that someone note the exact time of birth. I'd already learned my first two midwifery lessons: Weather matters; birth time doesn't—unless you're into astrology.

I sat hugging my knees as the scent of coffee, cinnamon, and burning logs filled the cozy room. I smiled and rocked back and forth, watching Carole pull a tiny white T-shirt over the baby's head.

I nibbled my toast. Two more weeks. Midwifery school would start in just two weeks.

~ *Adidas to Birkenstocks*

For years I'd heard about Gaia, a hippie lay midwife with ten years experience. Stories about her spread from woman to woman over the organic produce at Monterey Foods, through the waiting rooms of Feldenkrais massage therapists, at Black Oak Books on Shattuck Avenue, and under the billowing parachute at baby Kinder-Gym classes. Finally, our star-paths intersected. We were classmates in midwifery school.

Although light years of lifestyle differences separated us, our houses stood less than a mile apart. Carpooling, our ticket to the commuters' fast track across the Bay Bridge, bought me priceless hours of time with this urban legend. As I listened to her talk of artists, foreign policy, public events, and her antiwar history, I began to feel like a $10 Timex in a drawer of exotic ethnic jewelry. Politically correct opinions flowed from her like cream, too obvious to require explanation. My parents always voted Republican, but she'd never hear that fact from my lips.

Gaia epitomized my loftiest dreams: experienced, confident, worldly, and groovy. Most of all, groovy. I watched her closely, trying to discover the secret to her grooviness.

Hair. Mine fell around my cheeks in predictable, dark blond waves; Gaia's black hair coiled like Medusa's snakes. She gathered masses of it into a loose knot and braided a multicolored Guatemalan belt into the tangled heap.

Voice. Mine sounded eager and chirpy, even to my own ears; hers came out all languid and throaty. I figured others must look at us and think, Betty Boop and Marlene Dietrich.

And clothes. I wore jeans, sweaters, and Adidas. She wore denim skirts, embroidered Mexican blouses—and Birkenstocks.

Birkenstocks. I should have guessed. Even though the stainless steel January sky threatened rain, Gaia wore dark brown Birkenstock sandals. In a nod to the weather, purple socks scrunched between the straps. But still. Birkenstocks in January?

It was such a hippie thing. And I was such a hippie wannabe.

I tried. Had tried for years, actually, but it just didn't stick. In the days of tie-dye and Toklas brownies, I'd ironed my curly hair to look like Marianne Faithfull's, and I went braless and wore long skirts with sewn-on fringe, but it was a fashion statement with me, not a religion. I hid my hippie costume under the bed when my parents visited.

As Rog and I made a down payment on a two-bedroom Craftsman bungalow, Gaia moved up the coast with a group of back-to-the-earth idealists. They settled onto a piece of raw land in the middle of nowhere to raise bees and babies and to grow mushrooms and marijuana. The men stacked firewood and plowed. The women got pregnant and delivered each other's kids. Gaia fell into midwifery the way many women did back then. Unflappable and possessing more common sense than the others, it soon became her task to deal with rashes, burns, bad drug trips, and labor pains.

While she caught babies among the redwoods in Mendocino, I assisted laboring women in a white-tiled delivery room. While she named her children Sunrise and Arabesque, I named mine Colin and Jill. While she grew pot and nibbled peyote buttons, I planted parsley and ate the occasional porcini. Her husband came to the city to march on Telegraph Avenue and shout at red-faced Berkeley cops. Mine strapped our son into a Gerry baby carrier and walked to Dwight Way Hardware to buy childproof electrical outlet covers.

But times change. After years of living in a cabin, she wanted a real bed in a real house and a real midwifery license. And I wanted to get out of the hospital, become a groovy Berkeley midwife, and do home births. With very different backgrounds and motivations, we both wanted the same piece of paper: certification as a nurse midwife.

Our instructors, eight bright women and pioneers in the field, introduced themselves. They included one nun, two lesbians, one home birth practitioner, and only one who had given birth.

"They seem a little out of touch with real life," whispered Gaia.

In stark contrast to the instructors, our student group of twelve boasted a Communist, a Jehovah's Witness, and five lay midwives. Eleven of us were mothers, and half had given birth at home. Two women had rap sheets from years of political activism, several were single moms, and one commuted from the Santa Cruz mountains and still found time to meditate three hours a day. And there was me, the Timex watch of the group.

In short, all of us had been juggling multiple hats for years. So when our instructors said, "Forget holding a job this year—you'll be so busy you won't have time to make love or even empty the cat's litter box," we just rolled our eyes. Adding midwifery school to the act without dropping all the other hats was difficult but not impossible.

But while our particular group of students collectively had years of obstetrical and midwifery experience, we all had holes in our knowledge and plenty to learn. Our instructors may not have understood what made us tick, but they made sure we filled in the gaps in our knowledge. I'd never performed pelvic exams or Pap smears, and I'd certainly never inserted an IUD, figured out which brand of birth control pills to prescribe, or repaired an episiotomy. Gaia and I kept twine tied to a knob on our car dashboards, and we practiced one-handed suture knots as we sat in commuter traffic.

"Not bad," said my instructor two weeks later, as she watched me stitch up a woman's perineum. "You've been practicing." Gaia grinned and gave me a thumbs up.

During my prenatal clinic rotation, I had to prove all over again that I knew how to examine a pregnant abdomen. Having an instructor breathing down my neck while I struggled with a speculum that kept jamming made me sweat aplenty, but behaving calmly in the presence of San Francisco's flamboyant patient population often put an extra twist in my knickers.

When Vinnie and Rosebud waltzed into the exam room, I blinked rapidly and grabbed a blank chart to give me something to focus on. Vinnie sensed my discomposure.

"Honey, you're not in Kansas any more," he said, his fuchsia boa nearly slapping me in the face as he tossed it over his left shoulder. He couldn't possibly have known I'd lived in Kansas for nine years of my childhood, but I'm sure my astonishment glowed as brightly as Dorothy's yellow brick road when he introduced me to his pregnant girlfriend, a four-hundred-pound black prostitute named Rosebud.

She'd gotten pregnant by Vinnie two months before he began hormones in preparation for a sex change operation. New breast implants already bulged on his bony chest. Vinnie wore tight-fitting gold lamé pants, purple high heels, a snug, purple-knit tank top, and that six-foot fuchsia boa that he just couldn't leave alone. False eyelashes, impeccable makeup, and a short, androgynous hairstyle topped his flashy outfit.

"You like my earrings, girlfriend? I see you lookin' at 'em."

He shook his head so the lime-green, iridescent triangles caught the sunlight. Sparks of green light skittered up and down the cracked walls as he vamped back and forth for my benefit. Only the telltale bulge in his snug pants revealed his original sex.

Rosebud, an enormous women whose skin and face you couldn't help but admire, sat quietly smiling at his antics. Where Vinnie's skin glowed so black he looked almost blue in certain light, Rosebud's face and arms reminded me of coffee with lots of rich cream. Vinnie's cropped hair hugged his shapely little head, but Rosebud's long shiny curls tumbled around her moon-shaped face. Vinnie's lean body rippled with sinew and muscle. Rosebud looked amorphous beneath her floor-length African print dress. His makeup was flamboyant; she wore only a dark, reddish-brown lipstick on her beautiful face.

When Rosebud entered the hospital in labor five months later, she looked exactly the same. Her bulk easily absorbed a full-term pregnancy with no alteration in her appearance. A few hours later, an eight-pound baby slid from between her thighs with the ease of chocolate melting on a Chevy's dashboard in August. Vinnie pranced and danced in the background, garbed in a cowgirl outfit that would have made Annie Oakley blush. With the short skirt flaring around his slim thighs, I couldn't tell if he'd completed the sex change surgery. Although I'm sure he wouldn't have minded my asking, it didn't seem appropriate, given the circumstances.

Midway through our year of training, we spent one full morning watching X-rated movies designed to desensitize us to the wide range of lifestyle and sexual practices for which the Bay Area is so famous. By lunchtime we were calling it The Virtual Fuckorama. "I'd have appreciated these movies earlier," I said to Gaia. "I might have been better prepared for Vinnie and Rosebud."

Sister Margaret Marie, the nun instructor, led us in a brainstorming session after lunch. "Try to come up with as many words as you can for male and female genitalia and for all the different sexual acts we've watched in these movies."

In ten minutes flat, the blackboard was filled and we were all hysterical. "You guys are good," she marveled. "I couldn't have come up with half of these terms."

"I'll bet she knows more than most nuns," Gaia whispered to me.

"Well, if she didn't before, she sure does now."

As cool summer fog gave way to the warm days of autumn, one instructor asked me, "What are your plans for after graduation?"

"I'm going to apply for privileges at Alta Bates. I've worked there as a nurse for the last ten years, you know, and there are a few doctors who've been very supportive. I feel like I ought to get some practice doing more deliveries in a hospital for a year or so, before branching into home births."

"Personally," she said, "I think you'll find you're suckin' a dry tit. Those Alta Bates docs are devoted to preserving the status quo, which means all the money for them and none for midwives. Why don't you consider asking one to hire you, instead?"

"No way," I said. Dr. Clark's statement that normal birth is a retrospective diagnosis still haunted me, and I intended to distance myself as much as possible from that medical philosophy. Besides, after following doctors' orders for fifteen years, I wanted to strike out on my own.

But as I began the process of applying for privileges, I realized my instructor's prediction had been accurate: the barriers would eventually tumble, but certainly not by my graduation. As our December graduation loomed, I looked with more interest at the possibility of immediately opening a home birth practice. I mentioned my thoughts to Maria's midwife, Carole, and word quickly spread among Berkeley's pregnant women. Twenty-four hours later I had my first client, a nursing instructor at Cal State Hayward pregnant with her first baby, and by November I began receiving calls at the rate of one a week. It looked as if I was in the home birth business.

One morning around Thanksgiving, I glanced sideways at Gaia tying suture knots beside me in the front seat of my VW bug. She wore black tights, a tunic-length cable-knit sweater, and her Birkenstocks. I glanced down at my khaki skirt, knee socks, and LL Bean loafers. Pathetic. Even Carole, a middle-aged suburban mother of seven, wore Birkenstocks. She'd told me about a birth she'd done in a no-shoes-inside household.

"I left my sandals in a pile along with everyone else's. It wasn't till I got ready to leave that I realized everyone had worn Birkenstocks. And they all looked the same, about twenty of them in a heap."

"How'd you find yours?" I asked.

"Well, I'm not sure I did. I tried on sandals till I found two that felt right. As soon as I got home I inked the heels with red marker, and I never had that trouble again."

Finally just one week of midwifery school remained. I sat beside Gaia at lunch and unwrapped my chicken sandwich. She'd brought tabbouleh in pita bread. She sipped carrot juice while I popped the tab from a can of Diet Coke. I inspected her from her flyaway hair to her toes. If I was going to be a Berkeley homebirth midwife—and it looked like I was—I felt I had to at least look the part. I definitely needed to go shopping.

"Where'd you buy your Birkenstocks?" I asked her.

She turned her gaze on me, the gaze that always made me feel like Dorothy, clueless in Oz. "My Birkies?"

"Yeah, where'd you buy them?"

"Earthly Goods in Walnut Square. Why?"

"Just wondering." Later that afternoon I zipped up to North Berkeley and bought my first pair of Birkenstocks. But mine were purple. Well, Eggplant, actually. It said so on the tag. And as soon as I got home, I marked the inside edge of each heel with a red indelible pen.

It was a start.

PART III

The wine of astonishment

"Thou hast showed thy people hard things; thou hast made us to drink the wine of astonishment."

PSALMS 60:3
THE HOLY BIBLE, KING JAMES VERSION, 1611

~ *Rubber Ducky*

Sandi hosted her annual Christmas party three weeks after I graduated from midwifery school. Between the cassoulet and the caroling, she toasted me and my new career.

Then I offered a toast to her. Sandi would be my assistant at home births.

Two months later, I called her at four A.M., right after I hung up from talking with Nadine. "Sandi, it's Peggy. Nadine's in labor, and it's her fourth baby."

"I'll meet you there," she said, setting the standard for her level of response. Sandi always sounded as if she was just dying to leap from her warm bed and drive through dark streets with a hand-drawn map clutched in her hand. I knew I often interrupted her sleep or her children's bath or bedtime rituals, but she never made me feel I needed to apologize.

Since I'd started my practice, all the babies had cooperated nicely, and Nadine's was no exception. Just as the rising sun filled the bedroom with daylight, the three older children crept in to see their baby brother glide into the world. Sandi and I divided the duties as usual. She assisted while I managed the birth, then I dealt with the placenta, stitching, and charting while she took charge of the baby.

Nadine's little fellow nursed happily, and then each child took a turn holding him while their dad used up a whole roll of film. The baby showed admirable patience as they shifted him from one small pair of arms to another. Finally Sandi laid out her supplies for baby evaluation: tape measure, scale, thermometer, stethoscope. I unwrapped the baby from his cocoon of blankets—and laughed.

Nadine's son had pooped so copiously that it squished between his toes.

Wriggling around inside his flannel nest, he'd smeared the stuff so far up his back that it soiled the hair at the back of his head. In front, slimy meconium—the medical term for the bowel movement of fetuses and newborns—completely covered his genitals, legs, and feet. This little boy had viscous, black meconium plastered absolutely everywhere. I could have obtained a perfect footprint without using an inkpad.

He didn't care at all, but his three older siblings screamed and fell on the floor laughing. His four-year-old sister, the oldest child in this close-knit family, declared, "Oooh, that's yucky! We need to give him a bath right now."

I agreed. Leaving Sandi to supervise Nadine's shower, I said, "I'll take this little tar baby into the kitchen."

Nadine's bemused husband muttered, "Cripes, that stuff must have some commercial value. Do you think it'd be good for gluing roofing shingles?"

Hanging face down in the palm of my hand as I carried him along the hall, he looked like a little rag doll that had been rolled in stable muck and left in the rain. The three older kids skipped beside me, asking if they could wash his hair, did he know how to swim, could he blow bubbles, what if he peed in the water, and did I think he'd like to play with the yellow rubber ducky or the blue wind-up submarine? I ran warm water in the sink, and my three helpers pulled up chairs and stationed themselves on the counter or beneath my elbow.

It wasn't my usual practice to bathe babies soon after birth because of the difficulty of warming them up again afterwards. I did it for only a few reasons. Some mothers requested it. There were those who wanted a bath as a bonding ritual and a few who wanted their babies bathed and wrapped before they got up close and personal with them. An occasional infant launched herself into a full-blown temper tantrum after birth. If after an hour we still had an inconsolable baby on our hands, I usually suggested a bath to see if the little tyrant would calm down. A very poopy baby was the last reason.

As I listened to the three chattering kids beside me, I recalled the seventies when a phenomenon known as the Leboyer bath surged like a tidal wave through the childbearing community. Named after its French inventor, it called for the baby to be placed into a warm bath immediately after birth, the theory being that this would allow the newborn to relax and recover from birth trauma. Along with the bath, Dr. Leboyer emphasized gentle handling, low lights, and soft voices so that the child would be received gently into the world.

Parents, especially first-timers, believed such a practice would contribute to world peace, that a baby handled in such a manner would grow up to be healthy, wealthy, and wise. Those of us in the birth business thought the gentle handling and soft voices were probably the most important aspects of the whole affair, but those parts got lost in all the hullabaloo. People latched onto that Leboyer bath with ferocious tenacity.

We nurses had suspicions about that latest gimmick in a decade full of gimmicks, but in the interest of keeping new mothers happy, we tried to accommodate them. We developed a system that worked sort of okay, some of the time, for some of the babies.

We filled a seamless Plexiglas crib at the scrub sink with about four gallons of water, which was as much as we could lift without risking back injuries, and replaced it on its wheeled metal cart. Then we added more water to adjust the temperature just before pushing the cart into the delivery room. Something always seemed amiss—too hot, too cold, too shallow, too deep. Of course no one can predict the exact time of a baby's birth. While we waited, the water cooled to the point that it was often *not* a pleasant experience for the baby when we lowered him into the tub, and the babies often screamed till we took them out.

Always a messy affair, the bath water spilled and splashed. The floor needed mopping. Afterwards the tub had to be emptied, washed, and disinfected, and by then the floor needed re-mopping. Before long, we universally loathed the entire concept, groaning whenever we heard Leboyer bath mentioned.

But since seeing those hospital-born infants arch their backs to recoil from the cooling water, I'd seen a few mothers at home climb into a bathtub and stretch their arms out for their newborns. I remembered Debbie, who lay in a tub with her wide-eyed infant just an hour after delivering. Without a word, her two year old peeled off her Daffy Duck jammies and climbed into the tub. Tasha, the three year old, hopped in as well, saying, "We're Daddy's four little mermaids."

Sam, the daddy of this brood, said, "Too bad there's no room left for me."

Tasha pulled her sister closer, saying, "There's room, Daddy."

So we lowered the already-brimming water level, and Debbie skooched forward a bit. Sam stripped off his jeans and Jockeys and eased himself in behind his wife. She leaned against his chest with the baby in the crease of her thighs. The other two girls sat at her feet.

"Somebody get the camera," said Debbie. It's still one of my favorite photos.

The clambering children at my elbow brought me back to the present. They insisted the water in the sink must be ready, and they were right. I lowered their grungy little brother into the warmth and watched with pleasure as his tense arms relaxed, his eyes opened wide, and his spine uncurled and swayed. He paddled his feet enthusiastically in this familiar environment, soaking my shirt. His older sister squirted baby shampoo on his head, and one of his brothers squished it into a spiky Mohawk. The children screamed with glee.

Once they had washed the baby and finished zooming the rubber ducky back and forth across his little frog belly, the older kids settled down and just watched him. I lowered his ears below the surface to make him feel even more like he'd returned to the womb. He looked so calm, so curious and trusting floating in the warm water, bathed in the morning sunlight coming through the window. With so much to look at after months in a dim and static environment, the baby stared in wonder at his wonderful new world.

And I thought, This is how Dr. Leboyer meant it to be. The unnatural pressures imposed by the hospital setting had doomed the ritual bath to oblivion. In the proper setting, with three giggling helpers and a squeaky rubber ducky, it turned into something quite lovely.

∿ Good News and Bad News

I sat in the back of a speeding car with a half-born baby's bum in my hand. The baby's mother, Catherine, sprawled beside me with one foot in my lap and the other pressed against the window. Thoughts flipped through my brain like shuffling cards as the car again swerved too close to the ravine.

Would we get to the hospital in time? Would I deliver this breech baby in a speeding car? Would the baby be okay? Would we crash?

I also feared that my midwifery career, which had begun only five months earlier, might come to an abrupt end. I'd never needed to take a mom to the hospital before, and I had no idea how I'd be received, especially since I'd missed diagnosing this breech presentation. As soon as we arrived at the hospital, my mistake would be exposed.

Catherine's husband, Todd, looked over his shoulder as Catherine screamed. Again we skewed dangerously on the winding road leading down from Grizzly Peak Boulevard. Another half-inch of the baby's hind end oozed into my hand, but Todd's erratic driving scared me more than the prospect of a backseat breech delivery.

"Todd, just drive safely. If the baby starts to come out, we'll stop and you won't miss a thing. So, don't look back here again, okay?"

Catherine's yells sounded normal to me, but it must have been hard for Todd to disregard her heart-stopping cries. However, he managed to drive us out of the hills and onto the freeway without looking back again.

Catherine, athletic and trim with close-cropped blond curls, was three weeks from her due date. The last time I had seen her prenatally, I prodded her belly, perplexed. Hard round mass? Or softer, irregular mass? Sandi and I poked and palpated for a good ten minutes, trying to tell the difference between the head and the bum.

Finally we decided it was the head floating just above Catherine's pubic bone. Just to be sure, I scheduled her next visit with Dr. Stallone, my backup doctor. But Catherine started labor the day before the consultation and called me at seven that morning.

"My bag of water broke half an hour ago, but I'm just having a few cramps."

Remembering my flicker of doubt the previous week, I said, "I think I'll come check you when I get my kids off to school, just to be sure your baby's headfirst."

"What if it's not? Will I have to go to the hospital?"

"Yes, breech births aren't safe at home. Things can go downhill quickly at the end, when it's too late to get to the hospital. The head comes last, and the cord can get squished between your pelvis and . . ."

"Oh, between me and the baby?" she interrupted.

"Exactly, but don't worry. I just want to double-check before you go into active labor."

Ninety minutes later, I wound my way to the top of the ridge and parked behind Catherine's car, a red Jag with an "I Wanna Be Barbie. That Bitch Has Everything" bumper sticker. Suspended over a hillside of ivy, wildflowers, and manzanita, her redwood house clung with incomprehensible faith to the edge of the ravine.

Twenty irregular stone steps led down to a blue front door. I rang the bell and bent to pet a friendly calico who materialized at my feet, but no one answered the doorbell. I rang again, then knocked twice. Nothing. Trying the door, I found it unlocked and stepped inside. The cat scooted past me and disappeared down a long flight of stairs leading to the bedrooms.

I listened. Silence except for a teakettle hissing on the stove. The sports page of the *Chronicle* lay open on the kitchen table beside a half-eaten English muffin.

I heard the watery splashes of someone showering and understood why they hadn't heard me knocking. But then came the roar of a laboring woman, and I ran, hitting the bottom step just as Catherine, stark naked, burst from the shower and flopped onto the bed.

I grabbed a sterile glove from my small home visit bag, my mind racing with impossibilities and improbabilities. She'd been in labor only two hours!

Todd, also naked, followed Catherine from the shower. When he saw me, he spun around and pulled on a pair of khaki shorts. "I don't get it," he said, zipping his fly. "Catherine's really good with pain. The contractions started an hour ago, but I had no idea she'd be so noisy from the very beginning."

My fingers hadn't gone two inches into Catherine's vagina before they bumped into the soft, irregular, rounded shape of a baby's bum. My mouth went dry. Catherine was ready to deliver. It was coming the wrong way. I was alone, except for a clueless husband. We were on top of a mountain. And I was a very new midwife.

It's amazing how quickly a brain sorts out priorities and options, accepting some, rejecting others, reviewing emergency procedures, choosing what to do first and what to skip altogether. In the scant seconds it took me to remove my soiled glove, I performed mental gymnastics. Speed counted most. Summoning 911 would take too long. I'd call the hospital and ask them to alert Dr. Stallone and prepare for a breech delivery. Todd would drive us—and I'd deliver Catherine in the car if I had to. At least we'd be closer to the hospital if the baby needed assistance.

I grabbed the phone and dialed. As it rang, I turned to Catherine and Todd and said, "I have good news and bad news. The good news is your labor's nearly over. The bad news is she's breech. We have to go to the hospital. Right now."

Catherine froze, eyes wide.

Todd said, "She . . ."

Just then the clerk answered the phone. Fearful of the repercussions my words might have on my budding reputation, I took a deep breath to compose myself. "Susan, this is Peggy Vincent, and I'm on Grizzly Peak with an undiagnosed breech. The mom's complete, and it'll be close, but we're coming by car. Please call Dr. Stallone for me and have him meet us in the ER. And . . ."

"Got it. We'll have everything ready for you. Good luck, Peggy."

I wanted to kiss her. I couldn't believe it. She didn't sound horrified or dismayed at all. But she was the clerk. I'd still have to face the nurses and Dr. Stallone.

Todd still stood in his skimpy khakis, hands hanging limp at his sides. "She? It's a girl?"

I hadn't even realized I'd disclosed the baby's sex after my exam, but Todd picked right up on my inadvertent reference, and the news paralyzed him. "Yes, it's a girl, but . . ."

At that moment another contraction began. Catherine grabbed her knees and started to push, but I shouted, "No!" I held her face with both my hands and enunciated each word. "Catherine. Yell. Roar. Scream. Blow. Just. Don't. Push."

She tried. She really tried.

"A girl," whispered Todd, starry-eyed and smiling, lost in space.

"Todd, get something for Catherine to wear. We've gotta go." He picked up his keys.

Catherine glanced at the stairway. "How am I going to get up all those steps?"

"As fast as you can, that's how," I said.

Todd started up the stairs, and I shouted, "She doesn't have anything on, Todd!"

He turned and snatched something red from a chair. Then he pounded barefoot up the steps, neck and neck with the freaked-out cat.

Catherine started talking to herself. "Okay, Catherine, you can do this. You have to do this. All the way before the next one starts. Here I go."

She took a big breath and began running, sheer determination carrying her up to the front door. Todd sat in the car with the engine running and the rear door open. The little cat crouched halfway up the stone steps near a clump of pink impatiens. Fur fluffed out, body tense with wide-eyed panic, she looked ready to run either way, depending on Catherine's next move.

Catherine paused to take a breath, and then, still naked, she dashed up those smooth stone steps, past the impatiens, past the cat, past the ivy, all the way to the car. I turned off the teakettle, locked the front door, and ran after her. She grabbed the open car door and moaned through another contraction, trying not to push.

I put my hand out and fluttered my fingers at Todd. "Dress," I muttered, and he tossed me the dress.

But it wasn't a dress. Not even close. It was an exercise crop-top, bright red, and when I pulled it over Catherine's head, it didn't even come to her belly button. Too bad, I thought, and climbed in back where Catherine lay with her head against the driver's-side door.

She draped her legs across my lap, and we were off on that wild ride out of the Berkeley hills and into the flatlands. One glance between her legs convinced me we'd never make it. Bruised like a plum by the speedy trip through her mother's pelvis, the baby's purple butt protruded a good two inches. As I placed my hand beneath it, she pooped a glob of meconium into my palm.

Although most babies don't expel meconium till after birth, about 25 percent do. Usually it's no problem, but occasionally it indicates fetal distress. However, in breech births, meconium is expected. The pressure of the birth canal squeezes the tar-like stuff out as if it were toothpaste.

With every contraction, Catherine's back arched and her hips lifted into the air. She hollered just as I'd told her to, but even without her pushing, the contractions themselves forced more of the baby into my hand.

Dr. Stallone, his dark eyes fixed on our speeding car, waited with a wheelchair outside the ER as Todd zoomed up the ramp. The doctor's olive complexion blanched when he saw the baby's whole rear end in my hand.

Somehow Catherine again did the impossible. She crawled from the car and perched on the edge of the wheelchair seat. Dr. Stallone grabbed the handles and began running. Completely exposed, Catherine held her baby's bottom with one hand and the armrest of the wheelchair with the other. Mouth wide open, she threw her head back and screamed nonstop as we barreled through the emergency room. Visitors and staff came to every doorway. I heard a nurse yell into the phone, "Woman with half a baby hanging out on her way up" as we zipped past her desk. An ER attendant held open the door to the lobby and then ran for the elevator.

We passed an empty gurney. Thinking of Catherine's nakedness, I yanked off the sheet, flapped it into the air, and brought it down on top of Catherine, covering her completely. She looked like a screeching Halloween ghost flying through the corridors.

Into the elevator, up to the third floor, down another hallway, through some double doors, and straight into the delivery room we zoomed. Everyone was ready for us. Many hands lifted Catherine onto the delivery table. Other hands pulled covers over Todd's bare feet and wrestled him into a gown and mask. A pediatrician checked resuscitation equipment while an anesthesiologist started an IV in Catherine's arm. It all happened between one contraction and the next.

Dr. Stallone gowned and gloved and moved the Piper forceps to the front of the table. These are special forceps to deliver the head of a breech baby, which may be too big and round to pass easily through the mother's pelvis.

The unknowns of a breech delivery, not to mention our dramatic arrival at the hospital and the speed of the entire labor, created a high level of anxiety as the baby's legs, abdomen, and chest quickly emerged. At that point, her arms, too, should have been out, but they extended over her head, causing further delay.

With the umbilical cord—the baby's lifeline—squeezed between the baby's head and Catherine's pelvic bones, every second counted. Dr. Stallone manipulated his hand into Catherine's vagina, slipping two fingers beside the head until he felt an elbow. He flexed the arm and pulled it out. With the limp torso lying on his forearm and a leg dangling off each side, he repeated the process for the other arm.

"Okay, Catherine," he said urgently. "I need you to push harder than ever. We need to work fast. Come on, Catherine. Push!"

She pushed. She pushed like a silent, efficient machine. She pushed so hard the veins in her neck bulged like bell ropes. Todd hovered to one side, hands pressed to his mouth, eyes wide with fear. I took his elbow and led him closer, and he put his hand on Catherine's sweaty arm, seeming to take courage from her strength.

But the head didn't come.

The room grew quiet. Reaching behind him, Dr. Stallone picked up the forceps. I held the floppy body aloft with bare hands while the doctor knelt to slide the forceps into place. "Push!" he urged, and one gigantic push later, a limp baby girl flopped out, her body completely white, her head as purple as a ripe eggplant. Sightless, wide-open eyes stared unblinking into space. She flopped in my hands like a tattered rag doll.

I held the baby as Dr. Stallone cut the cord, and then I passed her to the resuscitation team. The clamp swinging at the end of the cord stump clattered against the side of the metal cart as the pros went into action.

Sobbing, Todd buried his face in Catherine's neck. I leaned down and whispered an explanation of what they were doing to the motionless baby. But all the while I talked to Catherine, another refrain played in my mind.

Breathe, baby, breathe, breathe, I chanted to myself as I stroked Catherine's hair. *Breathe for yourself, breathe for your momma and daddy.*

And breathe for me, a small part of me prayed. For five months I'd done home birth after home birth with no need to bring a mother to the hospital. But now I'd missed diagnosing a breech, and the baby lay pale and motionless on the warming bed.

I heard the staccato comments of the pediatrician.

"Heart rate 95. Pupils react to light."

Great! I thought, and my heart lifted.

"That's good news," I said to Catherine and Todd. I moved closer to the resuscitation cart and watched the baby turn pink as the nurse forced quick bursts of oxygen into her lungs. Half a minute later she began breathing on her own.

"Heart rate 120 . . . 140 . . . 150 and steady."

She coughed once, took a big breath, and held it as she blinked her eyes. A spark of interest came into them. She squinted under the bright lights and released a mighty cry, sounding a lot like her mother when we were halfway down that steep ravine.

For a moment I laughed along with everyone else, but then tears filled my eyes, tears of joy and thanks, tears of relief for the sake of the baby and her parents . . . and tears of relief for me. I might lose face. I might lose credibility. I might even lose my backup doctor. But the baby was fine.

Later, with the infant tucked into Catherine's arm and Todd standing beside them with a dazed look, I sat next to Dr. Stallone while he finished charting. He glanced at me and smiled, took a sip of coffee, and filled in another line on the form.

"Thanks, Bill," I said, and it sounded so inadequate that I continued. "You were great. I know I probably missed the breech prenatally. And it was a scary delivery, but you made it look almost easy. I just can't believe I missed it. The breech, I mean."

He leaned forward, pushing his wheeled chair back from the desk until he stretched almost flat. He stared at me, and my insides flip-flopped. Here it comes, I thought.

"I've backed a few lay midwives over the years, and now there's you, and I really like it. When midwives call with problems, we docs get to do what we're good at, the emergencies, the drama, the flashy stuff. I like swinging from the branches a bit, playing hot-dog obstetrics, and I know you do, too. But that trip through the halls took years off my life. Just give me a little break before you do it again."

Do it again? Had he said, Do it again? I nearly burst into song.

"You mean, after this, you'll still back me?"

He laughed. "Aw, hell, Peggy, we've all made mistakes, missed breeches, missed twins, you know that. Shit happens. As a nurse, you've saved my ass more than once. It's just pay-back time."

"Wow," was all I could muster. Maggie and Rita, two of my nurse friends, grinned from behind his back and lifted their thumbs.

I was still in business.

We Couldn't Have Done
It Without Him

I always asked my pregnant couples to invite another person to attend their home births, a person we dubbed the "housemother," regardless of gender. This housemother, a real job-juggler, might serve as babysitter for older children, gofer, photographer, extra coach, chauffeur in case of hospital transport, whatever. We also expected the housemother to hang around for a while after the birth to do laundry, cook a meal, and run the household while the new mom and dad napped.

Most women chose a mother, sister, aunt, or best friend. Many asked more than one extra person. Sometimes a whole crowd assembled, and then I knew we'd party afterwards.

At most births, women outnumbered men ten to one, but one of the very best housemothers I ever worked with was Steve, a gay guy who eventually attended about five births. His flawless intuition made him more priceless than rubies, and he won my heart forever when he slow danced for four straight hours with an exhausted woman, helping her endure a long, long night of hard labor.

Occasionally prospective grandfathers received an invitation, but their responses were sometimes less than enthusiastic. Unsure of their exact place in the whole affair, these gray-haired men tended to seek comfortable chairs in far corners of the room or look for something to tinker with in the garage.

Sofia's dad, however, had a different agenda. Glancing through the doorway of the bedroom where she labored, he said, "That's it, Sofia, you're crowning. Just a little longer and you'll be finished. I'll put the blankets in the oven."

Sofia stared at me in astonishment. Having examined her just ten minutes earlier, I knew she was only six centimeters dilated, nowhere near ready to begin pushing. And crowning, the moment when the baby's head completely fills the vaginal opening, wasn't even an issue.

"He's mistaken, Sofia," I said. "You still have more work to do."

In the background, I heard the squeak of the oven door. I knew the six baby blankets, wrapped in pairs in aluminum foil, would burn if they went into the oven this early.

When I ask someone to warm the receiving blankets, it's a signal to the laboring mother that the birth really will happen at home, just as she had dreamed. As a leap of faith, an act of affirmation, a vote of confidence, this business of timing when to warm the blankets mustn't be taken lightly. It's an important moment in a woman's labor. It tells her the midwife really believes the baby will come soon. Put in too early, the scorching smell can discourage the perspiring woman, making her feel she's not performing as quickly as the midwife expected.

One of ten children in an Italian family, Sofia had invited a sister and her mom and dad to attend her second child's home birth. Her father, a physician who still maintained a private practice at an age when most of his peers had retired, clearly considered himself in charge.

I looked over my shoulder at Sofia's sister. "Donna, those blankets will burn. Take them out of the oven, please, and tell your dad it's way too early."

Donna slipped into the kitchen and removed the three aluminum-wrapped packages. The oven door squeaked horribly, and her father reappeared. "What are you doing?" he asked her, frowning.

"Peggy says it's too soon. They might burn."

He grumbled but retreated to the living room where his wife sat knitting.

Sofia heard his grouchy retort and smiled at me. "He's really not comfortable with my having this baby at home, but he couldn't stand the idea of not being here, either. I'm sorry if he's a pain in the ass."

I tried to relax my tense smile a notch or two. In truth, he *was* a pain in the ass, but I felt sure I could handle him. Ordinarily I'd have asked Sofia's husband for assistance, but he was busy caring for their toddler in another room.

When Sofia's labor stalled at seven centimeters, I encouraged her to walk along the hallway to bring the contractions closer together. She leaned on my arm and shuffled toward the living room where her parents sat. Actually, only her mom sat, her knitting needles clicking as she worked on something in pale yellow wool. Sofia's dad paced. He smoothed his thinning hair with one hand while he rearranged books, pens, and other small items on a desk. When he saw Sofia grimacing in the doorway, he rushed toward her, pushing me aside to grip her by the shoulders. "Sofia, what are you doing out of bed? Get back in there right now. You shouldn't be on your feet. What if the baby comes?"

Sofia gently removed his hands and started back down the hall, speaking over her shoulder to him. "Daddy, that's the idea, isn't it? If this kid wants to be born in the hallway, that's fine with me."

Patting the cushion beside her, Sofia's mother said, "Ernest, come sit down. When the fruit is ready, it will fall."

Her knitting needles clicked faster as her husband sighed and flumped onto the couch. Moments later he bounced up again, saying, "I'll go deal with those blankets."

Again came the squeaking hinge. This time, I just glanced at Donna, and she went to the rescue.

In spite of our vigilance, he eventually put the three packages into the oven without our noticing. All too soon, the smell of toasting flannel wafted into the room, and I appointed Donna the official blanket monitor.

"Don't be too obvious," I told her, "but listen for that squeak. I don't think he's gonna give up easily."

I heard him later, grumbling, "Someone keeps taking these out." He succeeded in popping them into the oven three more times. As soon as he turned his back, Donna whipped them out.

"Leave them in. I'll keep an eye on them," he assured her once.

"Peggy says it's not time yet, Daddy." Her patience amazed me.

The issue about who was in charge of the blankets irritated me, but even more troublesome was his insistence on trying to manage his daughter's labor. Most of the time he crouched beside her, telling her she had only a few more contractions left. Sometimes he paced in the hallway, muttering to himself and shouting commands through the open door. The rest of the time he loomed over me, saying, "It's taking too long. The baby should be out by now."

I felt my blood pressure rising, and I knew I hovered on the verge of saying something rude. All my old feelings left from years of doctor-nurse communications surfaced. I took a deep breath and clenched my hands. "Doctor, her progress is normal, and Sofia and the baby are fine. I'm not concerned."

From the living room came a serene grandmother's voice. "Ernest, come in here. You're like a nervous old hen, and you're even starting to get on *my* nerves!"

The next time Sofia's dad barked, "Push, Sofia. It's almost out," I looked at her face to gauge her reaction, and realized she'd tuned out his incessant kibitzing. It had probably been more than thirty years since he'd delivered a baby, and she knew it. I wished I could ignore his presence as easily as she could. He buzzed, buzzed, buzzed in my face like an irritating mosquito, always there, always too close.

As the tumultuous final phase of dilation began, Sofia grew noisier, and her dad matched her volume. "Come on Sofia, push. Push hard!" he shouted, ignoring the fact that I'd just told her not to push quite yet. "Don't stop. Push, and it'll soon be over," he yelled.

"Dad," she groaned, rolling her eyes at him. Soon she found a spot that made it impossible for him to get in her face. She boxed herself into a corner behind an overstuffed chair, holding onto the back of it and swaying with each contraction.

"Listen to me, Sofia, you've got to push," he insisted, yanking on the chair. With equal determination, Sofia pulled it back, preserving her fortress.

I swear I heard my jaw pop as I unclenched my teeth. "Actually, she's not fully dilated yet," I said with what I thought was admirable control, "and I don't want her to push for at least another ten or fifteeen minutes."

He's just an old man, I told myself over and over, like a mantra. He's not used to being in a secondary position, and he's not comfortable with the whole idea of home birth—but I still had a strong desire to tie him to a chair and put duct tape over his mouth.

"Oh, perfect, Sofia, it's crowning!" he crowed.

Sofia turned her eyes toward me, and I shook my head. To her dad, I said, "It's *not* crowning. She's not even completely *dilated* yet." My fingernails dug into my palms.

He replied cheerfully, not at all put out by my testiness, "Oh, I know, but it'll give her courage."

I started to argue, but something stopped me. All eyes focused on Sofia. Everything ticked along like clockwork. A perfect birth awaited us if I could control myself—because I clearly couldn't control her father.

He was no fool. He knew Donna whisked those blankets out as fast as he put them in. It wasn't bothering him. It wasn't bothering Donna. It sure as heck wasn't bothering Sofia, barricaded behind her chair. I was the only one having difficulty with this man.

Suddenly I just . . . let go. I quit trying to prove I was in charge of everything, including the baby blankets. If slightly scorched blankets and my bruised ego were the only bad outcomes of this experience, it was a small price to pay. I turned to him and said, "Dr. Genovese, would you do me a favor? Would you please put the baby blankets in the oven?"

He bolted. I thought I heard him cackling with glee.

Donna raised her eyebrows at me, but I said, "It's still a little early, but it's close enough. Just sniff around now and then, in case they start to burn."

"Maybe now he'll be happy," grinned Donna, throwing her arm around his shoulder as he trotted back into the room.

"What? What?" he asked, seeing everyone smiling at him.

"Nothing, Dad. The blankets will be perfect, and we're about to watch Sofia give birth to your sixteenth grandchild."

About forty minutes later, just as the smell of over-baked blankets began to make my nose itch, Sofia's big baby boy plopped out, looking so Italian I thought we should dress him in something with an Armani label.

"Doctor, would you get one package of blankets for me, please?" I asked, and as he zipped away, I hollered, "Leave the other two in the oven, but turn the oven off. They'll stay warm, and I'll need them later."

Bearing the hot blankets in his outstretched arms like Melchior offering precious frankincense, Dr. Genovese returned to the bedroom in triumph.

Having successfully survived one skirmish, the doctor now moved on to another field of combat: the kitchen. Assuming the demeanor of a military field commander, he began preparing breakfast for everyone. As I walked through the kitchen to get ice for Sofia's swollen perineum, I watched her father turn his manic energy once more toward the stove. Like a short order cook on amphetamines, he turned burner, broiler, and oven knobs at random, finally succeeding in getting three burners lit and three frying pans in action.

While I helped Sofia's baby begin nursing, I heard her dad barking out orders. "Donna, start toasting this bread. We'll need at least sixteen slices, and make sure they stay warm under a towel. No, don't come near the stove. I absolutely do *not* have the fire too high. I've got everything under control here. There's plenty of bacon, and I think twenty eggs will be enough for, how many are we? Eight? Yes, eight. Mary, don't touch that pan. I know how to scramble eggs, for God's sake. Your job is to make coffee. Hurry, hurry! Someone make orange juice. Donna, set the table. Hmmm, the eggs are cooking a lot faster than I expected. Hurry up, everybody."

The sizzles and smells of bacon, eggs, toast, and coffee filled the house. I inhaled, then sniffed again. Burning baby blankets!

Running into the kitchen, I couldn't believe no one had noticed the smoke curling from the oven door. Experimenting with the stove's dials, Sofia's dad had set the broiler on High and failed to turn it off. Yanking open the door, I found the aluminum foil charred and falling away from four flaming blankets. Leaping forward, Sofia's dad pushed me aside and plucked them out with his bare fingers—*zip, zip*—onto the linoleum floor. He kicked them out the screen door where they promptly set the wooden porch on fire.

Three of us stomped on the burning blankets and smoldering decking for several minutes. Sofia's mother ran relays with a pasta pot, pouring water on the charred mess.

When danger passed, I glanced at the nimble-footed old man beside me. A look of pure pleasure spread over his face. It had been a good day: he'd put the blankets into the oven in time for his grandson's birth, he had organized breakfast for eight, and he'd saved the house from burning down.

From his perspective, we couldn't have done it without him.

~ Huh?

As I drove around Berkeley, I regularly spied bumper stickers that made me feel part of an elite, by-invitation-only underground movement.

SEE A MIDWIFE FOR A SPECIAL DELIVERY
MIDWIVES DO IT AT HOME
MIDWIFERY: A LABOR OF LOVE

The license plate on my VW Bug read MITWIFE, and whenever I passed one of those other cars, I honked and exchanged a thumbs-up. Sometimes I'd catch puzzled glances from clueless drivers in other cars and feel pity for them.

I took pride in my profession and believed those bumper sticker slogans. As I knelt to catch each woman's baby, I paid homage to a miracle. Not just to the wonder of new life, but also to a woman's transformation from girl to woman to mother—and, for a moment, to goddess.

In some way, each birth is special. In spite of the years that have passed, I can flip through my birth record and recall something unique about nearly every single one.

But I forgot Cindy. The shock of staring into that abyss in my memory led to a permanent change of routine. I didn't ever want that to happen again.

I had one foot out the door when the phone rang that day. I paused, indecision pulling me both ways. Already a little late, I itched to go visit a new mom whom I'd delivered three days earlier. But perhaps someone was in labor. Sighing, I picked up the phone.

"Peggy? It's Miriam Bishop."

"Yes?"

"Umm . . ."

Tapping my foot, I checked my watch, hoping this soft-spoken woman would get to the point quickly. "How can I help you, Mrs. Bishop?"

"We were wondering, didn't you say you were going to visit Cindy?"

"Huh?"

Cindy, Cindy, I said to myself. Why does that sound familiar?

"Perhaps I misunderstood, but you delivered her baby four nights ago and . . ."

Cindy! My stomach plummeted. It came back to me like some familiar old movie. The two A.M. phone call, the fast drive, the faster delivery, the trip home and straight back to my bed. By the next morning, *nada*. Gone. Just vanished, as if my brain were a sieve with great big holes. Holes big enough to let the image of a nine-pound baby slip through. I'd forgotten Cindy's birth altogether. *Shit!*

"Oh, yeah, sure, *Cindy!* God, it just slipped my mind. Of course I'm planning a visit. How's she doing?" No, much too hearty a tone. Let's try to be more professional, I told myself. "Would it be convenient for me to come right now?"

I canceled my postpartum visit in the suburbs and headed toward Cindy's house.

Oh. My. God. Totally brain dead. But now, it came back, all right, every second of the missing memory. *Judas priest!* I muttered, pounding the steering wheel.

I drove through the tunnel beneath the Oakland Estuary, recalling the events of three nights before. A phone call at 1:53 A.M. awakened me, and I grabbed the receiver on the first ring. Rog slept peacefully next to me, hearing nothing.

"Hello?" Strange, snuffling sounds came through the phone, then a low moan. "Hello?" I repeated, a little louder.

"Peggy?" replied a shaky voice. "Miriam Bishop, Cindy's mom. I'm afraid we waited too late to call you. Cindy's having the baby, and I don't think you'll make it."

Rog didn't even twitch as I ripped off my nightgown, pulled on sweats, grabbed my clogs, and ran to my car.

The streets and sidewalks stretched empty ahead of me. A shuffling homeless man materialized from the shadows, but I didn't spot more than five cars as I flew toward Alameda. My car swerved around a huge pothole as I turned onto Cindy's street, and I concentrated on looking for the house with a wrecked Chevy in the front yard. I pulled into the driveway and glanced toward the rear cottage, a tiny one-room affair with no plumbing. Nineteen-year-old Cindy lived back there with her husband and son, but every window stared back at me, pitch dark.

All the lights blazed in the main house, however, so I raced up the front steps and banged on the screen door. A young teenager in baby-doll pajamas and hair rollers jerked it open and pointed me down a corridor toward the kitchen. Encumbered with boxes of birth supplies (see Appendix Two) in both hands, I wiggled in a two-step tango along the narrow hallway.

The kitchen looked like a silent movie set with six or seven people frozen in place. But no Cindy. Her husband, Tommy, held up his low-slung jeans with one arm and his two-year-old son with the other. Cindy's hollow-cheeked mother clutched a bloody towel in her hand. A girl in a magenta T-shirt and skimpy underpants stirred a cup of cocoa, while Cindy's father perched on the edge of a chair, toying with a Bud. A little girl of about eight wearing nylon jammies far too short for her skinny legs balanced on his knee.

I stopped in the middle of the bright room and swung left and right, then back again, searching for Cindy. Her little boy tipped up a bottle of red Kool-Aid, and the high-pitched *zzzzzzz* of air entering the plastic bottle whistled through the silent room.

I asked, "Where . . ." but before I could say more, a door burst open and slammed into the wall. Backlit by a bare bulb, mongo-bellied Cindy erupted from the stark light of the bathroom. Blue eyes glowing like gaudy dime store gems, she streaked across the linoleum, holding her crotch and bellowing like a Brahman bull. She shimmied past me and barreled down the hallway. I turned and chased after her.

Cindy did a quick right turn into a room with a king-sized bed that took up every inch of space. She sprawled on the edge of the bed, her legs high in the air. With lips drawn in a toothy snarl, she gripped her ankles, grunted once, and pushed her baby's head out.

I still had my supplies in my hands. Dropping everything with a crash, I caught the rest of the baby in midair.

"Whew!" I said as I held the screaming baby with my bare hands.

"Whew!" sighed Cindy. "I'm sure as hell glad *that's* over!" She pushed her fine, damp hair out of her eyes and smiled at me.

"Whew!" whispered Cindy's mother behind me. "I can't believe you made it."

"Just," said her father.

I turned and saw them, looking like a Norman Rockwell illustration as they crowded into the doorway to watch the birth. It hadn't been much of a birth, in my opinion. More like an eviction without due notice.

Someone handed me a towel, and someone else brought two warm receiving blankets and a pie pan. In the next few minutes, I dried the baby, cut the cord, and delivered the placenta. I inspected Cindy's perineum, which looked like nothing had happened, examined and weighed the baby (nine pounds), and tucked her into Cindy's arms. I hadn't been in the house ten minutes, and I was pretty much finished.

I fished a pen from my purse and did some charting, but there wasn't much to say. Half an hour after she delivered, Cindy bounced off the bed and showered. Her sister changed the sheets. Her mother heated a couple of cans of Campbell's chicken noodle soup, and I sipped a mug of it and watched everyone scurry around, doing all the housewifely tasks I usually did after a birth.

Tommy laid his sleeping son on the couch in the crowded living room where Cindy's father started on another Bud. Canned laughter from a *Gilligan's Island* rerun blared from the TV.

I checked Cindy's bleeding and blood pressure. Perfect. I checked her uterus. Firm and right at her belly button. Perfect. The baby checked out fine, too, all pink and puckered, sucking away in her sleep, eyes squeezed shut against the bright lights.

The first critical hour after the birth passed without a hitch. Everyone looked sleepy. I began to feel that only Gilligan and I were keeping these polite folks from their beds. And, really, I had nothing left to do.

So I went home, snuggled under the quilts, and fell right back to sleep.

I felt terrific when I awoke in the morning. Fresh. Well rested. I drove a car full of noisy kids to school and then filled a grocery cart at Safeway. In the afternoon I measured pregnant bellies and listened to the heartbeats of many unborn babies. I fixed tacos for dinner, helped Colin with a report, and did the dishes while Rog drilled Jill on multiplication tables. I flopped into bed with a clear conscience.

The next day, more of the same. And the next.

Then came Miriam Bishop's apologetic phone call, precipitating the biggest guilt trip of my professional life. I prayed to all the gods of every faith that I wouldn't find a jaundiced baby or a mom with hemorrhoids like walnuts.

I saw Cindy through the cottage's screen door. She crouched on the double bed, changing the baby's diaper. She stood up when I entered. I noticed her T-shirt tucked into the front of her jeans. Size six jeans, zipped up tight, four days after delivery. Jeez, teenagers!

"I didn't want Mom to bother you. You didn't have to come again. We're fine."

She was apologizing to *me*. My guilt deepened. "No, I always visit moms and babies a few days after the birth," I assured her, feeling my cheeks flush. "Let me give you both a once-over."

They checked out perfectly, of course, and I tried to rationalize that surely they would have called had there been problems. But would they? Such self-effacing people, the Bishops. Working class, a little shy, not wanting to trouble anyone.

"I didn't want to get you out of bed too early," explained Cindy's mother when I asked why she hadn't phoned me sooner in the labor. "After all, it was the middle of the night, and you have a family and an important job." Good manners had waged war with good sense, and politeness had won. She'd waited way too long to call.

Once again, the truth of the old adage came home to me: It's better to be lucky than smart. But forgetting a baby's birth altogether? Uh-uh, I didn't ever want to risk its happening again. Rog usually asked me in the morning how a birth had gone, but it appeared I couldn't count on that any longer. After all, he never even knew I'd left home.

So I developed a method of ensuring that a birth never again slipped my mind. As soon as I returned from a middle-of-the-night birth, I placed the mother's chart front and center on my desk, and first thing the next morning, the sight of it jogged my memory. Never again did I forget I'd delivered a baby. And I never forgot Cindy. In fact, I thought of her every time I came downstairs for breakfast and saw a chart on top of all my other papers. No matter whose chart it was, I always thought of Cindy first.

~ Hallie's Reputation

In 1982, Rog and I took a family vacation to the Gold Rush country along Highway 49. Colin, ten years old at the time, frowned as he stared out the car window.

"Why does it look different here?" he asked as we traveled the narrow roads in the Sierra Nevada foothills.

"Maybe the mountains in the background?" Rog suggested.

"Or all these little towns with funny names like Volcano or Rough and Ready?" I offered. But he shook his head, still puzzled.

Then his face lit up, and he exclaimed, "Wheelchairs. That's what's different. Where are all the wheelchairs?"

Berkeley, handicap-accessible long before someone coined the term, probably has more wheelchairs than Guinness has records. Curbs at every intersection slope for wheelchairs, also delighting cyclists, rollerbladers, and skateboarders. Once I spotted a seeing-eye dog pulling Georgia, a disabled woman I know, in her broken wheelchair up to the Center for Independent Living to have her wheelchair repaired. In Georgia's lap sat the dog's blind owner, and both women manually spun the wheels to assist the gallant dog.

Tom, a young author I met at a writing workshop, married Darcy, a paraplegic woman. Their wedding announcement featured a delightful photograph of her in her wedding gown, her veil flowing in the wind. She was powering her wheelchair down a sidewalk and towing her tuxedo-clad, top-hatted, champagne-toting husband on his skateboard.

Hallie and Ian belonged to this very-Berkeley, very-iconoclastic group of disabled individuals and their partners. I'd met Hallie a couple of years before I became her midwife. She'd been present as a housemother when I delivered several of her friends, and I'd been impressed with her calm, straightforward attitude. Nothing seemed to be too much for her. In any crisis, you would want Hallie beside you.

But her lifestyle would have made her father, a career military man, disown her if she hadn't left home first. As a teenager, Hallie packed a 75-cent Salvation Army suitcase and took a Greyhound bus from Virginia straight to a tattoo parlor in San Francisco's Haight Ashbury. Still dragging the old suitcase by a broken handle, she walked out with her first tattoo, a blatantly erotic purple, black, and pink orchid on the back of her calf. It would have embarrassed Georgia O'Keeffe.

Hallie threw herself headlong into the counterculture's sexual and political revolution of the early seventies, trying to put herself through college with her earnings as a tarot card reader, masseuse, and tattoo artist while living in a communal household with no bedroom doors. When she found it impossible to make ends meet, she took a job as a live-in attendant for Ian, a partially disabled, soft-spoken Irishman confined to a wheelchair by an auto accident.

As an attendant, Hallie found herself surrounded by "crips," as the disabled often refer to themselves. She made friends with other young women working as attendants, and soon she and Ian moved into a commune led by Bjorn, a charismatic quadriplegic with a pointer stick strapped to his forehead. Unable to speak clearly enough to be understood, he used the stick to operate his wheelchair and to tap instructions to his housemates on a keyboard mounted in front of him.

By this time, Hallie's body sported at least twenty tattoos, and within Berkeley's disabled community she and Ian were known as the couple who finally ended Bjorn's autocratic leadership.

"Yeah, in the beginning it was one big free-for-all," Ian explained during a prenatal visit, "and Bjorn was kinda like the conductor of the whole flamin' orchestra. Only then Hallie 'n' me fell in love. Not what either of us was lookin' for, no indeed. But it happened, and so I bought a bedroom door and put a lock on it."

"Bjorn didn't like that challenge to his authority," Hallie added.

"Yeah, he left a couple of weeks later, and then others split off. Four couples and a bunch of kids stayed here, but all in separate bedrooms."

This had happened more than five years before I met them. During those years, Hallie finished college, had her first baby, and became a political activist, a fixture at Berkeley and Oakland city council meetings as a spokesperson for the homeless, the crazies, and the disabled. "Hallie gets things done," said one councilman.

But I didn't know her independence extended to childbirth until I missed the birth of her second child. When I asked why she'd waited so long to call me, she explained. "I didn't want to bother you too early. My first baby took more than twenty hours of hard work, so I thought I had tons of time left."

"'Tons of time.' Ha!" Ian snorted, slouching in his wheelchair. Hallie's biceps bulged beneath a tattoo of barbed wire and roses as she shifted him upright, never losing her grip on her toddler, Jonah.

"But you live with gazillions of other people," I said. "Where were they?"

"Gardenias," said Ian.

Seeing my blank look, Hallie explained, "When labor started, I wanted to be surrounded by gardenias. So I sent everyone out to buy all they could find."

Alone together in the big house, an hour passed as Hallie rocked to the rhythm of her labor. Then she disappeared into the huge communal shower, and Ian watched from the doorway. "Hallie, girl, shouldn't we be callin' the midwives?"

"No, no. It's way too soon," and she gyrated to the other end of the tiled space.

However, when her singing changed to a lower pitch punctuated by long pauses as she boogied and high-stepped in tight-lipped silence, Ian wheeled himself to the hall phone and called me.

"Well, now, Peggy, it's thinkin' I am that you'd best be comin' along. You see, Hallie's been singin' in the shower for quite a while, but now the contractions are makin' her dance a bit."

I tensed as he described her behavior. If the contractions were making Hallie "dance a bit," I needed to be there. I called Sandi and drove off.

Sandi and I arrived within moments of each other and hustled up the zigzag wheelchair ramp to the front door. Pushing it open, we were greeted by what looked like a nativity scene in a church pageant—except for the wheelchair and the nudity, of course.

Ian slouched in his wheelchair in the middle of the room. Hallie, naked except for a string of coral beads at her throat, knelt on a plaid flannel shirt beside him. She hummed, rocking back and forth as she stared at a newborn in her arms. Her soft blond hair fell back from her face as she looked up, those blue, blue eyes shining with pride. Ian's round face bent toward her, his heavy, dark-framed glasses sliding down his nose. His hand rested lightly on Hallie's head, and tears made little tracks on his cheeks as he pushed his glasses up with a blunt fingertip.

"Ah, sweet Mother of Christ, I couldn't even help her," he said.

The baby curled peacefully in his mother's arm, waving his fist like a drunken conductor. Sandi dried him off and covered him with a clean blanket while I helped Ian cut the cord. Then I started to deliver the placenta.

Hallie put her hand on mine and said, "I'd really like to finish this myself. Do you think I can?"

"Hallie, I think you could do your own root canal at this point. Of course you can deliver the placenta."

Hallie handed the baby to Ian, and Sandi wedged him in place with a pillow. Then Hallie squatted over a lasagna pan, and with a determined push and a little traction on the cord, the placenta plopped out.

We expected the return of the whole noisy household, loaded down with gardenias, at any moment, and Hallie wanted to put some clothes on. She stood, but paused beside Ian's wheelchair. Standing proud, still naked except for the coral beads shining against her fair skin, Hallie kissed first the baby's head and then Ian's. Placing her hand against his cheek, she held him within her Madonna gaze.

Ian raised his weak left hand with some effort and cupped her breast in his palm. They remained like this, eyes locked, until it seemed they would dissolve into each other. He finally spoke in a voice thick with emotion. "Hallie, girl, it's lovin' you I am, I am!"

So Hallie's reputation for independence gained mythic proportions. When she conceived her third child and came to me for the first prenatal visit, we talked about that solo performance of hers. "Did you intend to use me like a fire extinguisher, handy to have tucked away in the closet, just in case? Did you plan it that way, so I'd arrive moments after the delivery?" I asked. She denied a hidden agenda, and I think I believed her—but I remained just a little suspicious. "Hallie, it's fine with me if you do it yourself again, but just get me there. If there's a problem, I don't want to arrive too late to help."

Hallie's third labor started on a gray afternoon as the cold summer fog rolled under the Golden Gate Bridge and crept across the bay to Berkeley. As I'd requested, she called me immediately. With mild contractions more than fifteen minutes apart, we both knew I didn't need to be present. But I cautioned, "Hallie? Remember?"

"Yeah, yeah, I know. I promise."

I loaded everything into my car, and then I sat by the phone, picking it up now and then to be sure it was working. Four hours later it jangled at my elbow. Ian's deep voice boomed, "Ah yes, well now, Peggy, Hallie's getting' on with the singin' again, but she hasn't got to the dancin' part yet, so I think you've got a bit more time this go round."

In less than fifteen minutes I parked in their driveway. The house and yard looked much tidier than on my visit three years earlier. Since Hallie's last birth, the household had shrunk. Only a gaunt man with severe cerebral palsy named Rick, his wife, Artemis, and their three children remained as house-mates.

We pushed open the door, and it was déjà vu: Ian in his wheelchair in the middle of the room, and Hallie on the floor beside him, naked. But this time, Hallie was still pregnant, and they were better prepared. Hallie crouched over towels and absorbent Chux, a commercial waterproof product. A small pile of birth supplies sat on a low table within arm's reach.

Limited by his wheelchair and his disabilities, Rick looked overwhelmed by the five children, his own three as well as Hallie and Ian's two boys. Artemis rose from Hallie's side, tossed her long brown braid over her shoulder, and hurried toward Rick and the kids. Her gauzy skirt puddled gracefully around her hips as she settled on the floor, and within seconds all five children engulfed her. She looked like a Navajo storyteller doll.

When I examined Hallie, none of us were surprised that she was almost ready to deliver. "You still want to do this yourself, Hallie?" I asked her.

She nodded but didn't speak. She was too occupied staying calm for the sake of the children who tumbled over each other like puppies, trying to see what was going on. Rick passed out Fruit Roll-Ups to keep them occupied, and soon the sound of ripping plastic wrap followed by sucking was the only noise in the warm room.

Hallie grimaced with the first urge to push. I knelt beside her, and she threw her arm across my shoulder. Putting her other hand between her thighs, she shifted her legs till she crouched on one knee. She pressed her face to mine, and I whispered, "That's it, keep your hand there so you'll know when the baby's crowning. It's already coming fast, you don't have to try to speed it along. Think of it as steering rather than pushing."

Ian patted her head and murmured, "Ah, girl, yer doin' a fine job, you are."

A few contractions later, Hallie froze. A quick look between her legs revealed that most of the baby's head had just filled her hand, and a glance back at her face told me she didn't quite know what to do with it.

"Just the tiniest little push, Hallie, and the rest of the head will come right out. It's teetering right on the brink. Press against it just a little so it doesn't come too fast."

"Ah, Hallie, I can see it myself, luv. 'Tis grand, oh, 'tis."

"Perfect. The head's out and the eyes are open. Can you see its face, Ian?"

"Aaah, Jesus, Mary, and holy St. Joseph, yes, I can, I do. Oh, blessed Mother of Christ, Hallie, it's a wonder, you are."

Hallie had made no sound since my arrival. I glanced at the children and saw five wide-open pairs of eyes riveted on her. Five sticky little mouths rounded into perfect Os. Not a single piece of plastic wrap crinkled.

With the intense pressure eased, Hallie relaxed, took a few quick breaths, and looked at me with a "what next?" expression.

"Ah, Hallie, Hallie," crooned Ian, placing his palm on her cheek.

Sandi came in, glanced between Hallie's legs, and went straight to the oven for the baby blankets. She set them next to me and then got more Chux and towels to make a little dam for the gush of fluid that often comes after the baby.

"Hallie, squat back on your heels and let the head rest on the floor. Now, take your hand off the head—don't worry, it can't drop or get hurt. I want you to feel up inside and see if there's a loop of umbilical cord around the neck."

She didn't move.

"You can do it," I assured her. "It just takes a second or two, but if there's a cord there, you must slip it over the head before the body comes out."

She just looked at me.

"Can you do it?"

She shook her head and breathed a single word. "You."

So I eased one bare finger up into the slippery, corduroy vaginal folds, up beside a soft seashell of an ear, over the baby's cheek and jaw, and into the silky warm folds of the neck creases. I found no cord hiding in the rolls of baby fat, and the final contraction started as I slipped my finger out.

The top shoulder slid under Hallie's pubic bone with ease. "Perfect. Slip your hand along the baby's other shoulder, Hallie, and lift up as it comes out. Can you use both hands?"

Sandi stood behind Hallie and let her lean against her legs. Hallie took her arm off my shoulder and, using both hands, cradled the baby's body as it dropped with a soft thump onto the toweling.

"Ah, sweet Jesus, Hallie, it's a girl. We've got ourselves a girl! Come here Jonah, Michael, come see your little sister. Ah, now, 'tis a miracle for sure."

The sweet cries of a newborn filled the room. Sandi wrapped her and fluffed up her downy black hair with an oven-warm blanket. As the five children crowded round, Ian reached out a finger to touch his daughter's wrinkled hand. Hallie pushed damp hair off her forehead and looked at me. Beaming, she said, "Well, I got you here in time."

"Yes, just barely, but indeed you did. Are you ready for the placenta? You have to preserve your reputation for independence, you know."

She thought for a moment and then tilted her head and laughed. "Nah, you can do the placenta this time. I've had enough independence for today."

Only What's Necessary

Janelle, one of my very first home birth clients, introduced herself by saying, "I'm a Christian Scientist." I didn't know what that meant except that she probably believed in the healing power of prayer instead of doctors and drugs. When Janelle's labor began, I realized that lessons I'd learned in my fifteen years of working with laboring women wouldn't apply to her. She didn't respond to contractions the way other women did, and she exhibited none of the usual clues of advanced labor. Janelle just didn't seem to feel her contractions at all.

When she had pushed five or six times, her intact bag of water bulged between her legs like a fortuneteller's crystal ball. I could see the baby's hair floating back and forth like seaweed in the ebb and flow of the tide. Janelle chatted with her husband and commented on a neighbor's noisy barking dog.

Suddenly the bag broke with an audible pop, and we all jumped.

"Oh, my goodness," Janelle said, looking at me with mild surprise. That was absolutely her only response to the entire labor. Ninety seconds later, she lay back with her arms behind her head and observed her baby's gentle birth as if she were watching "The Mary Tyler Moore Show."

Many other Christian Scientists came after Janelle. They didn't all act like she did, but they definitely didn't act like my other, non-CS clients. I threw out my usual rulebook and tried to figure them out based on other criteria, but I'm not sure I ever really got a handle on them. I just learned to watch them more closely, to be very, very alert.

So when Susannah said her labor had begun, I knew enough not to trust her. She was, after all, another Christian Scientist.

Her husband, Paul, had delivered their first three children at home with no preparation except his faith, two manuals on emergency childbirth, and the boundless blessing of having married a woman born to have babies gracefully. But they went shopping for a midwife for their fourth baby because the Christian Science church had been criticized for policies relating to the well-being of babies and children. Legal issues arose when parents made decisions not to seek standard medical care for underage children, and in a few instances the state had made children temporary wards of the court to treat them for conditions like pneumonia and meningitis. So, perhaps feeling under some pressure, Susannah and Paul began interviewing midwives, and a Christian Science practitioner gave them my name.

Susannah said, "I don't need doctors to have babies. Will you do only what's necessary, only what's required by law?"

I agreed, but when I explained that I wouldn't cross the bay to attend births so far from my backup facilities, they decided to have the baby at Susannah's parents' house in Oakland. This would require them to drive an hour from their home in Marin County.

On a balmy, late summer afternoon, Susannah called from her home high on the slopes of Mt. Tamalpais and said her water bag had broken and labor was beginning. They would round up their boys and drive across the bay. Hmm, I said to myself. Three previous easy births. Christian Scientist. An hour's drive ahead of them. I decided to leave right away and wait for them at her mother's house.

I drove over the hill to her parents' spacious modern home in the Oakland hills. I had all my equipment set up in the guest bedroom long before Susannah and Paul's gray Subaru station wagon pulled into the driveway. As the car stopped, three noisy towheads tumbled out the rear doors, shrieking, "Gramma, Grampa, we're here, and Momma's gonna have her baby today!"

Paul opened the wayback, behind the rear seat, and unloaded a bag of groceries, a diaper bag, and a Port-a-Crib. Susannah brought up the rear, carrying nothing but a bouquet of cosmos and freesias for her mother. From a distance, she could have passed for eighteen. Wearing a beige and pink floral maternity dress tied above her enormous belly, pink leather sandals, and a wide-brimmed straw hat with silk flowers spilling over one edge, she looked like a picture on a Hallmark Easter card. Her long blond hair blew around her face as she breezed into the house with the graceful walk of a ballerina. You'd never have known she was pregnant, let alone in labor, from the way she moved. Only the stupendous belly gave her away.

In fact, I assumed the contractions had stopped. She greeted her parents, settled the boys in the TV room, and fixed herself a cup of herbal tea. I saw no evidence of contractions. She talked animatedly and steadily. She never paused to hold the wall or rub her stomach. She didn't breathe deeply or sigh—or anything.

"How's the labor going? Did things slow down on your way over?" I asked.

"Oh, not really. It's all progressing according to God's plan," she answered with a vague wave of her hand.

Her fair skin glowed, but she wasn't perspiring. She removed her hat and set it on the gleaming console table in the entryway. Then she pulled a storybook from the diaper bag, scooped up her squirmy two year old, and headed to the bedroom where my supplies lay on the walnut dresser in order of anticipated need. The French doors stood wide open, and beyond them a willow tree trailed drooping branches into a creek that meandered through a Japanese-style garden.

Susannah kicked off her sandals and sat on a towel on the edge of the bed. Her son nestled against her and sucked his thumb while she read a story about a mother cat named Snowy having four little kittens. She never missed a word. Once she shifted slightly and stretched her back, twisting to one side as if to work out a kink. Nothing more.

As I lifted aside the loose folds of her dress to check the baby's heartbeat, I saw that she wore no underpants. Fully dressed as if for church, but no panties. How interesting. I looked at her face. She smiled placidly and continued the story of the frolicking kittens.

About four pages remained in the book when she closed it and handed it to her son. Puzzled, he started to protest, but Susannah set him on his feet and said in a tone that brooked no dissension, "Take it to Gramma, Peter. She'll finish it."

He backed away, keeping his eyes on her face till he reached the doorway. She sat still as stone with her hands in her lap, watching him. I heard the splashing sounds of the untamed creek at the back of the property. It was so quiet. A muscle twitched in Susannah's temple. She blinked, and I saw her teeth clench.

Peter still hesitated. She looked hard at him and said, "Peter, go see Gramma. Now." He turned and ran.

"Paul!" she shouted, and I jumped.

As Paul appeared at the far end of the long hallway and headed toward the bedroom, Susannah spread her feet on the floor and pressed her fists to the bed on either side of her hips. She lifted her bottom a couple of inches above the towel and crouched over the bed.

For a moment I didn't realize what was happening. But something about the way she held her breath, the deliberateness of her movements, the careful way she lifted herself higher—something made me pull her dress aside again.

A baby's face stared at me, bubbles coming from the pink lips.

As she continued to stand up, the rest of the baby was born. Not born, really. Not born in any active, dramatic way. It seemed more like Susannah just lifted herself off the baby that was already lying on the bed.

"Oh, for heaven's sake," I muttered. I pushed the baby back from the edge and covered her with the towel. My birth supplies were fifteen feet away. "Why didn't you say something?"

"It wasn't necessary," she said, pulling her hair off her neck, twisting it, and securing it on top of her head. She smiled like a cat with a saucer of cream and blotted two drops of sweat from her upper lip.

"What?" asked Paul, appearing in the doorway.

The baby made a tentative cry as polite as the manner of its birth. Paul's eyes grew wide, and he froze, listening.

Susannah stood on an unblemished expanse of soft, jade wall-to-wall carpeting with the umbilical cord looping back to the baby. A single drop of blood no larger than a nickel fell to the carpet, but any minute there might be a real gusher. I yanked back the bedspread and sheets and pushed Susannah onto the plastic.

"But . . . is that the baby? Susannah, what on earth?" Paul stared at the mewing, towel-wrapped bundle behind his wife.

"Paul, of course it's the baby," she said.

"But—"

"Heck, Paul, don't feel like the Lone Ranger," I said as I clamped the cord. "She didn't tell me she was having it either."

"*Sus—AAAAN—nah!*" he cried.

"What? Everything's fine. It was like laying an egg. Now I know how chickens do it."

The placenta slid out with the same lack of fanfare as the baby had. I placed it in a pie pan and said, "But chickens at least cackle, and you didn't make a sound. You didn't even flap your wings—or anything."

"It wasn't necessary," she insisted, pulling the baby onto her chest.

"Well, what is it?" asked Paul, creeping closer.

"It's a girl, honey, a little girl. I already told you."

"Did you even look, Susannah? You've been telling me it's a girl for five months. Are you sure?" he asked, and I wondered the same thing myself, knowing I'd covered the baby with a towel before Susannah had turned around.

"It's not necessary. I know it's a girl."

Paul turned to me with a desperate look, and I put him out of his misery.

"She was right all along, Paul. You've got yourselves a daughter."

Ninety minutes later, Susannah had showered and dressed—underwear and all. We sat in the garden sipping tea and nibbling macadamia nut cookies. I don't think little Peter ever heard what happened to Snowy's kittens, but in the excitement of meeting his baby sister, he didn't seem upset. I checked Susannah and the baby a few more times and then drove home.

I found Rog sitting at the kitchen table slicing peaches for homemade ice cream. He stared at me in surprise. "That was fast. I didn't expect you back so soon. I guess she wasn't in labor, huh?"

"Oh, she was in labor, all right."

"You mean you delivered the baby already?"

I picked up a juicy peach slice and popped it into my mouth. Then I smiled at him as I licked my fingers.

"It wasn't necessary."

The Perineal Cry

When my dentist accused me of grinding my teeth, I knew my efforts to "make nice" during hospital committee meetings had gotten to me. As a firm believer in the adage that a camel is a horse designed by a committee, I have the tolerance of an irritated gnat when it comes to the negotiations typical of such official groups. But it was important, so I had to smile and look sweet—and grind my teeth.

Alta Bates, the Mt. Everest of the medical community, had been considered unconquerable by a mere midwife. Then Dr. Joe Weick, always a champion of the underdog and my backup physician since Dr. Stallone had moved to southern California, raised his hackles. Joe lodged a complaint with the Fair Trade Commission, charging Alta Bates with restraint of trade for refusing to grant privileges to midwives. Faced with possible loss of federal funds in late 1983, the OB department quickly hammered together some guidelines.

I read the document and then threw it onto Joe's desk. "This is offensive. With their hands tied by rules like this, midwives in some cases would have less authority than nurses. No midwife would want to practice at Alta Bates under these rules."

"That's their objective, Peggy. They've complied with the law, but they're hoping no midwife will actually apply. You've got to do it."

"Oh, no, not me. I'm the wrong person. I have a short fuse when it comes to bureaucratic shenanigans."

"You're exactly the right person. At least they know you, and most of them liked and respected you when you worked here as a nurse. Now that you're a midwife, you're an enemy, but at least you're a known enemy."

"But . . ."

"It has to be you. They may not like your being a midwife, but they know you're a safe practitioner. Once you're in, you can work to change the guidelines into something that will actually allow you to practice."

So I did it. But by merely challenging the status quo, I alienated doctors with whom I'd previously had good relations. With folded arms, they sat across the long table from me, unwilling to meet my eyes as they challenged my right "to practice obstetrics."

"I don't practice obstetrics," I countered. "I practice midwifery."

After eighteen months of grueling meetings, acrimonious negotiations, and nit-picking work on the protocols, I finally agreed to a document that would eventually allow me to deliver babies without constant supervision.

But I knew their magnifying glass would exaggerate my every action. Until I'd proven my skills to even the most antagonistic of the doctors, I could expect intense scrutiny, hostile stares, and frequent chart reviews by oversight committees. I knew my future—and that of other midwives who would inevitably follow me—depended on my performance.

This was especially true during my first ten deliveries, during which a physician would observe each birth and complete an exhaustive evaluation for the department chief. Everything had to be perfect.

Kati would be among those first deliveries. She called me early Sunday morning and said, "My bag of water just broke, and it looks like there's maybe a little meconium in it." She wanted to delay hospital admission until her labor was well underway, but, since meconium can indicate fetal stress, I needed to check her baby's heartbeat right away. I parked in front of her cozy bungalow, hoping I'd be able to reassure her that it wasn't meconium at all, just some brownish mucus mixed with the amniotic fluid.

As I walked through the fairy tale garden leading to the front door, I glanced through the window and saw Carl sitting on an opened futon. In front of him stood Kati, and the sight of her astounded me.

Her mass of tangled dark hair lay wet with sweat against her face and shoulders, and her bare buttocks showed below a cut-off T-shirt. Only twenty-five minutes had passed since her phone call saying labor hadn't started, but now she looked like a woman in heavy labor. Then I saw her grimace, grip Carl's shoulders—and squat.

Galvanized, I bolted through the unlocked door and ran into the living room, nearly falling over three-year-old Alyssa, who was sitting in a red rocking chair. As I dodged her, two rabbits scuttled under the futon.

A puddle of dark fluid pooled on a white towel between Kati's feet, the very kind of meconium I'd hoped not to see. Blotches of bloody mucus stained her thighs. She watched me rip open a sterile glove and said, "I'm sorry I'm carrying on like this. I've only been in labor for forty-five minutes, but I'm not handling it very well."

I knelt to check her and confirmed what I already suspected: Kati was about to give birth. A quick check of the baby's heartbeat reassured me, but there could still be serious complications at the delivery.

"Actually, you're doing great," I reassured her. "In the last half hour you've coped with progress that takes most women ten to twelve hours, but . . ."

"This is my new dress, Peggy. Do you like it?" Alyssa stood beside me, admiring her blue-flowered smock.

I ignored her when I saw Kati headed toward the bathroom. If she reached the toilet, I might never get her out of the house. Steering her past the bathroom, I said, "You're ready to deliver, Kati, but there's lots of thick meconium. We have to go to the hospital right now. You don't need the toilet. It's just pressure from the baby."

I put Alyssa into her father's arms and said, "Carl, load Alyssa in your car while I call Alta Bates. I'll lock up and bring Kati."

Another contraction brought Kati to the floor. She grabbed me around both knees, nailing me to the spot and still out of reach of the phone. Carl gave me a strange look, and I sensed he felt both Kati and I were being drama queens. Sighing, he walked out with Alyssa on one hip and a heavy duffel bag loaded with all their hospital paraphernalia in his other hand.

Meanwhile, Velcroed to Kati by her grip on my thighs, I inched my way another few feet down the hall. A curious rabbit hopped along behind. I lunged for the phone and dialed labor and delivery.

As I listened to the phone ringing, I marveled at how quickly Kati's and my plans for this birth had gone awry. Due to a rare complication, her first birth had ended with an emergency cesarean in the seventh month. Now pregnant with her second child, she had carefully planned the birth. She and Carl had written an elaborate list of requests that included staying home until the onset of heavy labor, low lights, soft music, privacy, a quiet atmosphere, and a Leboyer bath for the baby. When she'd called me less than an hour earlier, I'd heard the concern in her voice, concern not just for the baby but also for the loss of autonomy this would mean.

I thought about how much we both had at stake in this birth. Scrutiny by the OB staff would be intense, but now I sensed Kati and I were on the verge of losing control of the situation.

At last the ward clerk picked up the telephone.

"Susan, it's Peggy. I'm bringing in a lady on the fast track, nine centimeters, thick meconium, previous cesarean. I'm under the observation period, so Dr. Weick has to supervise me. Would you please call him? We'll be there in fifteen minutes."

I hauled Kati up and pulled a pale blue maternity dress over her head as she slipped on heavy clogs. Then I pushed a bunny away, steered Kati outside, and locked up.

We made it almost to the car before another contraction hit. An elderly man in overalls walking his beagle paused in amazement as Kati fell to her knees on the sidewalk, right between the blooming cosmos and the blue Corolla. As her moaning filled the air, the beagle howled in harmony.

I climbed into the back seat, expecting to pull Kati in beside me. But there sat Alyssa, buckled behind the passenger seat. Kati crawled in front and Carl pulled away. There I was, in the back seat with a chatty three year old to my right and Kati way too far away.

As we turned onto Shattuck, still about two miles from the hospital, Kati arched upward and yelled. I squeezed in front of Alyssa, pushed aside masses of Kati's hair, and spoke into her ear.

"Just breathe out. Try not to hold your breath. We're gonna make it. Yell or blow, just don't push. Great, you made it through another one." Then I spoke to Carl. "Blink your headlights, blow your horn constantly, and don't stop at red lights unless you absolutely have to."

Beside my hip, Alyssa said, "What's your favorite color?"

Carl asked, "You really want me to go through red lights?"

"Absolutely."

Kati howled again and I said, "Blow! Let your breath out. Breathe with me. Like this. Huh-huh-huh. Keep making noise, Kati."

Alyssa chirped, "Do you have sandals on? I do."

"Is this really necessary?" asked Carl.

Kati reared back and groaned, "Oh, my God . . ."

Alyssa asked, "Do you have bunnies?"

"Good going, Kati," I said into a cloud of hair. "Reach down and tell me if you feel anything different."

"No. Well, it's swollen. Ooh! Ungh . . . hunf!" and she gasped.

"Come on, Kati, don't push. Holler!"

"See that sign?" said Alyssa. "That's an S for STOP."

"Carl, don't stop. Just go on through. No one's coming."

"Christ."

"It's coming!" bellowed Kati. "Ungh . . . hunf!" She slid forward until her buttocks rested at the edge of the seat.

I leaned over with my butt right in Alyssa's face, yanked Kati's dress to her waist—and saw her vagina gaping. Praying Carl wouldn't brake and send me through the windshield, I stretched further, slipped a bare finger inside, and bumped right into the baby's head.

The next contraction began as we approached a grocery store just a block from the hospital. The baby was minutes from birth, and I teetered over the back seat with both hands between Kati's legs. I couldn't see anything because of Kati's hair.

I was trying to manage a delivery in a moving car with no visibility and a three year old somewhere beneath me saying, "This is where my mommy buys me jelly beans. I like blue jelly beans best. My dress has blue flowers. Do you like my dress?"

This is insane, I told myself, spitting out a mouthful of hair. "We're not going to make it, and I can't work like this. Pull into the Co-op parking lot, and I'll deliver the baby there. Then we'll go to the hospital."

As Carl started to turn in, Kati whined, "Oh, it's a new car. I don't want to get blood on the seats. Please let's try."

Carl zoomed through the intersection.

Thirty seconds later we screeched up to the main entrance. I jumped out and ran around to Kati's side. As I jerked the door open and started to swing her feet around, another contraction began. She slammed one foot down on my right hand, grinding it into the floor pad with her clogs.

As I writhed in agony, an orderly appeared with a wheelchair. I wished he'd brought a stretcher, but Kati sat down, scooting forward till her bottom hung over the edge. Instinctively, she pressed her hand between her legs.

Knowing this baby might be mere seconds from increasing the population of Berkeley by one, I said, "Kati, don't take your hand off that baby, no matter what."

Alyssa admired the marigolds and lobelia in a round planter as I yanked her from her car seat. I threw her into the arms of a perfect stranger, a balding, middle-aged man who stood gawping at all this activity at nine o'clock on Sunday morning. Saying, "Follow us and hurry!" I trotted toward the front entrance with the wheelchair.

Carl left the car illegally parked and galloped after us with the duffel bag and Kati's purse. My own purse and the home visit bag tangled in the wheelchair's wheels, jerking it to a halt. I threw them at the stunned stranger struggling to stay abreast of us, shouting "Hold these, too!" Alyssa praised his choice in eyeglass frames.

The orderly held the elevator doors open and kept everyone else at bay. To the morning visitors and employees, we must have looked like a disorganized, ragtag street circus.

All six of us wedged into the elevator, me kneeling between Kati's legs. As the elevator doors closed, I heard Alyssa's surreal monologue again. "Why are lights behind those buttons? What's your name? I'm Alyssa."

Carl took my bags from the bewildered man.

Midway up the elevator shaft, another contraction began. Kati gripped the arms of the wheelchair and produced what is known in obstetrics as The Perineal Cry. It's a sound that cuts across all cultures. It's the scream of utter disbelief that women make as the biggest diameter of the baby's head fills the vaginal opening. It's a cry that galvanizes experienced nurses and doctors. They know it's the last sound before the baby comes.

The nurses told me later that, as Kati's cry echoed throughout the entire third floor, the delivery room staff scattered, trying to find the woman who was having a baby somewhere in their department. One ran to the public bathroom, another to the waiting room, and several disappeared into various labor rooms.

The Birth Goddess smiled on me that day. If I could have requested one person to greet us, it would have been Bonnie, my friend and occasional home birth assistant. When the elevator doors opened, there she stood. She had chosen to check the elevator as her best guess for the location of that incredible sound.

Carl, finally grasping the urgency of the situation, hurled himself from the elevator and spun in circles with purses twirling like berserk satellites. The pale and sweating stranger followed with Alyssa. Bonnie helped me upright, then pulled the wheelchair down the hallway and into a procedure room. Meanwhile, scuttling backwards, I delivered the rest of the baby's head. Bonnie shouted to another nurse, "Get me a precip pack and suction stuff!"

Carl became wedged in the doorway by the wheelchair. The duffel bag flopped onto Kati's belly. Bonnie and I were the only ones actually inside the small room. The stranger with Alyssa stood directly behind the wheelchair with a slow grin spreading over his face as, at last, he began enjoying his ringside seat at the greatest show on earth.

Craning their necks in the background were a crowd of nurses, visitors, and patients. And Frank, a tall, Jamaican nurse-anesthetist with a lilting accent and calm manner. He was why we had come to the hospital. His job? Baby resuscitation.

Then Dr. Weick's head appeared at the edge of the crowd, a look of astonishment on his tanned face. I cringed at the bizarre impression I knew we made.

Kati reached over the duffel bag and touched her baby's head as the little body fishtailed into my hands. Rivers of meconium and blood gushed out, soaking me from the knees down. A precip pack, a bare-bones tray of emergency equipment, was passed overhead into Bonnie's hands. She ripped it open, hooked up a suction tube, and began sucking thick meconium from the baby's nose and mouth while I cut the umbilical cord. Within seconds the baby went hand-to-hand in reverse into Frank's upstretched hands. He dashed away with the limp but gasping little baby.

Alyssa's voice floated above the hush that followed the birth. "Those are pretty flowers in that garden, aren't they, Mommy?"

Bonnie had just finished piling absorbent flannel sheets on the floor when Frank loped back with the now-pink baby girl in a nest of blankets. The crowd in the doorway parted like the Red Sea, and Frank placed the infant in Kati's arms. Carl hauled the heavy bag from his wife's lap and took Alyssa from the man who now seemed like one of the family. Alyssa instantly climbed into her mother's lap and put her finger in the baby's palm. She looked thrilled when her sister grasped it tightly. Her high-pitched voice squeaked, "Look, Mommy. The baby's blanket has blue flowers on it, just like my dress."

Kati had wanted peace, quiet, serenity, and privacy at her birth. I had wanted a picture-perfect delivery, a birth so routine that every aspect could be examined under the microscope of the obstetrical overseer committee members—and they would find nothing amiss.

In actuality, her chaotic delivery had played out in the presence of ten or eleven total strangers on a brightly lit public corridor. I wondered how she would reconcile her dream birth with reality, and I wondered how Dr. Weick would feel about continuing to back me, after what he'd seen.

My concerns about Kati faded when she beamed up at me and said, "Well, it was certainly nothing like I planned, but I have no complaints."

Then Dr. Weick's voice came over the crowd. "I'll bet it's nothing like Peggy planned, either, for one of her first hospital deliveries. If this is what backing a midwifery practice is like, I'm going to have many interesting experiences."

He was smiling. So was everyone else.

PART IV

Not only with our lips but in our lives

"... and that we show forth thy praise,
not only with our lips, but in our lives,
by giving up ourselves to thy service ..."

A GENERAL THANKSGIVING
BOOK OF COMMON PRAYER, 1928 VERSION

~ Spirit Baby I

Colin, my twelve-year-old son, discovered me late one rainy afternoon sitting at the kitchen table, a damp Kleenex crumpled in my left hand, wiping my eyes as I tried to compose myself for his sake. It was the third week of January, two months after I'd miscarried a pregnancy, but I still found it impossible to get through a day without at least one meltdown into misery.

Stunned when the test came back positive, Rog and I had stared at each other with doubt and ambivalence. At forty-one, my professional life consumed me. I'd just achieved what some had predicted was an impossibility: I'd been granted delivery privileges at Alta Bates, and as a consequence, my midwifery practice burgeoned. Some months I delivered twelve babies, and no one ever knew if or when I'd be home. Rog, too, felt stretched to his limits, keeping his business afloat while picking up the slack for my frequent unscheduled absences. Colin and Jill approached their challenging adolescent years. How could we fit an infant into our lives? But when I lost the pregnancy and all hope for resolution dissolved with my tears, I fell in love with the baby that was not to be.

Colin asked, "Are you crying about the baby?" and when I nodded tearfully, he said, "Well, you just have to have another one, Mom, because it's a Spirit Baby, and you should be its mother."

I must have looked puzzled because he said, "Don't you know about Spirit Babies? How could I know about them if you don't? I mean, you're my mom!" But he could see my perplexity.

So my first child, this not-yet-teenaged boy, pulled a wooden chair to my side and draped his thin arm across my shoulders, saying, "Well, Mom, here's how it is. See, I was one myself, so that must be how I know. Anyway, every woman has a circle of babies that goes around and around above her head, and those are all the possible babies she could have in her whole life. Every month, one of those babies is first in line. If she gets pregnant, then that's the baby that's born. If she doesn't get pregnant, the baby goes back into the circle and keeps going around with all the others. If she gets pregnant but something bad happens before the baby's born . . . now listen, Mom, because here's the really cool part. It goes back into the circle, but it becomes a Spirit Baby, and all the other babies give it cuts. Each month, it's always first in line. Isn't that great?

"So you just have to get pregnant again, and you'll have the same Spirit Baby. If you don't, though, then the baby circle will just beam that little Spirit Baby over to some other woman's circle, and it'll be first in line for her. It keeps being first in line somewhere until it finally gets born.

"But it'd be a shame for you not to have it yourself, because I know how much you want it. So you just have to try again. Mom, remember that baby you lost before I was born?" I nodded wordlessly. "Well, that was me. Really. I've always known I was a Spirit Baby. I mean, I know what I'm talking about here, Mom."

In spite of Colin's certainty that our household, so often bordering on chaos, lacked only an infant to make things perfect, Rog and I demurred. But Colin didn't give up and even enlisted his sister's support. Driving with them in the car one evening, I looked at my son in the passenger seat beside me. He stared out the side window and tried to hide his tears, but I saw the flush on his face, the shaking of his shoulders, and the surreptitious swipe of hand across cheek.

Six months had passed since my miscarriage, and I had just finished yet another discussion in which I'd told my pleading son that having a third baby at my age was out of the question. I reached over the space between us and squeezed his fingers. "Colin, I don't understand this passion you have for a baby. Why do you want one so much?"

He tore his gaze from the distant hills and looked at me with swimming eyes and trembling lips. In a choking voice, he put all of his twelve-year-old passion into his reply.

"Oh, Mom! Oh. Just for the *joy* of it!"

Jill stretched forward from the back seat and placed a hand on each of our shoulders. "Yeah, Mom, just for the joy of it."

It was my turn to look out the side window and struggle with misty vision.

So, at a time when most women eye the empty nest at the end of their branch on the family tree with something approaching relief, I gave consideration to laying just one more egg. Several months of discussions peppered with doubt and disbelief followed. Although Rog and I made the final decision, there's no denying that a big part of our decision to have a third child began with the insistence of our adolescent children that we "needed a baby in the house." Rog and I took a deep breath, looked at each other across the blond heads of those two wishful children, swallowed—and made a giant leap of faith.

I conceived my Spirit Baby a week later. Just for the joy of it.

Practice What You Preach

"Everything hurts," moaned Mary Anne. "Two more weeks? I can't stand it! My legs are swollen, I have indigestion, I've gained sixty pounds, I'm constipated."

Eight months pregnant myself, I nodded sympathetically as I rested my hands on my own belly. I'd heard those words hundreds of times, the common laments of pregnant women everywhere. But I took a secret pride in the knowledge that my pregnancies weren't like hers. I'm one of those women—obnoxious, some would say—who love being pregnant and would happily spend the rest of my life about seven months along. I waken every morning feeling like the Queen of England in a new hat. I lose my taste for chocolate, coffee, and alcohol as I begin craving broccoli, nutritional yeast, and brown rice. My hair shines. My skin glows. I smile at nothing, at everything.

"Try to do something special every day," I advised Mary Anne. "Make a date to see a movie for the day after you're due."

"You think I'll go overdue?" she wailed.

"No, but it'll keep you from focusing on that particular day, just in case," I trailed off lamely.

"Impossible," she declared. "I'll just die."

As I made an appointment for her next visit, I patted my belly and knocked on wood. I'd wondered if my being forty-two would make this pregnancy harder, but I couldn't see much difference from my other two. Sure, hauling an unborn baby around in an internal front-pack twenty-four hours a day grew tiring. Yes, my back ached most nights by eight P.M. And leg cramps, oh boy. Rog became adept at waking from sound sleep to wrestle with my calves as I screamed, "Left one! No, I mean the right one! Pull harder!" And my ankles, swollen to obscene proportions, could have won a prize in the Guinness Book of Records. But for the most part I skirted the major complaints of pregnancy. I even considered inventing heartburn or hemorrhoids that I never had, just to increase my credibility.

In everyday life I shy away from gardening like a snail avoids salt, but when ripe with child I want to plant radishes and roses. Of course, as soon as I have the baby to tend, the budding sprouts get neglected. But for those few months before fresh diapers appear on the backyard clothesline, we have fresh vegetables on the kitchen table.

Then on a Friday morning two weeks before my due date, just one day after I delivered Mary Anne's baby, I rose from my pillow more slowly than usual. I drank my tea and ate my cranberry bagel in thoughtful silence. It took me most of the morning to run three loads of laundry. I felt as if I'd gained thirty pounds overnight. I definitely didn't feel like the Queen of England. More like the Wicked Witch of the West on a bad hair day.

I dragged myself out the door for a full afternoon of office hours. The box of patients' charts felt like a wet sandbag as I hoisted it into my car. I found myself chanting, Not two more weeks, God, please, not two more weeks of this.

The afternoon dragged on. I rubbed my lower back long before my first client mentioned hers. I peed every half-hour. My ankles felt like balloons, and as I glanced at other women's feet I realized none could compare with mine for sheer shock value. Blinking back fatigue, I found it hard to remember ever feeling really good.

Although Jill and Colin both boogied into the world before their due dates, I had to acknowledge that this could last fourteen more days, and I really didn't see how I'd cope. Smiling, smiling, smiling, I tried to make each woman feel as special as she deserved to feel, but I waged an uphill battle. All my smug thoughts of easy pregnancies disappeared.

Finally the last pregnant woman left, and I locked the office. My list of complaints now stretched miles behind me, unwinding like a tattered typewriter ribbon as I drove home.

As soon as I entered the house, I flopped into an armchair in the darkest corner of the living room and stared at the watery February sun dropping behind the rim of the bay. I stretched my melon legs out and sat there, waiting for someone to notice me. To notice how tired I looked, how great with child, how miserable.

Just waiting, really, for the pregnancy to end.

The house smelled good, chicken something. Louder than necessary, I cleared my throat. Rog poked his head out the kitchen door. "Hi, honey, I didn't hear you come in."

"I don't want any dinner," I interrupted, although he hadn't actually offered.

He blinked, pressed his lips together, and pulled his head back.

"I just want to be quiet," I warned, although no one said a word.

"I don't want any music," I grumbled, although no one approached the stereo.

They ate, a hushed voice now and then interrupting the scrape of fork on plate. Half an hour later, my husband tried again, "Do you . . ."

"I want to be left alone," I said. I sat there glaring, fingertips steepled in front of me, forearms resting on my tight belly.

"Uh-huh, we've been here before," he muttered, nodding like a sage. "I'm going to put plastic on the bed. We're gonna have a little baby soon," and he trotted upstairs to deal with sheets and Chux and towels.

"Umph," I snorted. Unwilling to admit he might be right, I glowered when he glanced over his shoulder at me with a fond smile. But some part of me acknowledged that my sour mood felt slightly familiar. Suddenly I knew what other pregnant women felt like. I'd just forgotten that it happens to me only at the very end. Groaning as I shifted in the chair, I forced my mind thirteen years into the past. Twenty-four hours before Colin was born, my happy hormones took a dive and forgot to come up for air. I'd slumped to the floor and declared that within the previous ten minutes my pregnancy had become intolerable.

When I awakened the day before my second child careened into the world, I waltzed around the house to songs from *My Fair Lady*. I could have danced all night, but by noon I'd decided that pregnancy was not at all my cup of tea. Pour the dregs down the drain, wash the cup, and put it away.

My family had come to expect my constant sunny skies during the past months, so the sudden clouds gathering on the horizon made them run for cover. Perhaps Rog showed wisdom to prepare for a hurricane.

I heard him upstairs opening the creaky linen closet door, his footsteps going back and forth. Then he paused. "Honey?" His voice sounded cautious. Smart man.

"Mmm."

"Where's the plastic sheet?" Why did he have to be so nice?

"Cedar chest."

"Thank you," and off he went. I could just picture him bustling around like a mother hen, busy, busy, busy with the bed, the plastic, the towels. Any minute I expected him to start clucking. Maybe he'd like to lay this egg himself, I fumed.

Colin and Jill tiptoed past. They'd been warned.

I sat and stared at my sausage feet. The cat jumped on my lap, prepared to stay all night. I sat in the darkening room as the kids at the kitchen table murmured to each other about long division and compound verbs. I dozed.

When they again crept past me and headed up the stairs, it was dark. I faked sleep, but through slitted eyes I watched them. Rog stood on the bottom step, willing me to tell him how he might help. I kept my eyes lowered till I heard him on the squeaky third-from-the-top step and then in the bathroom. Wishing for a good cry, I listened till all footsteps ceased and the hallway lights dimmed. Then I levered myself from the chair.

Not even trying to be quiet, I clomped upstairs, pried off my shoes and dropped them on the floor. I splashed and brushed, flossed and flushed, pulled my nightgown over my head, and turned off the light.

Passing the armoire mirror, I stopped and looked at myself. Old. Tired. Swollen. Grouchy. Still two full weeks from my due date, but I wanted it over right now. How did other pregnant women stand feeling like this, some for months on end? I felt connected to every other woman with leg cramps, backache, depression, and fatigue. It didn't lift my mood, but it made me feel as if I had company. Then a horrible thought occurred to me. What if I went overdue?

I'd die.

I eased into bed and pulled my greater-than-usual share of the covers over my bigger-than-usual body. Struggling through the nightly ritual of getting all the pillows into place, I only snorted "pffffh" when Rog laid his hand on my hip and whispered, "You'll have the baby tomorrow. You'll see."

He kissed my neck. I reached down and gave his hand the barest squeeze required by common courtesy. Moments later he jerked once, and his fingers grabbed at my nightgown in that reflexive twitch of deeper sleep. Left alone with my thoughts, I listened to his steady breathing as I squirmed and tensed, stretched and groaned, trying to get comfortable, trying to relax. Trying to achieve an attitude adjustment, if nothing else.

Two more weeks of this? Impossible, just impossible. Eventually, I slept.

What was that? A sharp tweak of pain lasting only a nanosecond zipped through my pelvis. In a sleepy fog, I knew I'd heard something as well, a subliminal *ping,* like a knuckle cracking. I peeped at the clock. Five A.M. Thinking the sound I'd heard must be some internal phone noise, I waited for the ring. Someone in labor?

But I waited much longer than the interval between telephone rings, and nothing happened. I rolled onto my back and tried to think clearly. As I did, a trickle of warm liquid dribbled from my body.

My eyes flew open. Okay! Bag of water breaking! I'm the one who's in labor!

I wiggled from bed and hobbled into the bathroom with my knees pressed together. Enthroned in triumph, I expected a gush of water the moment I relaxed.

Nothing happened.

I'll just wait here a little longer, I thought. I know there's more than that puny teaspoon. So I waited, rocking this way and that, leaning forward. Nothing.

Definitely weird. I knew it wasn't pee, because of that little *ping* of pain. I kicked the rug aside and stood up. Bounced on my toes once or twice. Tried a jump. Another one.

A drip the size of a garden pea ran down my thigh. Before it could slide away to nothingness, I scooted downstairs. I needed my roll of Nitrazine paper.

I stored my home birth equipment six feet from the front door, always ready for a quick getaway. In the tackle box was a roll of magic Nitrazine paper. Amniotic fluid turns the lemon yellow paper the color of unfaded 1950s Levi's, and I wanted to press the tip of that paper into this minute dewdrop.

I squatted to open the box, and it came again: *ping.* But this time it tweaked my back, as well. I straightened to relieve the discomfort and immediately knew I had no further need of the Nitrazine paper. I became a Niagara Falls. Wave after wave of fluid gushed from my body, smacking noisily against the hardwood floor.

My God, I thought, staring between my feet. That's a whole lot of water. The splat of the water hitting the floor brought an image to my mind: my tiny Irish grandmother tossing buckets of wash water onto the alleyway behind the tall, narrow house where she raised five children. She had birthed all of them at home.

But no time now to dwell on Grandmother Mac. Legs spread wide, nightgown above my hips, marooned in a five-foot-wide sea, I stood stranded, soaked, and speechless. Then I heard the children coming from their bedrooms.

"Did you hear that?" asked Colin.

"What on earth . . . ?" murmured Jill, confused by the unfamiliar sound that had awakened her.

I hollered, "Come here and help me."

"Where are you?"

"Here. Bring towels."

"Oh, wow! Dad, you've gotta see this. Hurry."

At eleven and thirteen they considered themselves quite grown up, but they tumbled down the stairs like two clumsy puppies and then collapsed, hugging each other in laughter as they watched me straddle the spreading pool.

"Get towels! Hurry!" I begged.

From the middle of the humps of quilts in our warm bed, Rog muttered, "I knew it last night. What did I tell you?" He appeared with a small, pink hand towel, took a look at the flood, and turned toward the utility room closet where we keep beach towels.

So today would be the day, I mused, as my kids crawled around wiping the floor. Saturday, February 20, 1985.

Then I remembered my promise to Sandi. After four years as my assistant and a year of midwifery school in South Carolina, she'd returned to California just a month earlier, and I would be her first client. After not seeing much of her four children the previous year, she'd planned an overnight at a coastal B&B with the youngest two. Talking on the phone a few days earlier, she'd said, "Just don't have your baby on the nineteenth or twentieth," and of course I'd promised.

Well, I figured, that's Murphy's Law of Midwifery, and the sooner she learns it, the better: Babies come when it's most inconvenient for the midwife.

Finally the floor looked dry, and Rog rigged me a sumo wrestler's loincloth from a sanitary belt and a bath towel. By 5:30 A.M., three pairs of eyes looked at me, and I read the same message in each of them: Do something, Mom.

"Let's go back to bed," I said.

"You expect us to go to sleep after this?" groaned Colin.

Jill looked at me in disbelief and said, "No way."

But Rog, older, wiser, knowing how little sleep he'd get in the weeks ahead, turned without a word and headed upstairs. Sighing, the children straggled behind. "Just promise you won't let us miss it, okay?"

I assured them I hadn't had even one single pain yet, but as I reached my bedroom door, I felt the first one. Light, tight, just a half-hearted attempt, over and done with before I'd reached the bed. But it hurt in a familiar, once-experienced-never-forgotten way.

I changed into a clean nightgown and lay on my side as the contractions rolled in like small waves on a sunny day at Stinson Beach. A surfer waiting for The Big One would have been bored, bored, bored. But I gave up thoughts of sleep and gathered together the pillows I'd collected as pregnancy advanced, the pillows that had forced Rog to huddle ever closer to his edge of our bed. One night, fighting for an extra inch of territory, he muttered, "I don't see how your belly can still be so big. I swear you've already given birth to a whole litter of pillows."

So I pulled my fluffy little pillow family around me and scrunched under the quilts, trying not to fidget as the contractions continued. Throwing my leg over Rog's thigh to rake in his warmth, I lay wide-eyed, pondering my dramatic change of attitude from yesterday. My hormonal storm had passed out to sea with the breaking of the water. The tidal waves of amniotic fluid had swept away my depression, my impatience, even my aches and pains. I felt lighter, too, not surprising in view of how much water had surged from my body. I breathed easily, and I just couldn't stop grinning.

I drummed my fingertips against my belly and signaled to the baby within, to my third child, my little spirit baby: today, little baby, today is your birthday.

A few hours later, the house began filling with guests: my parents, several midwife and nurse friends, Sandi and her two kids, a photographer, and Aggie, our Swedish *au pair*. All morning I stayed on my feet, busy doing laundry and preparing food for the post-birth party. By noon, I looked at the stairs and thought, I'll have to crawl up those steps if I wait much longer, so I filled a glass with iced tea and headed for my bedroom. All the women followed in a little parade. The three guys, Rog, Colin, and my dad, hovered in Colin's bedroom, trying to figure out how to program our new answering machine.

With contractions closer and harder, I timed my bathroom trips carefully to avoid being caught neither here nor there. But once, just as Colin came into the hall, I realized I wouldn't make it back to the bedroom. I set my tea on a bookshelf, grabbed my belly and turned toward my young son.

"Oh no, Mom, not me," he moaned.

"Hold still," I said into his ear. A silly grin crept across his face, and I felt the heat of his blush as I clutched his knobby shoulders and nailed him to the wall.

He wasn't embarrassed at my semi-nudity, he wasn't humiliated at the reality of a pregnant mom, he wasn't put off by the idea of a home birth, and I knew the prospect of a baby brother thrilled him. He was simply embarrassed by his own adolescent male self in a house full of women. A boy just teetering toward his teens, he found himself pushed to the wall by 160 pounds of moaning, sweating mom, while ten women watched.

As the contraction pushed ahead like the wind preceding an avalanche, I spread my feet apart and let the pain rock me. Seconds later the full force of it hit. I pushed my forehead into the top of his head and groaned, "Just stand still. Let me lean on you." Breathing between clenched teeth, I heard myself making a "ssssss-huh–ssssss-huh" refrain as I swayed side to side.

Then, like a gift, I felt him relax. His thin boy-hands touched my hipbones, and he held me the way he'd seen me hold Sandi six years earlier, the same way I'd supported countless women over the decades. Locked together, we rocked like two trees in the wind, limbs swaying to the same breeze, the same dance. As the contraction eased, I opened my eyes. He lifted his face with a quick, shy smile and kissed the tip of my chin.

"Thanks, honey," I whispered.

"Mmm-hmm. Your breath stinks," he said. He hiked up his jeans and ducked into his bedroom where wires, screwdrivers, microphones, and digital displays spoke to him in a language he understood.

I brushed my teeth, picked up my tea, and headed back to my sunny bedroom. Back to cold washcloths, acupressure points, and the fragrance of plum blossoms floating through the open windows. Back to the soft voices of wise women who spoke to me in a language I understood.

My son had been surrounded by the facts of childbirth all of his life. Daily conversations included words most children rarely hear spoken aloud, and he'd seen one birth. But I understood his ambivalence. The house teemed with a kind of primal, feminine energy. He and his dad and grandfather held fast to a rickety raft of testosterone in a surging sea of estrogen. No wonder he felt overwhelmed.

Rog divided his time between Colin and my dad, keeping them occupied as my labor dragged on. Now and then he came into the bedroom with a fresh pitcher of tea, and I grabbed him, hanging from his belt loops as I hula-danced through another contraction. It felt good to cling to his masculine body, to feel his strong arms and rough whiskers. I could lean all of my weight into him, and his hands at my waist felt familiar and sure.

But mostly I wanted the women. The women with heartbeats that pulsed on my wavelength, their touches that felt just right, their inner music that already knew the dance I danced. The pitch and timbre of their voices hummed an ageless birth song with me. The knowledge of our shared profession, the intuitive gift of women who care for women, of knowing when to speak, when to be silent, when to laugh, when to hug, when to be pliant, and when to stand firm. How to be "*mit wife*." With woman.

My daughter already knew. A year earlier while Rog and Colin went camping for ten days, I'd taken Jill to eight births. By the end of the week, she'd learned how to massage, touch, and verbally support women in labor. Now she stayed at my bedside, her eleven-year-old gaze fixed on me. One contraction brought me to my knees beside the bed, and I flung my hands out. I felt small hands in mine and heard my daughter's voice through a fog of pain, "That's it, Mom, you can do it. Great, keep it up. Don't forget you're having a baby." When I opened my eyes, she smiled shyly.

But it hurt so much. Jill's birth had been painless, and for eleven years I'd congratulated myself on having learned to labor painlessly. I knew now I could claim no credit for the ease of her birth. Luck, not smarts, had made it a cakewalk. This one hurt. Ah, well, I was just proving another old midwifery adage: First births are hard, second ones easy, and thirds are unpredictable.

Like most laboring women, I had shed one item of clothing with each centimeter of dilation. By one P.M., I was nude, standing at my bedside surrounded by women. Mijo rubbed my calves. Claire stroked my hair. Jamie took pictures. Mother suffered. Maggie pressed on my lower back, and once I felt her lips press a cool kiss to my waist. Carole, with artsy, metallic triangles dangling from her ears, stood at my side, and with each contraction I pushed my face against her cheek and rubbed, rubbed, rubbed. She removed her left earring, afraid I'd lacerate my face.

Sandi rested her hands on my shoulders. Sandi, my first assistant, now my midwife. I, her teacher—and now her patient. Surrounded by my family, her children, other midwives, and all those nurses, I knew the pressures she must be feeling.

She knelt on the floor to examine me. Nine centimeters. Soon, soon.

Ten minutes later I felt that curling-over at the top as my uterus began to bear down like a giant toothpaste tube being emptied, squeezing all the toothpaste toward the small opening at the far end. I began pushing.

I pushed standing at the bedside. I gulped half a glass of iced tea after each contraction and then swooned, leaning into the wall of women, sure that wherever I flung myself, they would support me.

Without preamble, my left hip cramped, and within a few minutes it felt like a railroad stake being driven into the joint. I threw myself onto the bed, scrambled into a curled position, and screamed into a push. It felt wrong, all wrong, and I heard myself rivaling some of my noisiest clients.

My unquenchable thirst for iced tea was nearly as unbelievable as the hip pain. "Tea. Tea, tea, tea, quick! More tea," became my refrain, and Aggie ran downstairs to make another half gallon.

I struggled to find a path around the pain. If not around it, then under it, or over it. I ground my knuckles so deeply into my hip that bruises remained for a week afterwards. Nothing helped, and I fought the forces of my body.

My son appeared and stroked my cheek, whispering, "Come on, Mom, you can get him out."

As each contraction ended, he held the glass of tea to my mouth. I drank six quarts of it—one and a half gallons—during the last hour of my labor. That's twenty-four cups, and still I shouted and begged for more. "Tea, tea, more tea. Hurry!"

An hour passed. More than an hour. The baby didn't come. I sensed a stillness, a heightening of tension, lowered voices. I snatched brief glimpses of the knowledgeable, loving women, my friends, my nursing cohorts, my sister midwives, my mother, my daughter. I saw their concern. My mother muttered, "Mmm-mmm-mmm," and pressed her lips together. Maggie whispered to Claire. Mijo looked at Sandi. Sandi stared at my crotch. Jill pushed her face into Bonnie's hip. Carole said, "Humph," and muttered something to Rog, who rubbed his chin, worried.

Aggie just kept brewing tea. My dad kept rocking in his chair in the corner. Colin held the glass to my lips.

"Don't you need to go to the bathroom?" asked my mother.

I shook my head and heard Carole explain how absorption slows down during heavy labor, how blood supply goes to the uterus instead of the stomach. I only know the tea entered my belly and stayed there, sloshing around like bilge water, but still my thirst raged. Maggie poured, Mijo passed, and Colin held it for me. I gulped another full glass and sank onto the pillow.

Eighteen people stared at me, hoping I'd get my act together before the baby became distressed. Then Sandi leaned forward and peered between my legs. "I think . . ." interrupted immediately by Colin's jubilant voice.

"Yeah, hey! That's gotta be the head."

They all got so excited I expected the baby to pop right out. Three or four contractions later I grew suspicious. I asked for a mirror and watched as I pushed. "Shit, is that all? It's no bigger than a nickel," I snarled. I threw the mirror across the bed and then almost smiled as my mother pounced on it before it slid to the floor. A mirror caught unbroken spares seven years of bad luck, her relieved expression said. She had the grace to look sheepish.

"Tea, more tea!" I shouted. I sucked down another six ounces as Aggie slipped from the room again, shaking her head at the empty pitcher.

Damn, his head was right there. I just needed to push it maybe another two inches to get the biggest part out. But it hurt so much I feared I'd break something. Could my tailbone have re-fused? Could my pelvis actually fracture? Did this child weigh twelve pounds? What the devil was taking so long?

The next contraction came grinding down on me, but it felt different. A white-hot hole of knowledge opened in my pain. I saw that in my effort to get around or under the pain, I'd been avoiding that central point of intensity, staying on the brink of the primitive surrender that's required to get a stubborn baby out. I'd talked hundreds of women into taking that leap of faith, that shut-your-eyes-and-jump moment of bravery. Like a girl standing on the high dive, walking back and forth the length of the board, shivering, going to the brink again to stare down into the water so far below—and then she's off, airborne. Free.

With sudden clarity, I knew it would have to hurt more before it got better. I wouldn't be able to circumvent the pain. I had to go through it, enter willingly into the void, holding nothing back. I had to jump off the diving board.

I took my fist away from my hip, and with a roar that must have sounded like Godzilla shoving over a skyscraper, I pushed into the center of my pain. Suddenly the whole room erupted in a communal yell.

"Yeah! All right, now we're rolling!"

"Okay, Peggy, you've got the little sucker on the move!"

"Oh, Mom, here he comes!"

"Move in close, Rog, so you can catch him. It's coming fast now."

As Rog knelt between my legs with Sandi's hands on top of his, I felt that impossible moment when what is already stretched to the max stretches more. And then just a little bit more.

"Flex the head, Sandi. Flex his head more."

Yeah, good idea, I thought, as the contraction eased. Who said that? But everyone laughed, and Carole said, "Oh, quit midwifing yourself, Peggy, and just push the baby out."

I'd said it myself.

In a red blur, I watched through two more contractions as the rest of the head oozed into Rog's cupped hands. Colin's cheek pressed against mine. Jill stood behind Rog with her hands on his shoulders, her lips slightly parted, a rapt look on her face. My mom stood to one side with her face all crumpled in tears, pressing a Kleenex to her lips as my dad put his arm around her. And all the rest of them, all around me.

As the baby's arms untangled and slipped free, I pulled his body out myself, lifting him above my head as the room erupted in cheers. I felt like Jerry Rice receiving a perfect Joe Montana touchdown pass.

Jill clamped the cord. Colin cut it, saying, "Okay, little bro, you're on your own."

I cuddled him to my chest and stared into his face, my baby boy. Putty nose, slate eyes, no hair, and surprisingly calm considering the noise level in the room. Like mothers the world over, I sniffed him and peeked into all his crevices. Skin like satin and pillows of down. Unfolding his fists, I showed Jill and Colin his tiny fingernails, iridescent chips of mother of pearl, but soft and pliable. So beautiful, so perfect in every way. Another example of the chinless, neckless, wobbly, big-eyed bundles that we women find so appealing—and that our men smile at politely, hiding laughter behind their hands.

Dewy champagne bottles and tall-stemmed glasses appeared, and everyone drank a toast. I saw Mijo dip her finger in her glass and touch a droplet to my baby's lips. When she saw my glance, she ducked her head and said, "It's a French blessing. Anyway, my mother always did it."

Soon it was time to weigh him. I put a finger between his gums to slip my nipple from his mouth, and Sandi swung him aloft in the flannel pouch that had been used on more than five hundred other babies: seven pounds, twelve ounces. Mom and Jill dressed him in a long white gown with blue ducks marching around the bottom edge. He lay drinking in his new world of color and sound, surrounded by smiling faces. My son. My Spirit Baby.

Soon everyone left us alone and trooped downstairs to celebrate. I felt a wave of tea hit my bladder, and as my mother murmured, "It's about time!" I dashed to the bathroom and peed like a stallion. I did it twice more in the next half hour, but then I feared I was missing the hazelnut torte. I speed-showered, picked up my sleeping baby, and headed downstairs to the party.

The blood drained from my father's face when he saw me. "What are you doing?"

"I want a piece of cake," I answered, wondering what could be so wrong with that. Jill scampered through the crowd and cut me a piece.

"But, the stairs. You shouldn't be out of bed," Daddy stammered.

"Oh, Bill," said my mother, "things have changed since our girls were born."

Sandi and Carole nodded and smiled at him. Some color came back into his face.

Jill brought me the cake and a fork. "Do you want something to drink, Mom? Milk? Coffee? Champagne?"

"Just some iced tea."

Conversation stopped. "Did she say 'tea'?" whispered Mijo.

Aggie rolled her eyes and turned toward the kitchen to put the kettle on.

~ *My Little Helper*

Blissed out on lactation hormones, I finished nursing my two-day-old baby, Skylar. I shifted him against my chest, focusing on a pale vein meandering across his fuzzy head and down his forehead like a blue highway on a road map. His soft spot pulsed, and his milky, kitten breath smelled so sweet that I leaned forward to inhale it. As I started toward his cradle, the phone rang. I smiled, glad that no matter who it was, I wouldn't be dashing off to do a birth. Sandi was carrying my pager for the next seven days, and she would catch all the babies.

"Peggy, it's Corinne. Surprise, surprise, I'm early this time. My labor started an hour ago." Just then my beanbag-limp baby snorted and squeaked, arching his back and waggling his head like a too-heavy tulip on a fragile stem. Corinne laughed and said, "Oh, you beat me."

Our due dates had been identical, but I'd delivered first. Corinne and I had matched each other milestone for milestone during our tandem pregnancies. I palpated her lightly freckled abdomen one afternoon and felt the bubbly flip-turn of a baby with plenty of room to maneuver in its watery world. A moment later my own baby executed an aquatic roll, as if pushing off one side of a pool and floating across the width to repeat the new trick at the opposite side. I placed her hand against my bulging waistline. She pushed her strawberry-blonde hair behind her ears, and we smiled at each other, sharing the moment of mutual awe. Later we looked in dismay at each other's swollen ankles, and she said, "Gee, yours are even grosser than mine."

But Corinne envied me all the help I would have after I delivered, with an *au pair* and two teenagers to share baby care with Rog and me. I had to agree that her two-year-old son wouldn't be any help at all. Probably just the opposite.

"My pains aren't strong yet, but they're pretty regular," she said into the phone.

Sandi would have plenty of time to return from the symphony in San Francisco. I yawned, anticipating curling up in bed with my nose pressed to the spot on my son's head where he smelled so sweet, like warm biscuits.

"Allan just got home," Corinne continued, "and he's having a heck of a time getting Joe-Joe settled." Suddenly she shrieked and dropped the phone. At first I thought her son had thrown their cat out the window or something, but I gripped the phone when I heard heavy breathing. Corinne gasped, "Oh, gosh, Peggy, my water just broke."

My expectation of a quiet evening vanished. Once I paged Sandi, she'd need more than an hour to get to Corinne's.

"Oh, my goodness, that contraction was *so* different. Oh, God, here comes another one."

"I'll page Sandi and have her call you, but I'll get ready, just in case."

As I dialed Sandi's pager, a niggling suspicion pricked me: I would not be going to bed any time soon. My parents, still in town after my delivery, were puttering around getting ready for bed, but they stared at me, and my father said, "You're going to deliver someone's baby when your own child is just two days old?"

"I may have to, and I'll need some help. Mother, don't get undressed yet. I might need you."

Her eyebrows shot to the top of her forehead, and her mouth formed a big O. "Me?" she squeaked. One hand clutched her throat, and the other toyed with a pearl button on her blouse.

"I'll need an assistant, and you used to be a nurse."

"Oh, my goodness! Well I, oh, dear. Are you sure? Oh, my." She turned in a circle a few times like a dog on a blanket and then reeled away, muttering as she disappeared around the corner.

I gathered a change of clothes for the baby. Rog hooked the infant seat into the car. Then we all sat and stared at the telephone. When it rang ten minutes later, I answered on the first ring. It was Allan, and in the background I heard a child's voice, thin and reedy. "Daddy, I want juice."

"Wait, Joe-Joe, I need to talk to this lady."

"Allan? Is Sandi on her way?"

"Juicy-juicy-juicy," chanted Joe-Joe.

"Uh, yeah, but she's probably not gonna make it."

"Not going to make it?" My pulse pounded. Rog took the car keys from his pocket, and Mother sat up very straight.

"Uh, no. Joe-Joe, leave Mommy alone. Um, Sandi's still inside Davies Hall in the city, and her car's parked fifteen minutes away. It'll be over an hour before . . ."

"Aaaaaaagh! Umff! Umff!" howled Corinne in the background.

"Juice, mommy. Needa juicy, juicy."

"Peggy, what should I do?"

"I'll be right there," I said. Rog went out the front door.

"But Corinne said you just had your baby."

"I'm fine. Leave the door unlocked and put blankets in the oven. If Corinne starts to push, call 911. I'm coming."

Rog drove and I sat beside him, what-ifs ricocheting through my brain like summer lightening. I started planning. I'd jump out of the van with my basic supplies and let Rog bring the rest later. He'd hold Skylar while Mom helped me.

Mother, beside Skylar in the back seat of our ancient VW van, clucked, "Now, what exactly do you expect me to do? Do you think this is a good idea? How will I . . ."

I ignored her. Too busy thinking.

Glancing down, I realized I still had my nightgown on. Five years had passed since my graduation from midwifery school. I felt like I'd hit my stride. I had launched one apprentice and tucked two more beneath my wings. Having scored privileges at a prestigious Bay Area hospital, I could mobilize an entire operating room crew with a single phone call. In a field famous for longhaired hippie midwives, I knew I generally presented a professional image. Yet here I was about to attend a birth wearing nothing but a flannel nightgown and a maternity Kotex.

Ducky, just ducky.

I sighed. My brain must still have been in that foggy postpartum zone where it functions with the efficiency of a scrambled egg. Well, at least my nightgown hung to my ankles, so I had a chance of preserving some shred of modesty if I found Corinne on the floor.

Holding a penlight over Corinne's hand-drawn map, I directed Rog left, left, second right, and so forth, peering into the darkness. We made one wrong turn and then an illegal U-turn before stopping in front of a duplex. I grabbed my birth kit, pulled my voluminous nightie to my knees, hopped out, and galloped up the cracked sidewalk.

Two doors faced me. I had no idea which was Corinne's. I twisted a doorknob at random. Locked. Before I could try the other one, the first door exploded outward.

A startled elderly man in loose pants and a sleeveless undershirt looked even more startled to find a woman in a long white nightgown holding a fishing tackle box standing on his porch. His gaping mouth snapped shut as he leaned forward to peer at me in the dim porch light.

"Corinne's place?" I asked.

He scratched the few hairs on his head. Moving slowly, he held me in his gaze as he pointed toward the other door.

"Upstairs," he mumbled, and I clattered through the door.

Hunched sideways on the floor—of course, where else?—Corinne lay with her back to me. Joe-Joe sprawled beside her, sucking a bottle of juice. Between Corinne's thin legs I saw signs of imminent birth, and I suspected that with a good contraction the oval slit would reveal a patch of shiny, birth-slick baby hair.

Allan knelt nearby, rigid and wide-eyed.

I put my blue tackle box down and hurried to them. Corinne's moans changed to a wail of relief when she saw me. Joe-Joe never broke the rhythm of his sucking, and Corinne patted his back. Her other hand clutched the wooden leg of a chair behind her.

The bare wooden floor glistened with a slippery, five-foot-wide puddle of amniotic fluid. I thought of my mother and my newborn. Visions of broken hips and dropped babies muddled my thoughts. "Allan, put some newspaper on top of all this water so nobody slips," I ordered.

Allan seemed relieved to have a job. He skirted the amniotic lake, went into the kitchen, and reappeared with an enormous stack of newspapers. He began to spread them on the wet floor, the task utterly absorbing him. He laid them down symmetrically, edge to edge, overlapping just so, patting them to soak up the fluid, checking to be sure nothing seeped around the edges.

Then my mother came in with Skylar and settled into an armchair.

Before I could tell Mom what to do, Corinne screeched with another contraction. The high-ceilinged room filled with amazing sounds that soared high, caught, and turned into a series of yelps—then a single shriek as the baby's head stretched her open. A long, wailing decrescendo began as the pressure eased off, and the glistening head slipped back, but only a little. Once the head remains visible between contractions, progress is dramatic. I put my hand on the head and knew I couldn't take it off till the baby slid out.

Allan fiddled with his newspapers. Joe-Joe sucked on.

Rog clumped up the stairway with the rest of my gear. "Where do you want me to put all this stuff?" he asked, sounding a little winded.

"Just anywhere and take the baby from Mom. I need her."

He put down the three cases and reached for the baby. Mother met him with a stare, clutching the baby to her chest.

It was my first clue that my mother really just planned to watch. I should have left her there and asked Rog to assist me. But, *damn,* I thought, she's a nurse—even though it'd been twenty years since she'd worked in a hospital—and she'd just observed the birth of the very baby she held so tightly. Most of all, she was a woman. I figured Allan or Corinne might have an objection to a strange man attending their birth.

So I fixed my mother with a glare as stubborn as her own and said, "Give the baby to Rog, Mom, and come help me."

Grudgingly, she handed over the baby, and Rog took him toward the dining room. Before he disappeared, I saw him pull a lint-covered pacifier from his pocket. He licked off the fuzz and pushed it between Skylar's lips.

"Now, what is it you want me to do, dear?" asked my mother. "What's in those boxes? Is that the head showing already?"

"Open the tackle box and take out the package wrapped in the green towel."

"Which box?"

"The blue one."

"How do these clasps work? Do you push them, or pull?"

About three inches of the baby's head showed.

"Pull out on them, and then up and over, like ski boots."

"I've never skied, dear. Heavens, skiing," She fumbled some more. "Does it go up first? No, it must be down, I think."

"Allan, open that box for my mom."

With a wistful glance at his newspapers, Allan opened the tackle box. Then both he and my mother seemed to believe they'd done all that could be expected, and they backed off to watch from the corner. The open box still stood ten feet from me. The baby's head surged lower. Corinne buried her nose in Joe-Joe's curls. She closed her eyes and breathed loudly into his hair as the rest of the head emerged and lay in my palm. It turned to one side, and two big eyes opened wide.

"Oh, he's lookin' fer me!" said Joe-Joe. "Here, little baby, I'm right up here. Look. It's me, Joe-Joe!" His bottle of juice clattered to the floor.

I heard a choked sob and glanced over my shoulder. Mother held a weeping Allan in her arms, patting his back.

I still had no assistant, and I couldn't let go of the baby. "Joe-Joe, can you help me?" I whispered. His eyes popped toward mine, and he nodded his head. "Get the green package out of that box and bring it to me."

Joe-Joe scrambled to his fat, little baby feet and shuffled across the damp newspapers. He picked up the packet, set it on the floor next to me, and hunkered down to watch.

"Can you get the tape off that package, Joe-Joe? Are you strong enough?"

He grinned, picked it up again and yanked the autoclave tape off with one dramatic swipe. Then he retrieved his bottle and sat by my left knee, sucking juice.

I grabbed a rubber bulb and sucked mucus from the baby's nose and mouth. I squirted mucus onto the towel, and Joe-Joe squealed, "Baby boogers!"

Corinne flailed her arms overhead and grabbed both front legs of the large armchair. She bared her teeth in a grimace of pain and put her whole focus onto pushing her baby out. Pulling on the wooden legs, she moved the chair forward till it covered her head and shoulders.

"Why Momma unner the chair?" asked Joe-Joe, but I couldn't answer. As the shoulders came into view, I saw that the umbilical cord had wrapped three times around the fat little chest, and the overall length wouldn't permit further progress of the infant. As the cord cinched tighter and tighter with the baby's descent, I maneuvered two clamps in place and cut between them.

The sudden spurt of blood riveted Joe-Joe's attention. "Oooh, my baby's hurted!"

Busy unwrapping the coils of cord, I muttered, "No, it doesn't hurt when I cut the cord." Then my hands were suddenly full of a floppy, stunned-looking Little Boy Blue. The baby's wide-open eyes stared sightlessly at the world. Nobody home yet behind those eyes, dark with enormous, dilated pupils.

"Mother, get the blankets from the oven!" I hoped my voice carried enough authority to make her obey, and, indeed, she scooted into the kitchen. But I couldn't wait. I could feel with my fingertips that the baby had a strong heartbeat, but about fifteen seconds had passed since his birth, and he hadn't figured out how to breathe yet. I dumped the rest of my instruments onto the newspaper and used the rough green wrapper to rub him down. Vigorous rubbing is often enough to jump-start a listless or stunned newborn.

Mother hurried back with a foil package, tossed it to me, and returned to Allan, folding him again within her arms.

"Joe-Joe, tear that open for me, honey. Just rip it. Attaboy!"

He shredded the package with glee, throwing pieces of foil over his shoulders before dropping the blankets in my lap. I used one of the flannel squares to dry and warm the pale body.

Time stands still when a baby doesn't cry. I'm always conscious of a fixed smile of crossed-finger confidence pasted on my face. Background sounds become loud in the silence of no crying. My skin feels cold no matter how warm the room, and I talk to myself and to the baby.

"Come on, little fellow, come on, you can do it, work with me here, you've gotta meet me halfway."

Still no sound from the boneless baby, jiggling like Jell-O in my hands. I rubbed his spine and flicked the soles of his feet with my fingernail, allowing him a few more moments to get his act together.

It's odd how babies appear to shrink when they're not breathing, and this little boy was growing smaller by the second. With no muscle tone, his arms felt flabby, and his thin legs hung over my forearm like overcooked macaroni. The head that had looked so big coming out now appeared tiny. No time to waste. I lifted him to my face and blew gently into his nose and mouth.

"Oh, my goodness," whispered my mother.

Allan murmured, "Oh no, oh God, oh no," over and over.

"Why you bite my baby?" asked Joe-Joe in a scared little voice.

Corinne pushed the chair away and whispered, "Is he all right? Peggy?"

After five or six puffs of breath, I felt the tiny body jerk once in my hands. His arms came together and banged into my ears. And as he filled his lungs with air, he began to fluff up like a sponge soaking up water. He howled, and then he grew bigger and stronger and more alive right before my eyes.

Then I heard clickety, high-heeled footsteps on the wooden stairs. A moment later, Sandi appeared in her black silk dinner dress, taking everything in at a glance. She turned on my oxygen, dragged it across the room, and put the mask over the baby's face. He immediately turned an encouraging bright pink with the added oxygen. He batted at the mask, screaming in fury. Corinne laughed and reached her hands toward him. I wrapped another blanket around his squirmy body and laid him on her deflated belly.

From the bottom of the stairs boomed a loud voice. "Allan? Corinne? Need help?" Oh, what I wouldn't have given for that offer ten minutes earlier.

Corinne said, "Hey, Eddie, come on up. We just had the baby."

Up the stairs came Eddie, the baggy pants man from the front porch. Sandi tossed a towel over Corinne's crotch, but Corinne didn't seem to care.

Eddie looked around and nodded. "Umm-hmm, I thought it might be something like this. But y'all had me right confused for a while. First comes a lady in a nightgown banging on my door and carrying a tackle box. I sent her upstairs. Then a granny-type woman comes along carrying a little newborn baby, and I just couldn't make no sense of that. But I sent her on upstairs, too. I sure didn't order me no take-out baby from Domino's Pizza tonight, nosiree. So while I'm standin' there tryin' to puzzle it all out, along comes a gentleman looking like an Amtrak porter, loaded down with all sorts of baggage. I seen him acomin', and I just pointed my finger and shouted 'Upstairs!' before he even asked.

"Then I heard Corinne here making some kinda awful sounds like a she-goat being fucked by an elephant. 'Scuse me, I didn't realize little Joe-Joe was still up. Anyhow, those sounds made me suspect, you know, that maybe Corinne was hatchin' her chick. Only I still couldn't make no sense of that older lady carrying the little, squished-up-lookin' baby *into* the house. You understand me?

"So after the gentleman with the suitcases headed up the stairs, I just stood there tryin' to puzzle things out, right? And then along comes someone else. Well, by that time I figured there weren't nothin' left that could surprise me. Whatever pulled up at my house, man or beast—or little skinny mite of a woman all sassied up in a fancy dress like she'd been to the, whaddayacallit, the Black and White Ball, whatever come up my sidewalk, I reckoned it belonged up those stairs. So I just pointed her right on up. Hell, I even waved her along with the flashlight I'd gotten after the baggage man came.

"So, now, how 'bout if I cook up some scrambled eggs and toast for everybody?"

All three men disappeared into the tiny kitchen and soon emerged with champagne, eggs, bagels, cream cheese, and coffee. As we held the glasses aloft for a toast, I said, "Joe-Joe, come here and gimme five!" He put all his toddler energy into smacking palms with me as I said, "You were my best helper tonight!"

~ *Spirit Baby II*

I've been up all night with light contractions, but things are starting to pick up now," said Tammy.

Her baby was ten days late and had scored A+ on surveillance testing the previous afternoon, but even though she insisted labor was just starting to get more active, it seemed prudent to check her. However, only thirty minutes earlier I'd delivered another woman at home. So while I stayed to help the newborn start breastfeeding, I sent Margaret, my assistant, to check on Tammy.

Margaret telephoned me an hour later, and I heard strangled tears in her voice. She could barely speak coherently as she stammered, "Peggy, Tammy's baby is dead."

My mouth went dry. Tammy hadn't even been in good labor when I'd spoken to her. My mind reeled with the enormity of the situation: a home birth, me not even there, a possible coroner's case, the implications for midwifery and the institution of home birth. But most of all, I simply couldn't focus on the image of Tammy and Arthur with empty arms.

"What happened?" I whispered.

"It's too much to tell on the phone. The coroner's van just took the baby away. Hurry," Margaret pleaded.

I sped across town, and she met me on the front porch.

"Tammy's upstairs with Arthur," said Margaret through the tears that flowed again when she saw me. We sat on the front steps while she told me the incredible story of Eliza's birth.

When Margaret arrived at 7:30 A.M., Tammy, wearing a Japanese kimono, stood at the sink filling a teakettle. Arthur, having slept soundly all night, tap-tap-tapped at his computer. Tammy had spent the night in a rocking chair, dozing between infrequent contractions.

Tammy offered Margaret a cup of herbal tea. Just as the teakettle whistled, Tammy paused and stared out the window, looking puzzled. Then she excused herself and went upstairs to the bathroom.

As Margaret poured the water into a pot, she stared sleepily at a row of English teapots lining the sunny windowsill. She had just poured herself a cup when she heard a shriek. An upstairs door crashed against a wall, followed by pounding footsteps. Margaret looked up the stairs and glimpsed Tammy rushing toward her bedroom. Margaret raced upstairs and saw Tammy, holding the kimono above her hips, hurl herself onto the bed. She landed with her legs wide apart, and Margaret saw a head slick with birth fluid glistening between her thighs.

Instinctively, Margaret stretched out her bare hands, and a baby with limbs floppy like a well-loved rag doll tumbled into her arms. Tammy grabbed the baby from Margaret's disbelieving hands. Clutching it to her chest, she rolled from side to side, crooning, "Oh, my baby, my beautiful little girl!"

Arthur had run up the stairs a few paces behind Margaret. Both of them could see that the baby was dead. With no muscle tone, her rubbery limbs flopped into impossible positions. Half-closed eyes stared at nothing, and her pretty, bow-shaped mouth hung slack. Her ash-white skin, hardest of all to look at, had already begun to peel.

But Tammy comprehended nothing. She knew only that when she'd gone to the bathroom, her bag of water had broken and the baby's head came out. Realizing her labor was ending instead of beginning, she ran to her bed where the rest of the baby emerged with virtually no pain. Ecstatically happy, she remained locked in disbelief as Arthur dialed 911. Margaret snatched the baby back from Tammy to give mouth-to-mouth resuscitation, knowing the infant had been dead for hours.

Somehow we got through the next several hours of questions that had no answers, sadness that had no hope, and tears that had no end. Margaret and I left at noon when Tammy's sister arrived to help deal with countless details and decisions.

The next week went by in a blur. Margaret and I wanted to pack away the baby clothes, sparing Tammy that pain, but Tammy insisted on doing it herself. She cried quietly as she placed delicate dresses and pastel jumpsuits into a storage box. Her faith, based on years of studying Eastern religions and a belief in karma and rebirth, sustained her in ways that surpassed my understanding.

Bereft, Arthur could talk of nothing but his dream of a week earlier. In this dream, he stood at the end of a hallway glowing with unearthly light. His beloved Aunt Elizabeth, who had died a few months earlier, waited at the end of the hall. Behind her stood an open door. His unborn baby daughter, Eliza, to be named in honor of this aunt, floated in the middle of the hallway, vacillating as to which way she should go. Arthur called her, but at the other end of the hall, his aunt beckoned from within a halo of light. As Arthur cried aloud in his dream, his daughter moved farther away from him and into the shimmering aura of his aunt. Sad as he was, Arthur found comfort in his belief that their little girl had reached a state of grace.

I shared with Tammy and Arthur the story of Spirit Babies, the wondrous explanation my son had blessed me with when I, too, mourned the loss of a baby. Holding back tears, Tammy walked to a glass-fronted bookshelf. Small antique dolls, none more than six inches high, filled the top shelf. Tammy deliberated briefly before selecting one. The cloth doll had an exquisite hand-painted face and a dress of faded blue silk with row upon row of bugle beads sewn at the neck, sleeves, and hem.

"Keep this little doll for me," she said, pressing it into my hands. "It's part of my grandmother's collection. I've always believed these dolls have spirits, and you should have one."

I demurred, trying to give the doll back, this doll with a soul. I felt intensely uncomfortable accepting a baby doll from Tammy, when it was I who should be handing her a squirming, happy newborn. But Tammy insisted. "No, I want you to have it. Think of it as my Spirit Baby."

To protest further would have been rude, so I took the lovely little doll home. But I couldn't find the courage to display it. It felt like I picked at a scab each time I saw it, so I tucked it into a pigeonhole in my drop-front desk. It eventually disappeared from sight in the clutter.

In spite of extensive testing, no cause for Eliza's death was found. The coroner released her body to the funeral home a week later. At a private memorial service, Tammy and Arthur indulged themselves in looking at her delicate features for the first time since those desperate, incomprehensible minutes after her birth. Tammy's guru, a brown-skinned Indian in voluminous white robes, gave the eulogy. We all held Eliza and blessed her, kissing her waxen cheek and admiring her perfection. Then Tammy laid her down on the small, pillowed table, an altar of sorts . . . and she walked away.

"Eliza's fine," she whispered. "It's sad for us who are left, but she's at peace."

I thought my heart would break.

When they went to pick up the ashes two days later, her guru and I went along. On the way home, holding the painfully lightweight urn on her lap, Tammy shared the Spirit Baby story with her teacher, who said nothing. He just nodded, looking out the window.

Tammy seemed to feel the story warranted some reaction, and she said, "Can you believe a twelve year old made up that incredible, wonderful story?"

At that, the wise man jerked his gaze from the golden California hills. He stared intently at Tammy for a few moments and then placed his thin, dark-skinned hand on her pale, freckled one, patting it as he spoke.

"Made it up? But Tammy, my dear, he didn't make it up. Open your eyes, my daughter. Does it take a child to show you such a simple, universal piece of the puzzle of life? He graciously shared the story of Spirit Babies with us because he knows it for the Truth it surely is."

Years passed, and they moved away. Then one day I found a small envelope with a Florida postmark in my mailbox. But I don't know anyone in Florida, I thought, as I removed a card. It was a birth announcement. A little girl had been born to Tammy and Arthur. They named her Elizabeth.

On the left side of the announcement, Tammy asked if I would please return the doll to her, now that her own Spirit Baby had been born.

For a moment I panicked. Because of the pain it brought me, that little doll hadn't seen the light of day for more than five years. What if I couldn't find it? But I walked to the desk, pulled out some postcards and old photographs, and once again held the antique doll in my hands.

I packed it in a box with a copy of *Goodnight Moon,* and I sprinkled confetti and tinsel stars over everything. With a joyful heart, I mailed the Spirit Baby back to Tammy.

When Mom Is
a Midwife

W hen my husband or children were asked what I did for a living, I wondered how they felt as they answered, "She's a midwife." Although a few of Colin and Jill's friends had lawyer or banker mothers who jammed onto the Bay Bridge with thousands of other commuters, most had flexible jobs that allowed them to juggle wage-earning with carpooling. But midwives for moms were as rare as udders on chickens.

When I first met people who knew of my unorthodox occupation, they usually said, "Oh, so *you're* the midwife." Odd, medieval images pop into people's heads when they hear that term, but I'm one of the sliced and packaged white bread variety. So I watched as these people looked me over, trying to adjust their preconceptions to the reality of just plain me: naturally curly graying hair, round Irish face with pink cheeks and light blue eyes, Lands' End cotton knits, and Gap sweatshirts. Yes, I wore Birkenstocks, and no, I hadn't pulled on a pair of panty hose in years, but I was neither a wizened granny with mysterious potions nor a tie-dyed hippie with exotic crystals or bundles of sage tucked in my pockets. I just didn't fit the stereotype.

I remembered my midwifery school classmate, Gaia's, comment: "Just think about it. As midwives, we meet wildly interesting people and stay up all night with them. We ask them questions about their sex lives, eat their food, feel inside their bodies, snoop around their houses, drink champagne at all hours, and best of all, we get to catch delicious little naked, wet babies. What I can't figure out is, why doesn't everyone want to be a midwife?"

I can't dream of a more satisfying way to earn a living, but when I evolved from salaried nurse to self-employed midwife, I underestimated the effect these changes would have on Rog and our kids. The profession of midwifery is tough on marriage and family life, especially if the midwife is in a solo practice and on call 365 days a year, as I was. Without Rog's flexibility and versatility, I couldn't have been the kind of midwife I aspired to be. Although he gave a rueful laugh when people addressed him as "the midwife's husband," I knew he was proud of me.

Rog received his MBA and worked in a bank during the early years of our marriage, but he hated the regimentation and the hours. Although a product of East Coast prep schools, he said, "I'm not cut out to be a Suit," and went back to school. After earning a fine arts degree in the seventies, he became a potter and glassblower. By the time I went to midwifery school in 1980, he had evolved into a carpenter/painter/contractor. He deliberately kept his schedule flexible and carried a pager for those times when I suddenly needed him to take over household affairs.

Often with little or no warning, Rog substituted for me on school field trips, baked birthday cupcakes, cooked dinner, and drove carpools. One time he solo-hosted a party for fifty guests at our house; when I arrived two hours late, everyone looked happy and well fed, but Rog looked happiest of all. He took off his apron, handed me a glass of wine and poured an even larger one for himself. Then he sat down for the first time all evening.

And for two years in a row, it fell to Rog to explain to three disappointed children why I wasn't home on Christmas morning.

"Midwives are risky dinner guests," he once said to a woman whose party we'd been planning to attend before a phone call from a client changed our plans. Many times I arrived late at some affair, left early, or just never showed up at all.

"Midwives are social hazards," Rog explained to a newcomer at our neighborhood Labor Day potluck. The woman's eyebrows had shot up when she heard me use the words "placenta" and "vagina" without whispering. Like many midwives, I'm inclined to discuss casually topics that most other people never hear mentioned outside of a doctor's office. Once during dinner at a restaurant with another midwife and her husband, Rog nodded in heartfelt agreement when the other guy said, "Do you think we could get through this meal without one single mention of anything having to do with blood?"

"Midwives are unreliable lovers," Rog growled as the phone rang when we were well on our way toward the conclusion of an evening of lovemaking. I tried to stay with the rhythm as I talked with a woman panting in my ear—and I wondered if she heard anyone panting on our end of the line—but it was no use. A minute later, scowling with guilt and regret, I was out of bed and pulling on sweatpants and socks. As I ran a brush through my hair, I heard Rog mutter something about "coitus interruptus telephonus." I headed toward the door, and he called after me, "It's okay to wake me up when you get home, you know." I winked back at him.

Carole, Sandi, and I were nearly kicked out of a fancy restaurant one afternoon when Carole told us about her son, Andy, mistaking a placenta for a frozen pizza. Carole said the placenta was very unusual, and she wanted to show it at an upcoming midwifery meeting. She had arranged it just so on a baking sheet, all spread out with the attached membranes tucked up at the edges, and then she covered it with aluminum foil.

"I walked in the door and sniffed," she went on. "Something smelled like the lion cage at the zoo, and I asked Andy what on earth he was cooking. He opened the oven, removed the foil, and screamed as if he'd seen Freddie from *Nightmare on Elm Street*."

By this time, many of the Ladies Who Lunch had stopped eating to stare at us, fingering their pearls nervously. The hostess glanced our way a couple of times, tapping her pencil eraser on the reservation book.

As Sandi and I gasped with laughter, Carole graphically described the shriveled remains of an overbaked, but very unusual, placenta. "I told Andy, 'That's what happens when you have a midwife for a mom,' but I'm not sure he heard me. He was in the den with a sofa cushion over his head."

I saw a flushed woman at an adjacent table push away her uneaten lasagna and begin fanning herself with her napkin.

Like Carole, I too sometimes had a spare placenta hanging around. But Rog hated coming across one in a Ziploc bag when he was delving in the fridge for a late-night snack.

"Can't you freeze these things and shove them way to the back?" he asked.

"Freezing changes them. They're so much better fresh."

"But, when I pick it up, it . . . moves," he said with a shudder. "It jiggles. And suddenly I know exactly what it is. I just can't stand it, Peggy."

So I froze them. Most of the time. But sometimes I forgot.

Placentas really were best when fresh, and they worked great for educational purposes. When I taught childbirth or sibling preparation classes, I always took one along. And when my children had sex education classes in middle school and again in high school, they usually volunteered my services for the pregnancy and childbirth section. I had a little lecture prepared, and I used my photo albums of women giving birth, a life-sized baby doll and bony pelvis, a speculum, and lots of other goodies. But the best moment came when I popped the lid off a Tupperware bowl and lifted up a placenta.

After the girls finished shrieking and flapping their hands and the boys finished blushing and shoving each other sideways, they fell silent as I went through the rest of my spiel. With gloves on, I showed my spellbound audience the liver-like side that attaches to the uterine wall. Then I turned it over and showed the shiny, purplish-gray side that resembles the Tree of Life when you arrange it with the umbilical cord masquerading as the trunk. I pointed out the spot where the membranes, "the bag" that holds the amniotic fluid, had broken and how it's really two membranes lying closer together than two sheets in a ream of paper.

By then, the kids were usually hooked. Donning disposable gloves, they took turns examining the placenta, handling it as if it were an exotic snake. For weeks after each of these classes, kids who saw me waiting in the lines of carpooling moms laughed and said, "Hi, Placenta Lady."

Throughout their childhood, my children heard casual discussions of sex, childbirth, breastfeeding, AIDS, herpes, and other medical conditions as often as they heard debates on such things as the installation of speed bumps on our street. But as they grew older, they realized this was not the norm. When Colin invited Nicholas, a twelve-year-old school friend who was the only child of Type A parents, to come for dinner and a sleepover, our house was torn apart for Phase IV of our endless home remodeling. The downstairs telephone temporarily sat at the end of our dining room table.

As the time drew near for Nicholas's arrival, Colin looked at the phone and fell silent. Then he looked at me and said, "Mom, if you get a call during dinner tonight, could you take it upstairs in your bedroom?"

"Sure, but why?" I asked, wiping sheetrock dust off the table and buffet.

"Well, it'll probably be one of your patients, and I don't think Nicholas is ready to hear you asking some woman about the color of her vaginal discharge or when she last had sex, you know? I don't mind it, 'cause I understand about all that stuff. But you've gotta admit, Mom, it's just not normal."

During the summer after Skylar was conceived, Rog accompanied Colin to Boy Scout camp for a week and a half. I figured Jill and I would have lots of time for girl stuff, but I hadn't taken the full moon into consideration. It seemed that every time I answered the phone, someone said, "My bag of water just broke."

With my patients' permission, I took ten-year-old Jill to eight births, and she soaked up the drama like someone seeing *Swan Lake* performed for the first time. By the time the guys came home, she had developed a sixth sense for the ballet of birth: when to move closer and when to retreat, when to speak and when to be quiet, when to touch the laboring woman and when to move back.

During my labor with Skylar six months later, I wasn't surprised when Jill held my hands in hers and guided me through several contractions. Lost in the fog of my pain, I heard her speak the same words she had heard me say to other women when they, too, lay in labor: "Good, Mom, you can do it, just a little longer. Take it one breath at a time."

Three months after Skylar's birth, a new couple moved into a house up the hill. The woman later told me that her new neighbor had introduced herself and told her who lived on our block: "an anthropologist, a general contractor, a librarian, a computer salesman, a midwife . . ."

I glimpsed her unloading groceries a few days after the moving van pulled away and noticed she had a pregnant belly that looked ready to pop. Indeed, she gave birth three weeks later, and when her husband brought her home from the hospital, Jill and several other girls were playing out front. As soon as they saw the tiny six-pound baby, they swarmed around, oohing and aahing.

"Oh, she's so tiny. How much does she weigh?"

"What's her name?"

"How old is she?"

"How was your labor?"

That last question made the new mother laugh, and she turned to her husband. "Peter, that last one just might be the midwife's daughter, don't you think?"

Then she sat on her front step and told Jill about her incredibly efficient five-hour first labor. A few days later, Jill brought the new family down to our house and introduced us to Sally and Peter. My Skylar and their little Ellen grew up like siblings, sharing wading pools, pacifiers, bowls of ice cream, bathtubs, bedtime stories, and a mutual dislike of tofu. And three years later, I delivered Sally's second daughter, Claire, while Ellen watched from the safety of Jill's lap.

A couple of years later, Sally and Peter loaned me their second car during a time when my primary car, my trusty little VW bug, had a mysterious malady that defied all of our mechanic's remedies. Midwives need reliable cars, but the idea of buying a new car offends all of Rog's remaining banker genes. He'd rather buy me custom-designed jewelry, saying, "Fine jewelry appreciates with age, but a new car is worth only two-thirds of its purchase price as soon as you drive it off the lot." Consequently, I wear beautiful earrings, but I haven't driven a new car since our marriage in 1965.

By the time Colin and Jill were in high school, we owned five cars, but a couple of them were just one muffler away from the junkyard. One of Colin's friends said, "Your sister doesn't even have her license yet, right? Only three of you can drive. Why do you have so many cars?"

"When your mom's a midwife and your cars are as old as some of ours, you need a few extras around," explained Colin.

"Spare cars," Rog called them. When some insidious virus spread from one to another, we needed every single one in order to play musical cars while we ran relays to the auto shop. On those occasions, Colin sometimes ended up driving my VW bug to school, simply because it was the last functional car in the driveway, closest to the street.

One day he came home, parked my car at the curb, and came inside with a disgusted expression on his face. He tossed his books on the couch and stood there just looking at me, shaking his head. Finally he said, "Your car is too much, Mom."

"Oh, no. What's wrong?" I feared it, too, had succumbed to the malady.

"No, it's running fine. It's that MITWIFE license plate and the *Midwives Do It at Home* bumper sticker."

"Ah, I see. Embarrassment is the problem?"

"Well, sorta. I can usually just blow it off, but today was outrageous. There were these two girls, really cute, walking out of school ahead of me. Turns out they were parked right beside the bug, and I thought, Oh no. Sure enough, when they saw the license and bumper sticker, they cracked up. You know, whispering and laughing."

"Oh, Colin, I'm sorry. I could peel off the bumper sticker, I guess."

"Wait, I'm not finished," and said, holding up his hand. "I just stood there, feeling stupid, and then the tall one said, 'Is your mother a midwife, or something?' And I nodded and kinda kicked at the tire, and she went, 'Ha! So is mine! I know just what it's like.'

"So we talked some more, and anyway, we're gonna get together this weekend, but get this. As they started backing out of the parking place, I heard her say to her friend, 'I can't believe I've got a date with the Placenta Lady's son.'"

I tried to hide my grin, but I think he heard my snort of laughter as he continued.

"So Dad's known as The Midwife's Husband, and now I'm known as The Placenta Lady's Son. Great, Mom. Just great."

But he was grinning.

PART V

Who walketh upon the wings of the wind

". . . who maketh the clouds his chariot,
who walketh upon the wings of the wind."

PSALMS 104:3
THE HOLY BIBLE, KING JAMES VERSION, 1611

One More Soul

Most people associate California, especially the Bay Area, with casual acceptance of unusual lifestyles. Working as a delivery room nurse in Berkeley, the epicenter of diversity, I thought I'd seen it all. But as soon as I became a midwife, women from esoteric subcultural groups of which I'd been previously unaware popped up like exotic freesias in March. They'd been there all along, hiding among the more common daffodils and tulips, but I'd never encountered them because most had chosen to deliver at home.

Ocean lived in one of Berkeley's many guru-centered communes, the kind that make tourists raise their eyebrows in disbelief. Considering her name, I shouldn't have been surprised that she planned a water birth. Born to hippie parents in a tepee overlooking the Pacific, she now labored in a hot tub behind an enormous three-story Victorian. In addition to the main house, five or six small cottages were clustered together behind the house, and the twenty adult residents spent their time studying how to read auras, clear negative psychic energy, interpret people's unconscious thoughts, communicate by telepathy, and give advice based on evidence gathered from these various sources.

I gained a clearer understanding of the inner workings of the institute when Ocean was seven months pregnant. During a routine prenatal visit, I asked how it would be for her, alone at night with her baby on the top floor of the big house.

"The cleaning crew is there all night. They'll keep me company."

"But won't the noise of the vacuum cleaner keep you awake?"

"Oh, it's not that kind of cleaning. It's a psychic institute, so they're perfectly quiet. The night crew is busy cleaning out leftover negative energy."

"Ah," I said, trying to hide my astonishment.

Now some of those night shift energy cleaners were supporting Ocean during her labor. I lounged by the edge of the tub, watching her drift and float. But concern clouded my ability to fully enjoy the serenity. Too much peace in labor doesn't always bode well, and as time passed, Ocean labored less instead of more. She'd been working on getting this baby out for a long time and was beginning to tire.

Other women from the institute supported her. I quickly thought of them as the Vestal Virgins. Mostly in their twenties, they shared a dreamy, ingenue quality. Thin, lithe, and graceful, only two had had babies themselves; the others looked awed by the process. Several of them, naked, supported Ocean in the tub. Others, in soft, cottony skirts and loose tops, drifted in the background like wisps of fog.

In spite of their inexperience, they shared an intuitive ability to help Ocean relax. In fact, I wished they wouldn't do such a good job. I wanted to get her stirred up, but they wanted to "keep her grounded." They devoted themselves to "aura maintenance," a system of hand dancing, arm waving, and finger fluttering to clear the atmosphere, channel the energy, and deflect negative vibrations. Finally, I intervened.

"Okay, ladies, I'm so grounded I'm nearly comatose, and I can see how relaxed Ocean feels. Could you direct some energy toward *boosting* the intensity a bit?"

They clustered to discuss tactics, and indeed, the style and tempo of the hand dancing changed. But another hour passed without any alteration in the labor pattern. I decided on some herbal remedies and asked the women to take turns doing nipple stimulation, which releases a pituitary hormone to strengthen contractions.

They raised their eyebrows slightly but took turns twiddling Ocean's nipples while she leaned against the edge of the tub, her hair floating like strands of kelp. Every fifteen minutes I squeezed a dropper full of cohosh tincture beneath her tongue and asked her to swish it around for ten seconds before swallowing.

"It tastes like leaf mold, dirt, and dead mushrooms," she said, wrinkling her nose.

Contractions became closer and stronger for half an hour, then fizzled. We walked her up and down three flights of stairs for nearly an hour. I stretched and stimulated her cervix. We even borrowed a nursing baby from another woman to suckle for as long as the baby stayed interested. But eventually nothing had any effect. Ocean's labor had stalled with no end in sight.

"It's not working, is it?" she asked, awakening from a fifteen-minute nap.

"I'm afraid you're right," I agreed. "There's no emergency, but we should start thinking 'hospital' and 'Pitocin' sooner rather than later. If you become much more exhausted, I'm afraid you won't have energy to push." She nodded.

The leisurely pace continued as we dried her off and dressed her. One woman collected Ocean's slippers, robe, and some personal items, and we trooped down the wooden stairs leading from the wide front porch—but there was no man among us.

When I'd taken Ocean's history on her first prenatal visit, I'd asked about the father of her baby, and she'd looked at me with a vague smile. She waved her hand in the air as if brushing away the last few strands of a cobweb as she said, "No, no father. My baby won't need a father."

"I'm asking more in terms of medical issues, Ocean. Is the baby's father healthy? Does he have any health conditions I should know about?"

"No, he's okay, but he's left the institute, and I won't be seeing him again."

So the feminine entourage tucked their diaphanous skirts into four dilapidated cars and drove to Alta Bates. Since the birth center's opening seven years earlier, the nursing staff had grown accustomed to large groups of support people. But as I watched the women stream from the cars and waft through the hospital corridors, I knew the sheer number of this bunch would probably set a new record. I prayed for an understanding nurse who'd be able to groove with the energy flow.

I relaxed when Bonnie stood up from the nurses' station. Bonnie, her long braid twisted into a bun and her warm brown eyes smiling in amusement at our little parade, had already attended many home births with me and felt comfortable with my style. Even thirteen Vestal Virgins didn't faze her. She settled Ocean in bed, pulled extra chairs and beanbags into the room for the support crew, and started the Pitocin drip with practiced speed. She managed to create a quiet atmosphere, even though chaos raged in the corridor. This kind of hyped-up, tense, noisy energy can be very contagious in hospitals, and Bonnie seemed determined that it not spread into Ocean's room. She closed the door and drew the blinds. When someone turned on a tape of Gregorian chants, it began to feel like Vespers in a medieval cathedral.

Ocean's friends reclined everywhere, their pastel skirts resembling a smeared artist's palette. No finger dancing, so I assumed everyone had been grounded. I left for an hour to eat lunch and see a couple of pregnant ladies in my office.

When I returned, Bonnie had plugged the IV pump into the bathroom outlet and Ocean was back underwater. With each contraction she sank lower in the bathtub till just her face remained above waterline. The surface scarcely trembled as she breathed, and the hypnotic tape still played in the background. I timed the contractions as I felt them with my fingertips: every two to three minutes and strong. The Pitocin had been successful. In spite of all the equipment, the atmosphere felt holy, so still and serene.

Bang! Suddenly the door flew open. The overhead lights flipped on high, and a lab tech blew into the room with flapping white coat and a metal box bristling with tubes, needles, and cotton puffs. Lab slips fluttered from his hand as he talked loudly over his shoulder to someone in the hallway. Silently and in unison, the Vestal Virgins surged into high gear, their fingers dancing frantically. The quick and urgent movements lost the lovely sinuousness of maintenance therapy. This was crisis intervention, Berkeley style.

The tech turned and did a double take, gasping, "What the hell!"

It appeared the psychic grounding waves reached him quickly, however, because he backed up, turned off the lights, and slowed way, way down. "I need to draw her blood," he whispered to me. "Will they let me?"

I nodded. "They won't bite."

Glancing at the still-alert acolytes arranged along all the walls—they seemed to have multiplied while I'd been gone—he sidled into the bathroom. Sitting on the toilet and balancing Ocean's dripping arm on his thigh, he quietly did the job in the space between two contractions. The man looked awkward and uncomfortable, but I suspected he didn't want to risk another dose of grounding therapy.

Very soon Bonnie and I saw Ocean's belly curl under at the top. Her uterus pulled in at the sides, pressed down toward her spine, and tucked under. With that first push, her eyes opened under the water. She looked like the Nautilus rising in *20,000 Leagues under the Sea*.

Ocean pushed intuitively and well, but she had difficulty directing the pushing forces while lying down. One of her friends tucked her skirts into her waistband and stood in the water so Ocean could lean against her legs to squat.

I'd had hospital privileges for only six months, and I knew some of the more resentful doctors still watched me closely, waiting for me to have a problem from some "weird midwifery stunt." So, although I'd considered delivering Ocean under water, I can't deny my relief when she spontaneously stood up and walked into the labor room.

All this time, she didn't say a word. Many pairs of ardent eyes turned to her in the dim light. Ocean overflowed with the raw energy of birth, a naked goddess radiating pride and strength, towering over everyone. She raised her arms over her head, tossing her wet hair off her face, and began swaying side to side, keeping time to her inner music. Her hands ran down the curves of her body, honoring each part: face, neck, breasts, belly, thighs, buttocks—and her silent swaying continued.

Staring into the far distance with wide-open eyes, she danced for us. No one spoke. No one touched her. The IV pole and tubing attached to her arm might as well have been in Canada, so little did they intrude. A cushion of inviolate space surrounded her, a force field that excluded everyone. Some would have called it her aura.

Then Ocean began dancing more slowly, making low, throaty noises. Shreds of mucus dripped down her thighs as she stood on an island of absorbent cotton blankets. Peeking between her legs, I saw the baby's head begin to fill the vaginal opening. I held steaming washcloths to her perineum to give support and help relax the tissue, and Bonnie listened to the baby's heartbeat with a hand-held Doppler.

Still no one spoke. We listened to Ocean's occasional grunts and *whoofs* of expelled air. Holding the hands of a friend, she stood in the middle of the room, still dancing and swaying between contractions, although her feet no longer moved.

On my knees before her, I could see very little, but I'd done births by Braille before. The baby's head surged lower. I looked into Ocean's face to gauge her reaction to this extreme stretching, a feeling that surpasses belief. Without moving her head, her eyes looked down at me, and she spoke at last.

"It's coming, you know," she whispered.

"I know. Let it." I never took my eyes off hers as the baby was oh, so gently born. When the shoulders slipped through, Ocean's hands joined mine. She crouched slightly and pulled the rest of the baby out herself.

Standing tall and strong, Ocean held the little boy to her chest. She looked at her friends and turned the baby to face them. The gauzy, pastel-clad women held each other, and their quiet sobs blended with the temple bells coming from the tape player.

Ocean began swaying again, and this time she accompanied her dance with a song. No words. Just humming and crooning, the sounds soaring high and then low, striking chords of familiarity. Gregorian chants. Tibetan monotones. The muezzin's call to prayer. Her song seemed timeless and eternal, and with each note, the world expanded to make room for one more soul.

~ *Pragmatism in Action*

I dreaded having a laboring mom refuse to go to the hospital when I advised it. Other midwives said it had happened to them, but I just couldn't imagine such a scenario—nor how it would feel to find myself in such an impossible position. To allow a woman to manage her own labor in an unsafe setting seemed unthinkable. But so did the other two options: taking her to the hospital against her will or abandoning her to protect myself.

Only once did I think I teetered on the edge of that impasse.

We could almost see the baby's head—birth was that close. But as I rose from the rumpled futon where Susie had labored for the last eighteen hours, I had bad news to deliver. The stress of this long but otherwise normal labor had caught up with the baby, and her spiraling heartbeat now stayed low after each of Susie's heroic pushes.

The amniotic fluid, clear as gin for hours, had turned the color of dead leaves on the forest floor. Susie and Vita's baby might require more equipment, personnel, and expertise than I could offer in this third-floor walk-up. I hated telling them their dream of a home birth would remain just that, a dream.

"Sorry, Susie, but there's meconium, and the baby's heartbeat is too slow. We need to go to the hospital right now."

Susie, face puffy from the effort of pushing, blinked her brown eyes and used both hands to sweep her long dark hair off her face, damp with the sweat of labor. The glitter in her blue nail polish sparkled in the candlelight.

I glanced around, trying to assess whom I could count on most. There stood Vita, a thin, ascetic woman with a striking resemblance to an icon of a medieval saint. Unable to bear a child herself, she had performed Susie's insemination with a turkey baster. She rejoiced at the positive pregnancy test, supported Susie through the discomfort of the last weeks before birth, and planned to adopt the little girl they had conceived in their own bedroom. She looked tired, now, as she stared at the brown goop between Susie's thighs, but I knew I could count on her.

Beyond Vita crowded the cluster of women who'd invested long hours in Susie's labor. They had made tea, given massages, fixed meals, and done laundry together, jazzed at the expectation of a home birth. A gruff-looking woman stood at the center of the pack, one hip cocked higher than the other. I'd heard her earlier, bossing everybody around the kitchen. An in-your-face type, I thought, and I hoped she wouldn't give me any lip.

I picked up the phone, punched Alta Bates's number, and talked with the charge nurse. "Judy, it's Peggy. I'm bringing in a first-timer who's about to deliver. In the last ten minutes there's been thick meconium and fetal distress. Can you have everything ready for us?"

Susie listened. She nodded once, rolled off the futon, and began searching for her Birkenstocks under the bed.

All the women stepped back and stared at me. Motionless in the dim light, they looked stunned by the authoritative tone in my voice. Stunned, too, by the realization that we'd be leaving the cozy ambiance of the apartment to hustle Susie down two flights of rickety stairs to face a drive through the cold February night to the brightly lit, hypertechnical world of the hospital.

I turned to ask Vita to get Susie's coat. Her expression stopped me cold.

Trembling, wringing her hands, she whined, "But we don't want the hospital."

My dismay increased when the square woman I'd picked as possible trouble stepped forward. Baggy denim jeans hung from her solid hips, and a noisy key ring jangled from one belt loop. Her Doc Martens clomped on the bare wooden floor as she hiked up her pants. But her comment surprised me.

"Oh, Vee, shut the hell up. You gotta do what you gotta do."

"But . . . but . . . Teri," stammered Vita.

"Just cool it. You're not in charge. Shit, that's what you hired Peggy for, right?"

She scanned the room, daring anyone to disagree. Despite my brain's spinning with the logistics of our sudden change of plans, I ducked my head to hide a chuckle.

Susie had found her Birkies, and a woman with a purple crew cut helped her put them on. Teri wrapped Susie in a huge quilt and steered her toward the doorway. "Do you have your insurance card?"

"My purse," mumbled Susie. A fearsome contraction doubled her, and she gripped Teri's plaid flannel sleeve.

"Where? Where's your purse?" barked Teri, snapping her fingers.

"Hall table," gasped Susie.

Vita covered her face, crying. A thin blonde with a weight lifter's chiseled muscles hugged her and buttoned a sweater up under her chin.

"But the baby's almost here," stammered Vita.

"Yeah, the baby will be born in the next half hour," I said, "but she needs to be born in the hospital. She might need help getting started." I grabbed Susie's chart and a few supplies. "Who's got the biggest car?" I asked.

"I do. I've got a station wagon," said Teri. She pushed Susie toward the purple-haired woman and turned to wrap up loose ends. Her eyes snapped with the composure of a quarterback, and her capable hands hung ready at her sides. With her short, dark hair sticking out at funny angles from her head, she looked like a five year old who'd been playing beauty parlor with her little sister. But I didn't care what she looked like. She had Attitude and a station wagon. She was my new best friend.

"Great. Put Susie into the wayback."

"But couldn't we just . . ." bleated Vita between sobs.

Teri spun her around and pushed her toward the door, shooting orders like bullets. "Kath, take Susie down. Vita, you get in front with me—and don't talk. The rest of you, follow me. I'll drive to the ER and leave the keys in the ignition. Kath, after you've parked, come park mine for me. Got it?"

Everyone nodded and moved off. I stared at Teri. The world needs more people like her, I thought.

Susie started down the steps. Teri hollered, "Baby clothes?"

"Middle dresser drawer," said Susie. Then she leaned against the railing, bellowing into the frigid, foggy night as another contraction nailed her.

A resident of a ground-floor apartment opened his window and hollered, "Quiet up there. It's past midnight already."

"Aw, kwitcherbitchin, asshole," shouted Teri. "She's havin' a baby, ferchrissake."

The window slammed shut.

Teri ran into the bedroom, pulled baby stuff from the dresser, and dashed to the landing. "Is the oven turned off?" she yelled, "And the space heater? Candles?"

"Jeez, no," said one of the last women out of the apartment. She turned back.

Susie and I jockeyed for position in the wayback of the car. Vita twisted around and stared at us through teary eyes. The baby's heart rate hung between seventy and ninety. Too slow, way too slow. My jaw clenched.

Then we heard Teri still on the landing. "Keys, where're the keys? Come on, you guys, we can't just drive off and leave the place unlocked. Jeez, this is the 'hood, ya know?"

"God," mumbled Vita. She struggled from the car and tossed the keys up to Teri. Moments later, Teri slammed the driver's side door and gunned forward, shooting from the small parking lot behind the shabby building. Avoiding a Dumpster, she barreled down the dark street through ghostly swirls of fog. "Which way? College or Telegraph?"

"Telegraph. And don't stop at lights unless you have to," I answered. I saw a tiny scrap of the baby's head starting to show.

"Righto."

I glanced at her reflection in the rearview mirror and thought I saw her grin at the challenge of hot-dogging it down Telegraph Avenue. My kind of woman, I thought.

"Susie, blow or yell or scream," I said as she sucked in a big breath. "Just don't push till we're in the hospital, okay?"

"I'm trying!" she shrieked, and I watched her perineum bulge.

Vita covered her face and leaned against the window. "Oh, God, do you think we'll make it?" she moaned.

"You bet your sweet bippy, girlfriend," snarled Teri under her breath, leaning on the horn as she slowed at a red light. She glanced in both directions and blew on through, negotiating a squealing right turn at the next intersection. The red and white Emergency Room sign glowed a block away.

The car bucked forward and bounced back as Teri braked at the ER ramp. She hauled up the hand brake before leaping out and disappearing through the automatic doors. She reappeared almost immediately, pushing a stretcher. A protesting nurse trailed behind, but she snapped her mouth shut when she saw Susie and me.

"Dear, dear, dear," she clucked, reaching in to haul Susie onto the stretcher. "Hold on, honey, and we'll have you upstairs in two shakes of a lamb's tail."

As we pushed Susie down the bright corridor, I looked back and saw Teri holding Vita's face between her palms, speaking to her with a combination of calmness and intensity. Vita nodded in numb agreement, and then the two of them came hotfooting after us. The elevator doors rolled shut and up we went.

"Did you leave your keys in the car?" I asked Teri, knowing there'd be hell to pay if she'd blocked the ambulance entrance.

"Sure," she answered. "I said I would, didn't I? Kath'll deal with it. No sweat." Then she squeezed Vita and said, "Hey, we made it, girl. What'd I tell you, huh?"

Susie yelled, and I saw more bald head push through the dark thatch of her pubic hair. "Hurry, hurry, hurry," I chanted to the elevator, and moments later we rolled into labor and delivery.

Two nurses jumped up from the curved desk and steered the gurney into an empty room. One of them hooked the baby to an internal fetal monitor while the other grabbed the chart from my hand and dialed the phone.

I donned a pair of sterile gloves and hiked my right hip onto the edge of the bed. The baby's head oozed down, centimeter by centimeter, with each of Susie's labored groans. The contractions continued in a slam-bam pattern, and sweat beaded from every pore of Susie's straining body. The first nurse, pursing her lips as she studied the baby's wavering heartbeat on the monitor, put an oxygen mask on Susie.

Vita held Susie's right leg, but her attention kept wavering. Teary-eyed, she stared in distraction around the bright room, and Susie's leg flopped at odd angles. Frowning, I pushed at her leg with my elbow while keeping my hands on the baby. I saw Teri at the head of the bed, her eyes snapping, taking in everything. She flashed me a quick look, raising her brows in an unspoken question. I jerked my head toward Susie and said, "Get her legs."

As a tennis ball–sized portion of the baby's head filled my palm, the pediatrician came through the door and stood beside me. Susie pushed through two more contractions, and then the baby's head slid out. Covered with slimy meconium, her face looked like a little brown mummy. A nurse passed me the suction catheter. As I manipulated the tube into the baby's mouth, her hard gums chomped on my finger, and I breathed a sigh of relief. That biting reflex meant the baby wasn't unconscious or flaccid.

The baby wrinkled her face and tried to dodge me as I nudged the catheter into each tiny nostril. I sucked on the mouthpiece, filling the container with meconium thick as sludge.

Feeling better as the baby grimaced and snorted, I relaxed as Susie, with a mighty roar, pushed the rest of the infant into my hands.

"She looks good," boomed the pediatrician.

And she did look good—good, that is, except for the muck covering every centimeter of her body. Bubbles of the stuff frothed from her mouth, and she was so slippery I was glad Susie wasn't on the edge of a delivery table. I've never seen a baby really get away from a doctor or midwife, but I've seen more than a couple bobbled like a cake of soap in the shower. This little girl would have been a candidate for the slipperiest critter in any mud-wrestling contest.

After cutting the cord, I grabbed her heels and held her upside down to keep her from inhaling as I transferred her to the infant warmer. Normally it's good practice to dry a baby off quickly after birth, but the rubbing stimulates breathing, and I didn't want her to breathe till the resuscitation crew had their turn. Their endotrachael suctioning was exactly why we'd come to the hospital. It's not a skill that home birth midwives are expected to have. It takes practice to be good at it, and we have no opportunity to get that practice.

Lowering her onto a pad of heated blankets, I stood back as the A-Team went into action. The pediatrician, a nurse-anesthetist, and the nursery nurse launched themselves into a high-speed drill that reminded me of the guys who change tires in the Indy 500. Before the baby gasped, they passed a flexible tube into her bronchi and sucked—and got nothing. We smiled at this further indication that she hadn't aspirated any meconium.

As soon as they removed the catheter separating her vocal cords, Susie's daughter screamed.

"All right! Way to go, kiddo," cheered Teri, smacking palms with a panting Kath who, after re-parking Teri's car, had arrived just in time for the birth.

Still the baby screamed. She yelled and thrashed, and we laughed. She screamed on and on, registering her opinion of the whole affair. Shaking her head, the nursery nurse left with her hands over her ears. The pediatrician raised his hands in an "I surrender" gesture and stepped back.

The baby arched her back and beat her bony little heels in a machine gun rat-a-tat-tat that boomed loudly through four layers of flowered flannel in the baby warmer. Then a nurse brought in more warm blankets and swaddled her like an enchilada.

Vita pressed her tear-stained cheek to Susie's, and together they stared at their daughter.

"She seems fine," said the pediatrician. "I can't find a thing wrong with her." He tucked the baby, still shrieking, into the crook of Susie's arm.

Teri turned to the doctor with her thumbs hooked into her belt loops and said, "Great. When can Susie take her home?"

"Oh, in the morning, I suppose. I don't see any reason to keep her longer."

"In the morning?" said about five women in unison. "The morning?"

For the first time the pediatrician seemed to comprehend that he was the Lone Ranger in a canyon full of rustlers. Lesbian rustlers. He backed up a step or two and looked between Susie and Vita. Teri and the baby. Kath with her spiked crew cut, and a platinum blonde with pierced eyebrow and lip. And more of the same in the background, about eight altogether.

The doctor licked his lips and turned to me. "Ah, I see. They were planning . . ."

"A home birth," completed Susie. "We only got here about fifteen minutes ago, and I want to go home now. Please?"

The doctor pressed his lips together and checked the baby again. The heir to the throne of England could not have been checked more thoroughly. "Hmm." He stalled for time, toying with his stethoscope. "Um, ah, who's going to be staying with you tonight?" he asked, looking at Vita lying limp on Susie's chest.

"I am," stated Teri in a voice that brooked no dissent. She hiked up her jeans and took two full steps toward him as if to say, You wanna make something of it?

He looked her up and down. "Good idea," he said.

"So we can go?" asked Susie, acting like she'd bolt from the hospital before I'd even wedged a sanitary pad between her legs.

"Jeez, could you just give us an hour to watch her? Please?" begged the doctor.

"An hour?" whined Susie, making it sound like eternity.

"Look, I'll tell you what," said Teri. "While they get all their shit together and check the kid a few more times, and you prove you can walk and pee and not bleed to death, I'll go to the apartment and get it all cleaned up, okay?"

Susie smiled at the idea of returning to a warm, tidy apartment with all signs of her long labor cleaned away. I saw the pediatrician relax as the prospect faded that this woman would spirit her baby from the hospital less than an hour after delivery.

Fifteen minutes later Teri zipped up her parka. Pushing her fists into the pockets, she asked Susie, "Is there anything you want me to bring back for you?"

Queen for a Day Susie sat propped in bed sipping tea while she began ticking off her requests. "Yes, my toothbrush, the blue one in the porcelain mug. And my hairbrush in the top right bathroom drawer. And my chenille bathrobe on the back of the door, and I think my slippers, the fuzzy white ones, are under the bed. There's a chartreuse Polartec, snuggy, zip-up thingy for the baby—bring that 'cause it's so cold, and some diapers and the white elf cap from the home birth kit. And my contacts are on the table beside the bed . . ."

She droned on and on. I looked at Teri standing there like a waitress memorizing the whole order for a party of eight. She nodded and smiled and didn't write anything down or ask Susie to repeat herself. Not even once. Then she turned to leave.

I whispered to her at the doorway, "Can you really remember all that stuff?"

Speaking from the corner of her mouth with a deadpan expression, she muttered, "Shit, no. She's gonna be home within ten minutes of my gettin' back here. Chenille bathrobe, my ass. I'm gonna bring whatever the hell I think she might need to survive a ten-minute ride in a preheated car. Jeezis, chenille bathrobe."

Grinning at her, I said, "Teri, you're invited to all future births I attend. You've got what it takes."

Blushing, she hitched up her denims and shuffled her boots on the linoleum like a shy cowboy confronted by the schoolmarm. She just clouted me on the shoulder and turned to go. As I staggered to regain my balance, I listened to her clattering keys and clomping boots fade away as she strode down the long corridor.

~ *Sneak Attack*

In my years of hospital nursing, I'd encountered many unusual situations, the stuff of which stories are born: a naked husband, several women who acted as if they were in labor when they weren't even pregnant, and identical triplets when everyone expected only one baby. Drunken visitors provided lessons in diplomacy, and a fight between two men, each insisting we list him as the father of the baby, kept us talking for days.

But no pets. Photographs of their four-legged family members, yes, but never the actual furry critter itself. No one had ever insisted on bringing Fido or Fifi or Fluffy along to "share the experience."

Home birth, however, allows everyone to participate. Dogs, cats, gerbils, rabbits, even birds. I once spent the night listening to an insomniac cockatiel converse with a mockingbird in the tree outside an open window. All night the cockatiel mimicked the rambling song of the mockingbird, who in turn did a stunning rendition of a squawking cockatiel. By dawn, I was screeching like a madwoman at both of them.

I've napped while awaiting labor's progress only to awaken at the edge of a narrow guest bed with two cats draped across my feet and a black Labrador retriever snoring in my ear. And no narrow-eyed, challenging doctor ever made me as nervous as Turk. The massive husky sat motionless, guarding his mistress with his eyes fixed on me as I delivered her baby. Those unblinking eyes, that purple tongue, the unwagging tail . . . well, I didn't turn my back on him.

Some new moms presented their newborns for the family dog's seal of approval, hoping that a baptism by the sniff and lick method would guarantee the baby's acceptance.

I usually bonded with the cats. Except for a rare tussle over possession of the placenta, we were cool. But that was before I met Samantha . . .

★   ★   ★

So new that I could still smell the carpet glue, Victoria's tri-level, triple-garaged suburban house hunkered in a sea of mud. She and her husband, Will, moved in months before the landscaping trucks arrived in their subdivision, so a path of 2 x 12 planks stretched across the muck to their front door. At midnight, I darted into a cold February downpour and navigated that narrow walkway, grateful to reach the entry without slipping into the swamp.

I pushed the doorbell and heard an electronic rendition of the opening song from *The Sound of Music.* As I waited for Will to answer, I swallowed hard, remembering . . . Victoria had a cat. Oh, yeah, a really, really big cat.

When I delivered Victoria's first baby, Gillian, in their previous house two years earlier, I had noticed unblinking, predatory eyes glowering at me from beneath a wing-backed chair. "What the hell is that?" I'd blurted.

"That's Samantha," Victoria replied with a fond smile. "A Domestic Calico Longhair. Dear Samantha, sweetheart, pussypussypussy," she crooned at the twenty-five-pounder.

I had my doubts about that pedigree, because five years earlier Victoria had taken one look at the orange, black, and white fur ball at the bottom of a dumpster, pronounced her the sweetest kitty she'd ever seen, and carried her home wrapped in a green sweater. So who's to vouch for the kitty's ancestors?

Midway through our first meeting, I peeled Samantha off my calf and dabbed Kleenex to the claw marks on my leg. I studied her flat face, broad paws, and slitted yellow eyes. Domestic Calico Longhair? I think not, I said to myself. Calico Maine Mountain Lion, more like.

After Samantha sank her claws into me that day, Victoria tossed her outside, but we later figured she must have returned through the cat door. Victoria and I walked down the hall toward her bedroom so I could check her baby's heartbeat and be sure the head was still in the right position. Without a sound, Samantha flew from her perch atop an open door and thudded onto my shoulder with the finality of a grenade. Assuming either warfare or earthquake, I hit the floor with the cat wrapped around my head like a muffler in a March blizzard.

Victoria bent to remove Samantha's claws from my head, face, neck, and shoulder. "Oh, naughty, naughty kitty," Victoria crooned, nuzzling the cat as she shook her finger in front of its insolent face. Samantha looked away.

Oh, that's really going to make a big impression, I figured.

So my thoughts centered on Samantha as I stood in the rain getting colder and wetter. Finally, the door opened and Will let me inside.

"Is Victoria in the back bedroom?"

"Uh-huh. I think she's sleeping, actually," he replied.

"And the cat?" I asked, peeping behind him.

"I haven't seen her all night. Probably went outside when Victoria's mum came to take Gillian away."

So I relaxed and thought about Victoria, whose first baby had exhausted all of us in her struggles to be born. Forty hours of electric shock therapy, Victoria said, would have been easier than that labor. Now, as I slipped into the dim bedroom, I remembered her histrionics of two years ago and decided she'd probably called me way, way too early this time. She lay curled on her side with a stuffed teddy bear under her chin, breathing like a napping toddler, eyes closed, cheeks pink, hair matted, skin sweaty . . .

Wait a minute. Hair matted? Skin sweaty?

Women in early labor usually act social between the pains and breathe quietly during them. But when they shift into the high gear of late labor, they tend to reverse that ratio. They look comatose between the contractions and go ballistic during them. Victoria looked comatose. And the matted hair and sweaty skin made me study her more closely. The smell of the hard work of birth hung heavy in the air—a feral smell of sweat and urine, the salty, bleachy smell of amniotic fluid, the charged air dense with . . .

Victoria gave a cosmic howl as she flung her teddy bear across the room, scaring the bejeezus out of me. She lurched upright, vaulted out of bed, and crouched on the carpet beside me. Unleashing another roar, her whole body convulsed into a push.

I yanked open my tackle box, pulled out my supplies, and dropped to the floor beside her. Barely getting a glove on one hand, I cupped the top of her son's head in my palm. Victoria let loose another yell, and the rest of the baby's head filled my hand.

At that moment, Samantha's shaggy head loomed off to my right. I thought of my legs exposed beneath my denim skirt just nanoseconds before she sank ten claws and God knows how many piranha teeth into my thigh. I should have known. Where does a bodyguard cat station herself? Under the bed, of course. All the better to bite you, my dear.

"Aagh!" I yelled.

"Aagh!" yelled Victoria, working at getting her baby's shoulders out.

"Cat! Cat!" I gasped, trying to concentrate on the baby but more interested, really, in coming up with a creative way to annihilate a Domestic Calico Longhair.

Will peeled Samantha off my leg, and I shouted, "Lock her up."

Victoria screamed again and distracted Will from his mission. He dropped Samantha with a thud and turned to his wife. The cat leaped and landed on my back, holding on with all four feet. She lost her grip and dug her claws in harder.

"Aagh!" I screamed again.

"Aagh!" screamed Victoria, and an eleven-pound boy child slid into my hands. I let the baby glide to the rug as soon as I saw him crying and flapping around.

I must have resembled a wild woman attacked by killer bees, swatting, spinning, smacking. But I couldn't get Samantha off. Desperate, I flopped on my back and smashed her to the floor beneath me, and I didn't get up till I heard something from her that sounded like, "Aagh!"

Victoria hunkered on the carpet with her gigantic son in her arms and looked at Samantha, who lay spread-eagled on the rug like a pelt pinned to the wall of a trapper's cabin.

"Oh, Sammysammy, pussy cat, sweetums kittykitty. Were you scared?"

Samantha didn't answer. Will looked catatonic, transfixed by the image of his wife and his huge, roly-poly son. He didn't even glance at the cat. I sighed and dabbed droplets of blood from my shoulder with a gauze square.

Victoria needed some stitches. I unwound the suturing thread and gripped the large, curved needle with a toothed clamp. The shiny, silver instrument glittered, sending points of light darting around the room.

Samantha lay still for quite a while. Then she rolled over, shook her monstrous head, and hauled her massive body to her feet. I kept my eye on her. All too soon, she laid her ears back and lowered her belly to the rug like a tiger in the bushes before it springs on a hapless antelope. Her rear end wiggled; she dug in those hind feet, preparing for another charge.

I spun around and, snarling in my best imitation of the MGM lion, waved the big curved needle in her face.

Samantha stopped. That must have been the biggest claw she'd ever seen in her life. Her ears came forward and she sat up. She looked away, studying a blank wall with rapt concentration. Then she began washing her face. For the first time, I felt safe in that house. I didn't know how long the feeling would last, but it was sweet, very sweet.

Two days later I wore thick Levi's and a heavy sweatshirt when I returned for a postpartum visit. The surface of the mud puddles had crusted over, so the trip across the planking didn't feel nearly as risky as it had two nights earlier. I paused at the front door.

The cat. Sweetums kittykitty Samantha. How much would she remember?

The chimes played "The hills are alive . . ." and Will opened the door. For what I hoped would be the last time, I walked down that long hallway to the bedroom, checking the top of each open door. Victoria lay in the king-sized bed, nursing her fat-cheeked son. Samantha, the tip of her tail twitching, sat on a down comforter at Victoria's feet, puffed out and alert. The cat and I locked eyes.

She blinked first. So far, so good.

I knelt at the bedside. No way was I going to sit on the edge of the bed with my back to that animal—my back which had just begun to scab over. I began examining Victoria. Then I heard a low rumble, like a threshing machine way out in the back forty, and I saw Samantha crouch and start her rump-wiggling rumba again.

I spun around and raised both hands with my fingers curved into claws.

"Oh, good kitty, poor kittykittykitty," crooned Victoria.

Ignoring her and the damage I might cause to our future professional relationship, I mustered a throaty growl and lunged toward Samantha. Her eyes grew huge, and, glory hallelujah, she launched herself off the end of the bed and bolted down the hall, her powerful hind legs churning the nap of the pale blue carpeting.

I almost felt sorry to see the proud and mighty animal so humbled.

Almost, but not quite.

～ *Uh-oh*

I knew Rachel's weariness when labor started didn't bode well for the outcome, and I was concerned. I always felt pessimistic when women were already exhausted at the onset of labor. A fatigued mother often has a fatigued uterus, and a fatigued uterus doesn't contract well.

Single by choice, pregnant by design, and wealthy by bequest, Rachel had bought a new house high in the Berkeley hills. Just two days after the moving van unloaded all her belongings and two weeks before her due date, labor caught her flat-footed.

"Shit!" she raged at me on the phone. "How dare this baby come early? I'm not even slightly ready. I need at least another week. I can't even walk around in this place. What can I do to stop these friggin' pains?"

"Rachel, if it's the real thing, you can't stop it. Drink a quart of water and lie down. If it's false labor, it'll probably go away."

"Forget resting. I've got too damn much work to do."

She called again at midnight. "Shit, shit, shit! I'm so pissed. All day these contractions stayed ten minutes apart. Annoying, you know? Like, shit or get off the pot. So I worked like hell and got the bedroom organized, but now when I'm exhausted, what happens? *Now* it kicks in. *Now* the bloody show comes. Oy, vey! Just bloody, goddamn great."

An earthy, profane woman at the best of times, Rachel had found a worthy target on which to aim her stash of colorful obscenities. Royally irritated, she would need patience and stamina to get through the night, and both were in short supply.

I stifled a yawn. "How close are the contractions?"

"Pretty damn steady at four to five minutes," she snarled. "Close enough to bug me and not far enough apart to let me rest. Just fuckin' ducky! But don't come yet. My friend Pru's here."

I slept all night. As sunlight streamed through the window, I checked my clock. 7:15 A.M. I couldn't believe she hadn't called back. At nine, I risked a phone call, praying I wouldn't awaken her. Pru answered, and I asked what was happening.

"The pains drove her nuts, and her swearing drove me nuts. We're both beat."

"Rats," I muttered. Worst case scenario: a tired uterus and no end in sight.

"I'll come check her," I said. "Maybe you can sleep a while."

"Not here. This place is a battlefield."

"Oh, I'm sure I've seen worse."

But that was before I saw it.

I parked on the narrow street made bumpy by decades of earthquake tremors that caused the concrete to buckle like the shifting plates of the earth itself. I walked through a gate in a stucco wall and stepped into an English cottage garden. Birds scolded a squirrel mounting an attack on the birdfeeder, and San Francisco Bay glittered in the background.

But all sense of peace and tranquility ended when, at my knock, Pru opened the front door. Stacked everywhere and towering toward the ceiling, boxes and packing crates transformed the house into a stalagmite-filled cavern.

"Do you believe this place?" Pru asked. With one hand, she held her straight, dark hair in a loose knot behind her neck. Tai chi exercise pants hung from her narrow hips, and she stretched left, then right, working out the kinks of a restless night. Wide silver rings encircled three of her bare toes.

I shook my head in amazement as I wandered through the bungalow. Pots and pans vied for space with cutlery, noodles, and spices on the cluttered counters. Coffee beans crunched underfoot. The living room looked like the Grand Canyon with cardboard buttes and mesas. Costco boxes filled the bathtub, and one bedroom was impassable.

But Rachel had decorated her own bedroom in cool, muted colors and organized it to serene perfection. A gray cat stared at me from a rocking chair. With scabs still fresh from Samantha's assault, I eyed her. She stretched her front legs, curled up again, and began purring.

I sighed in relief on two counts. No attack cat here, and at least Rachel had one well-organized space in which to labor.

"But where the heck is Rachel?" I asked.

Pru pointed toward a stack of crates at the end of the living room and said, "She's back there. I'm going home for a nap."

I found Rachel snoozing in a narrow space bordered by the fireplace wall and eight feet of teetering boxes. Her brown hair lay in ringlets against her freckled shoulders, and her foxy little face was relaxed in sleep. She wore a Depends diaper to deal with the bloody show and a jog bra to deal with her abundant bosom.

She woke up cursing. "Goddammit, why won't this baby cooperate? She must think I'm some *bubbe* with lotsa time for her lazy style. Oh. When did you get here?"

"Ten minutes ago. Boy, this place is a mess. Why not use your bedroom?"

"Mmm, I dunno. I like it better out here."

I shrugged and checked her cervix. Only four centimeters.

"Hell, it's like, what? Over twenty-four hours already? Fergeddit. I can't do this."

Dehydration is inevitable in a long, debilitating labor, so I forced nearly a quart of water into her and got her walking. Nipple stimulation usually brings contractions closer and stronger, but with Rachel, it required constant attention to keep them that way. Whenever I slacked off, so did her labor. She soon growled and pushed my hand away.

Morning became afternoon. Pru, her hair still wet and smelling of hibiscus shampoo, returned with bags of groceries. She stocked the refrigerator and filled the cat dish. Afternoon became evening. I napped, and when I awoke around seven P.M. I checked Rachel again. Just six centimeters. Since she faced another sleepless night, I broke her bag of water in hopes of speeding things up.

Many times she wandered to the bedroom door, but something stopped her on the threshold. She stood in the hallway swinging from the doorframe, then shook her head and walked back to the jumbled living room.

Thirty-six hours down. "Jeezus, when is this friggin' kid comin' out? I'll never make it. Thirty-six hours is about thirty more than I expected. My sisters all had fast labors. What's wrong with me? I deserve a fucking break. How much longer?"

"Don't know," I said. "Sometime tomorrow. The baby's heartbeat sounds perfect, the water's clear, and you're progressing. It's slow, but your biggest enemy is fatigue."

"And attitude," Pru sighed. "You need a major attitude adjustment, girlfriend. I've never heard anyone kvetch and piss and moan so much."

"Well, dammit, Pru, anybody would."

"No, don't go sayin' that," said Pru, shaking her head. "I've been with eight other women in labor, and you take the cake. Keee-RIST, what a princess you are."

Uh-oh, I thought. Cat fight alert. I wouldn't have dared confront Rachel in such blunt terms, but Pru had no problem laying it out. I expected Rachel to lash back, but instead, she laughed and stood up.

"Shit, you'd think I'd get a little more sympathy, but noooooo. The nerve, complaining about my attitude. I'll show you attitude, girlfriend."

She bent over and mooned us.

But the laughter and energy created by that exchange lasted only an hour, and by midnight Rachel looked near collapse. I suggested she go to bed for a while, and Pru said, "Yeah, what've you got against that room, anyway?"

She shrugged and said, "It doesn't feel right," as she slumped into her favorite space between the boxes.

Labor dragged on all night. Exhausting, slow progress, poor quality contractions, low energy. The works. All stacked up, it translated into a miserable experience, and Rachel complained and moaned throughout. I checked her at six A.M. "You're seven centimeters."

"Fuck!" declared Rachel. I had to agree.

Margaret, my assistant, arrived a little later, bringing fresh energy. She dragged a drooping Rachel up and down stairs, poured more juice and water into her, and started nipple stimulation again. I dribbled my nasty-tasting herbal remedies under Rachel's tongue, but nothing had a lasting effect. I even started an IV to hydrate her, but I couldn't see that it helped much.

We hunched shoulder to shoulder in that living room, four of us in a space so tight it felt as if we were trying out for a coffin-fitting. Rachel occasionally strolled into the garden, but all too soon she slunk back into her funky cave. Against all odds, she finally reached full dilation at noon.

But would she push? Not a chance. She wanted the contractions to do it all.

I coaxed and cajoled and berated and pleaded and begged and praised and sympathized and threatened and swore. Two hours passed. Three hours. The sixty-hour total labor mark loomed ahead, and she'd had no more than two hours of poor-quality sleep. Fortunately, the baby's heartbeat chugged along like The Little Engine That Could.

With each contraction, Rachel moaned into wimpy little pushes that produced nothing. But after nearly four hours, in spite of the lazy pushing, the baby's head began to show. "Dammit, Rachel, come on," I said. "I can *see* the baby. Push her out!"

She glared at me and went, "Umph," and that was the end of that push.

Then, out of the blue, she took a deep breath, held it, and pushed like a champ. "Sssssss ... Hunph ... Omigod ... Hunph! *Jeezis!*" The head surged all the way to her perineum and bulged half out. More progress than in the previous two hours.

"Great!" I shouted. "Five more like that, and you'll be finished. You go, girl!"

Another contraction began. Rachel went "Umph," and said, "That's one."

"Oh, hell," I said, rolling my eyes at Margaret. I'd said the wrong thing. "Rachel," I bellowed. "I said five more 'like that!' Not just any old five pushes. Five good ones."

"Tough titties," she snarled, and fell asleep.

Sixty minutes, fifteen contractions, and countless cuss words later, a baby girl oozed out.

Rachel glanced at the pretty baby on her chest. She yawned and closed her eyes while I delivered the placenta and took a few stitches. Rachel didn't say a word, nor did she make any attempt to cuddle the baby, a gesture that comes instinctively to most women. Alarm bells sounded in my head. She hadn't given much thought to the baby during labor, and after the arduous birth, it didn't look like her attitude had changed.

Margaret tidied up the umbilical cord and swaddled the little girl. "She's lovely, Rachel. Look at her fingers, so perfect."

"Mmm," murmured Rachel, looking out the window. Then she faced me with a flat expression and said, "Finished?"

"Yep. All done. Isn't the baby beautiful?"

"Keep an eye on her, will you? I'm gonna take a nap."

To our utter amazement, she stood up, toddled into her pristine bedroom, spread a Chux on the clean white sheet, lay down, and fell asleep. Margaret and I stared at each other, too shocked to speak. Appalled, Pru just shook her head.

What about bonding? Was Rachel a classic example of a mother rejecting her newborn? No interest in nursing the baby or inspecting the shell-like curves of her ear, the wrinkles on the bottoms of her feet, the way her eyelashes were so long that they stuck to her cheeks when she closed her eyes? If they didn't spend these next few hours together, would Rachel learn to love this baby she'd labored so long to bring into the world?

Pru did a load of laundry, peeked into the bedroom where Rachel snored away, and then left, frowning. Margaret and I fixed tomato soup and a salad for dinner, making sure there'd be enough for Rachel, if she ever woke up. Margaret tore hunks from a crusty loaf of French bread and spread Cambozola on top for me. The baby lay on my lap as I ate. I let her suck my pinkie, and she didn't seem to notice that her tummy stayed empty in spite of her vigorous sucking.

The sun set, and the sky behind the San Francisco skyline lit up with all the rosy purple, magenta, and orange hues for which sunsets are so famous. I began to think we'd have to waken Rachel so we could leave, but three hours after she'd passed out like a drunk, I heard the floorboards squeak. She walked into the kitchen.

She glanced once at the baby on my lap and then looked at the table with avid interest. She went to the refrigerator and removed a bowl of grapes, some deli ham, three bottles of Anchor Steam beer, and a cheesecake that Margaret and I had overlooked.

"I'm fuckin' starving," Rachel said. She devoured the soup and salad, half a baguette piled with ham and cheese, several handfuls of green grapes, a beer, and two pieces of cheesecake. Then she sat back like Henry VIII and patted her stomach.

"I know why I didn't want to go in that room before. I was saving it for afterwards. And it was awesome to just sleep, knowing the baby was taken care of.

"Now," she said, stretching out her arms. "Let me see this little pain in the ass."

I handed the peaceful baby to Rachel. Slowly she unwrapped the layers of blankets and began an inch by inch inspection of her daughter. We didn't speak as Rachel finally did all the things most new mothers do right after the birth.

"Check out these toes." Rachel whispered. "What a pretty face you have, girlie-girlie, and what delicate fingers. Maybe you'll play the piano like your gramma did."

The baby grasped Rachel's finger and held on with a monkey grip as her mother ran the back of her hand across a downy cheek. "Oh, God, her skin is so yummy." She picked her up and buried her nose in her daughter's neck, crooning, "Oooh, she's even better than cheesecake, and I never thought I'd say that."

Margaret and I had been praying for this, hoping it wasn't too late for the magic to occur, the magic of falling in love. We smiled at each other and went home.

～ A Friend

"How far along is your noisy patient in there?" asked Dr. Rider. He frowned and jerked his head toward Room 2 where Latoya sat cross-legged on her bed. We could hear her from the nursing station. She hummed a gospel tune between her contractions and moaned "Ow-ow-ow!" during the peaks.

"About seven," I answered, then wanted to kick myself. Why did I answer this guy? A week earlier he'd buttonholed me on a quiet corridor and asked me how many women I delivered each month and how much money I made. I answered his first question and almost answered the second. "It's none of your damn business," was what I wanted to say, but I just bit my lip as he spoke again.

"Jesus, what's with you midwives that you never medicate your patients? Is it some kind of ritual female bonding? Something about suffering?"

Oh, boy. "Look, she knows drugs are available. She's figured out her own method of handling labor, and it's working. If she's bothering your patient, I'll close her door."

I saw Holly and Rita, two nurses, shaking their heads to tell me my patient's sounds weren't disturbing anyone except Dr. Rider. But I already knew what was really bothering the doctor. Me.

There were just three of us midwives, Sandi and Lindy, and I—and about fifty obstetricians. Unspoken issues hovered beneath the surface of nearly every interaction we had with each other.

Doctors looked stunned, incredulous when pregnant nurses bypassed their services and chose instead a home birth with a midwife. Dr. Rider confronted Cherie, pregnant with her first child, and demanded, "How can you consider having your baby at home when you work here and see all that goes on?"

Without missing a beat, Cherie answered, "That's the point. It's because I see what happens in hospitals that I'm having my baby at home."

Doctors were naturally resentful if women already under their care switched practitioners late in pregnancy. Mailing the prenatal records to one of us confirmed the fact that they'd been rejected in favor of a midwife. We had a very low rate of complications, and lowest of all for our home birth clients. I once overheard Irene, the nurse in charge of the unit that day, say to Dr. Rider, "Do you realize that women who see our midwives have cesareans a third less often than women who are cared for by the obstetricians?"

Some of the doctors clearly resented our popularity and our success, but money was the bottom line, the issue always simmering on the back burner of every discussion between midwives and doctors. I charged less than the doctors, I did only half of their volume each month, and I didn't perform surgery. But the doctors knew I made good money. This realization festered with many of them, like a splinter under the skin. Midwifery practice had been forced upon them; they had to deal with us, but they didn't have to like it. Some showed their displeasure more than others. Like Dr. Rider.

I heard Latoya's "Ow-ow-ow" start up again.

"Aw, hell, just give her a shot. She's only seventeen, right?" It's a good thing he didn't wait for my answer, because I seethed with outrage. The only way he could have known her age was by reading her chart, which was a violation of patient confidentiality.

"She's just a little welfare kid," he continued. "Unmarried, no doubt, and you're torturing her. I can't figure out why, unless it's your precious statistics."

Oh man, I thought, he's really taking this to a new level. I had calculated the statistics for my first five hundred deliveries and shared the results with the nurses. One of them copied the report and posted it on the coffee room cork-board. Three days later, a nurse saw Dr. Rider bending forward with his head tipped back to peer at it through his bifocals. She said, "Then he ripped it off and threw it away."

Muttering, "I'll close her door," I walked stiffly toward Room 2, but I felt his eyes on my back. I hadn't liked him when I worked as a staff nurse, and I liked him even less now, but it wouldn't do to sink to his level of sniping.

I entered Latoya's room, pushed the door closed, and took a deep breath. She had a girlfriend with her, another teenager who'd had a baby before fin-ishing high school. The diaper-clad tot rode on her mother's hip, big eyes round and solemn. I didn't credit the girlfriend with helping Latoya much. I hadn't seen her interacting in any way—no back-rubbing, no cold washcloths, no hand-holding. Nothing except occasional sarcastic comments about the hospital, boys, or life in general. She paced back and forth across the room, chewing gum with her mouth open, bouncing her daughter on her hip till the colorful plastic barrettes at the ends of her cornrows jiggled and danced.

I studied Latoya. She sat cross-legged on the bed, fingertips barely touching her naked belly as she traced tiny circles over the surface. Eyes closed, she rocked and hummed a churchy-sounding melody. A contraction began, and her rocking sped up. She tried to keep up the circle tracing and humming, but soon the pain grew too intense. She braced herself with her fists on the mattress, threw her head back, and began the moaning howl that had attracted Dr. Rider's attention.

"Ow-ow-ow. Oh, lordy. Ow-ow, sweet Jesus, my strength," She sobbed once or twice, wiped a single tear from her cheek, and began to relax.

"Whachu close that door for?" barked her friend, standing still and glaring at me from beneath heavy eyebrows.

I jerked my attention from Latoya and looked at this other girl. Her hard face scowled, and it didn't look as if she spent much time smiling. Skin-tight denim shorts stretched over her high, proud rear end, and a cut-off T-shirt revealed an inked tattoo on her belly, a home job. From where I stood it looked like a spider. Worn-down-at-the-heel rubber thongs slapped on the linoleum as she paced. But now she stood still, fixing me with an unfriendly stare.

"Huh? Whachu shut the door for?"

She had me. I didn't want to make it sound like a judgment of Latoya's sounds or behavior. As I stalled for time, Latoya opened her eyes and looked from me to the door.

"Am I makin' too much noise? Is somebody complainin'? It hurts so much, and it helps a lot to do what I'm doin'. Lordy, it's all I can do to keep from screaming."

Maybe Dr. Rider was right, I thought. Maybe I should medicate her. I watched her rock into another contraction and try to be quieter, "mmm, mmm . . ." but the tears streamed down her cheeks. She hummed louder, biting her lips, but it didn't work. As her tears flowed, I wrestled with my philosophy.

I felt that offering drugs to a laboring woman sent a message that she wasn't handling labor well, and I didn't want to impose those feelings onto her. Besides, any woman who has her baby in the hospital certainly knows narcotics are in some triple-locked cupboard at the end of a hallway. With first-timers, I sometimes made a little speech at the halfway point of labor. It went like this: "You're four centimeters, and you can have something for pain at any point from now on. But I'm not going to offer it again or pressure you one way or another. It's your business, and you can deal with it any way you want."

So, although I felt Latoya was doing great, I wondered if I should give my speech. Maybe she needed to be older to understand all this, especially since her friend didn't seem to be helping.

I wiped Latoya's face. I cupped her cheek in my palm, her cheek all damp with sweat and tears, hot with the hard work of labor, and I said, "Latoya, I shut the door because there's a doctor out there who thinks the sounds you're making mean you're in too much pain. He got mad at me for not giving you drugs, so I want you to know you can have a shot if you want one."

From the corner of my eye, I saw her friend freeze. I looked at her and saw her angry scowl. She snorted and then kicked the metal bedside table with her thong, kicked it hard enough to slosh the water in the plastic pitcher.

"Toya, what I be tellin' you, girl? 'Bout them doctors? You hearin' this woman tell you what that doctor wants to do?"

"Uh-huh," Latoya mumbled. "Mmm-hmm, I hear you," and she waved her hand to hush up her friend. She raised her shy eyes to mine and said, "Do I have to have something? Am I doing it all wrong? That why you wantin' to give me shots?"

Oh, damn, damn, damn, I said to myself, this is just what I wanted to avoid. Exactly what I feared she'd think. "No, honey. You're doing beautifully, just fine."

Her friend interrupted, kicking the stand even harder.

"Sheeee-it! That's all them doctors want to do. They just wants to shoot us women up with drugs and keep us quiet. Drugs. Drugs is a big part of what's wrong with my neighborhood. Sheee-it, Toya, if everything be normal, you don't need no drugs, girl. No, sir. That ain't no way to start out your baby, high on dope before he take his first breath. And being a mother is hard." She paused, blew a bubble with her wad of pink gum and popped it loudly for emphasis, then hiked her baby over to her other hip. "Yeah, being a mother is hard work, and taking drugs when you be birthin' that baby ain't no preparation for being a good mother. I did it on my own, and Toya, you can do it, too, girl. Ya hear?"

Dumbfounded, I stared at this hard-edged, smart-mouthed, street-wise, young toughie. She might not be a back-rubbing, hand-holding kind of friend, but just by her presence, she gave Latoya courage and faith and self-confidence to have her baby naturally. I, a white professional, a middle-aged authority figure, never could have given her that kind of support.

But I could easily do all the other stuff. I climbed onto the bed and sat cross-legged in front of Latoya. When the next contraction came, I held her body against mine and whispered into her ear. "It's okay, Toya, hum with me. That's it, as loud as you want, honey. Pull your voice down low, keep it low, low. Uh-huh. Good girl."

"Other women make lotsa noise, too?" she asked.

Her friend spun in a circle and guffawed toward the ceiling, "Ho! Noise? Girl, you shoulda heard me. I was *yellin'* . . . mmm-mmm!" laughed her friend. It was the only time I saw her grin.

"Really? It's okay?" persisted Latoya.

"You bet," I assured her.

When the next contraction began, she clutched me and howled again. I stayed there on the bed, and pretty soon she crawled right into my lap. Facing me, she straddled my body with her legs like a koala on a eucalyptus tree, wrapping her arms around me and pressing her head to my shoulder. Her sweat soaked into the front of my scrubs, and I smelled the sweet, flowery scent of hair gel in her tight braids.

Her friend stopped her pacing and sat in the vinyl armchair, settled her baby into her lap, and lifted her crop-top to expose a full breast. The little girl scrunched down and wiggled her body like a happy puppy as she nursed, keeping her eyes on her mother's sober face.

It wasn't long before I felt Latoya's body heave and curl forward. Her breath caught in her throat with a ragged, strangling sound. If I hadn't seen and heard it thousands of times, I'd have thought she was about to be sick to her stomach. In my childbirth classes, I often compared pushing to vomiting, saying, "It's a little like vomiting, but in reverse. Instead of throwing up, you throw down."

Latoya's body began "throwing down" with vigor.

In my experience, young girls occasionally have difficult labors, but usually they go very fast. There doesn't seem to be a middle ground. Latoya went fast.

She hurled herself into pushing with a vengeance, gripping me so hard I thought she wouldn't let go to allow me to deliver her baby. As a contraction ended, I scrambled out of her arms and rang the bedside call bell to summon help—a nurse, birth equipment, the baby-warming cart, the works.

Latoya flung herself onto her back and gripped her ankles, looking like a primitive Inca statue, a fertility goddess. With each contraction she groaned and pushed so hard it looked as if she'd explode. Her friend plonked her daughter on the bed next to Latoya's pillow and stationed herself beside

Latoya. Finally, finally, she touched her. She grabbed Latoya's flailing hand and pressed it to her chest. With her other hand she made a fist and held it up in a Black Power gesture. She growled, "Be strong, girl. Be strong and fight them pains. You can do it."

Latoya nodded and pushed again. In no time she cuddled a little baby boy in her arms.

Five minutes later, before I finished putting a few stitches into a small laceration, before the placenta even came out, the girlfriend slung a blanket around her baby and said, "Okay, sister, I'm outta here. I be seein' you tomorrow after you git yo' ass home."

Bang! went the door. She was gone.

Latoya touched her baby's downy hair, pulling out the soft curls and smiling as they sprang back close to his head. She tilted her chin to line her face up with his and grinned even more when his random hand movements brought his fingers to her lips. She opened her mouth and sucked in his whole hand and then laughed as he pulled away.

"You gonna be Shanda's baby's boyfriend?" she whispered.

"Your friend, her name's Shanda?" I asked.

"Mmm-hmm, she my best friend. She told me all about labor and babies and nursin' and stuff. I don't know what I'd have done without her. I just know I wouldn't have been able to get through this day myself. She helped me so much."

"How do you feel now, Latoya, now that it's all over?" I asked as I took the last stitch and snipped the suture.

Those shy eyes came up and met mine with a new confidence, and I wished Dr. Rider had heard her soft answer.

"Proud. I feel proud. Yes, I do."

What Flowers Are These?

I walked into the crowded waiting room to call my next client. Bougainvillea blossoms pressing against the windows cast a purplish-rosy glow over the interior of the office, adding a surprising sunset quality to the mid-morning light.

One woman stood out from the others. Her belly looked as if she carried triplets, and she didn't look well. But even with the sallow skin and gaunt face, her composure reminded me of Mona Lisa's beauty. I guessed her age at about forty, but it was hard to tell.

She wore an old-fashioned, pale blue maternity smock, pathetically inadequate to cover her massive abdomen. The other women sat with open magazines resting on their average-sized bellies and tried not to stare at the quiet woman in the end chair. Eyes closed, she nodded slowly in response to the younger man whispering in her ear. He held her thin hand in his, but his Father Confessor demeanor convinced me he wasn't her husband or lover. I watched as he referred now and then to a passage in a small bound book that rested open on his knee. Worn and well thumbed, it looked like a priest's breviary.

"Patricia?" I called.

She opened her eyes and looked at me a moment, seeming to pull her thoughts from far away. Her first attempt to rise from the deep upholstered chair met with failure as the mass of her belly forced her back into the depths of cushions. The young man stood and helped her to her feet. Others in the waiting room watched her from beneath politely lowered eyelids. In spite of her huge abdomen, she moved in a long, loose-limbed stride, full of surprising grace. She walked as if she were floating, and her arms swung like a ballet dancer's, thin with tendons showing. The man stayed behind, and before I closed the office door, I saw him open his red leather book to a ribbon marker.

Patricia chose a straight-backed chair in the consulting room and tried without success to pull her smock over her exposed belly. She sat twisting her loose wedding ring, offered a cautious smile, and said nothing.

I introduced myself and opened a new chart. Patricia's husband's call that morning had been vague, so I had very little to go on.

"My wife is about to enter a facility," he'd said, "and, because of her appearance, they require verification that she's not pregnant before they'll admit her."

Thinking back on that ambiguous statement, the germ of a fear, still just a suspicion, began growing in my mind. Something was wrong with this whole picture. I realized that on some level I'd prepared myself for a grossly obese woman who wanted to enter a health spa. But this tall, thin woman before me occupied a league of her own. In more than twenty years of examining pregnant women, I'd never seen such a huge abdomen—and her husband said she wasn't pregnant. So why was she coming to me, a midwife?

I began filling in the blanks in the chart. Address, phone number, birth date. I calculated. She was thirty-eight years old. "Number of previous pregnancies?"

"None," she answered in a sad little voice. "Tim and I never had children, and when my monthly cycles stopped two years ago, we assumed I'd started the change."

She stopped menstruating at age thirty-six? More alarm bells.

I glanced at the next blank on the chart and hesitated. I needed time to compose myself for what I feared lay ahead. Her answer would tell me if my hunch was on target, but I stalled a moment. "That's pretty young to stop menstruating. Did you see a doctor?"

Pen held above the chart, I forced myself to look right into her serene face.

"No, I didn't," she answered with a steady gaze.

And the penny dropped. I could think of only one group of women who wouldn't seek a doctor's opinion under such circumstances. Only one answer that would make sense. I lowered my pen to the Religion line.

"Are you a Christian Scientist?"

"Yes, we both are."

And I knew she was dying.

Her grossly distended abdomen announced a belly full of tumors and fluid. Her pale skin with the underlying yellow tints spoke of liver or kidney metastases. Her wasted limbs revealed her body's final effort to survive by consuming itself. Cancer. Liver? Colon? Ovarian? I had no idea, but definitely cancer, and widespread.

Her avoidance of medical language, a reluctance to discuss the physical aspects of her condition, and the absence of medical care were all giveaways, clues I'd learned to look for from my many Christian Science clients. And sitting here before me was another one, only I wouldn't be presenting her with my usual parting gift of a downy little baby wrapped in soft receiving blankets.

She might be at peace with her condition, but I found myself battling images of all the gifts of life I would have wanted in her situation, time being the greatest. Time to heal, to love an adopted child perhaps. Time to hold the mast of a sailboat and feel the wind in her face, to express her heart through modern dance. Time to climb toward the daffodils of spring on a distant hillside, time at least to try.

I knew she didn't have much time left, and I tried to keep my knowledge from showing, but when I raised my eyes, I saw that she knew. The corners of her mouth turned up in a smile that felt like a blessing, letting me know that death held no fear for her.

"Is that your practitioner in the waiting room, or your husband?" I asked.

Her smile rose a notch, and she relaxed, seeing I wasn't going to criticize her faith or the choices she'd made.

"My husband's at work. And yes, that's my practitioner. He suggested we call you. You delivered a woman from our church, and she told him you didn't insist on all the medical procedures and tests. He thought you'd be able to give me something in writing so I can go into Arden Wood for a while." It was the most she'd said all at once, and the effort exhausted her. She tried to take a deep breath but had to lean back so her chest could expand. I watched as she closed her eyes, gasping.

Arden Wood is a large Christian Science hospital where members of the church can go for prayer, loving care, support, and help achieving a dignified death when the time comes. They used to deliver babies in such places around the country, but stopped a number of years ago due to pressure from the medical community around legal and licencing issues.

"Do you think you could be pregnant, Patricia?"

"No, I'm quite sure I'm not, but the hospital needs a letter, something in writing to protect them legally." Again she struggled for breath. A magenta sunbeam reflected off the golden clasp holding her hair.

"Are you in pain?" I asked.

"No, I just have a few digestive problems that started about three weeks ago, and I've been somewhat short of breath."

A few digestive problems? No doubt more than a few, I thought, imagining the cancer cells coiling around her internal organs, destroying her from the inside out.

"Okay, let me check you. I'm sure I can help."

While she undressed, I waited in the hallway with my back against the wall, staring at the ceiling. Thirty-eight years old. Midwives' patients aren't supposed to die at thirty-eight. Midwifery is a happy, life-affirming profession, by definition dealing only with the normal. And it's not normal for thirty-eight-year-old women to die.

When I entered the exam room, she sat on the table with her head turned toward the window, overgrown with bougainvillea vines. She stared at the brilliant crimson blossoms throughout the physical examination. Propping her with pillows to enable her to recline, I palpated her belly, so swollen it seemed transparent around her belly button where the skin stretched taut and silvery. Everything felt tight, so rigid I couldn't even indent the surface with my fingertips, much less feel deeply for the outline of perhaps a long-dead baby—or a large tumor.

"What beautiful flowers," she murmured, stretching her hand toward the purple sunbeams.

I picked up my audio Doppler stethoscope and listened everywhere. Nothing came back except the deep, regular, thrumming kawumph - - - - kawumph - - - - kawumph of her own aorta. Slow, about 80 beats a minute. No quick, euphoric, dancing pace of a baby's heartbeat, that rapid pocketa-pocketa-pocketa, the joyful rhythm that always makes me smile. I listened everywhere. No baby.

When I examined her internally, I first used a speculum but couldn't see the borders of her cervix because pink clusters of flower-like tumors filled the vaginal canal. I felt inside her body with my hand, but I was lost. I couldn't define any landmarks. It was like searching for a cotton ball in the middle of a bowl of pebbles and whipped cream. I removed my hand and stared at the sacs of bloody tissue filling my palm.

"Patricia, have you been bleeding much?" I asked, trying to hide my dismay. Not even forty yet. Maybe she could have been saved. But now? My image of her on the sailboat heading for the open sea would remain a fantasy.

"Just a little now and then, although it's been more in the last few days."

"What about after sex?" I asked.

"We haven't done that in a long time," she replied, still looking across her shoulder toward the glowing window, shafts of pink illuminating the visible vein network in her abdomen. "I think it's been over six months since we, well, you know." She paused and looked toward the rosy light. "What flowers are these?"

"Bougainvillea," I answered. "They're beautiful, aren't they? Bougainvillea."

But it seemed the saddest word I'd ever spoken.

After she dressed, I called her practitioner into the examining room, and I told them that while I didn't believe she was pregnant, neither could I rule out a dead baby, maybe two.

"I'd like you to have an ultrasound exam, just to be sure. It can be done right away, and you'll have your verification within a couple of hours."

Patricia spoke briefly, "I want to do whatever will make you feel comfortable." Then she began coughing and waved her hand for the earnest man at her side to carry on.

"Yes, Patricia and I want to thank you for seeing her so quickly and for being so understanding. If you would feel better having the—what did you call it?"

"Ultrasound," I repeated. "It's painless and shows what's inside."

"Yes, ultrasound. If you feel it's necessary, then of course we agree. We'll do whatever is required. I'm sure you understand."

I did understand. I had cared for enough Christian Scientists to know that most of them wanted nothing more from me than attendance at their birth. Most refused blood tests for genetic defects, and none took vitamins or iron. But they always tried to avoid legal issues or negative publicity.

Patricia's practitioner knew that while I might disagree with her decision to use only prayer to treat her illness, I would not force my opinion on her. They trusted me not to shame or censure her. However, they didn't want to put me in a position where some DA or medical examiner could point a finger and accuse me of failure to follow minimal obstetrical guidelines. Patricia would do what I asked.

They left for the radiology department with instructions to return after the procedure. I examined several other women but found it difficult to concentrate on their discomforts and complaints of heartburn, fatigue, and puffy ankles. Part of me wanted to scream, "Did you see that woman who just walked out of here? Her only complaint is a little indigestion and shortness of breath. She knows she's going to die, while you're going to have a baby, despite your backache and difficulty sleeping." I struggled not to let my impatience show, realizing that my own sadness colored my reactions. Patricia seemed at peace. But I wasn't.

The phone rang. "This patient, this Patricia Adams?" said the radiology tech. "Can you give us a little more information?" He sounded shocked and spoke in a voice you'd use in church.

"I'm sorry, I should have warned you, but I couldn't say much in front of her."

"But she's . . . well, it's just that we've never seen anything like this before."

"I know."

"You're a midwife, right? So, who's her doctor? Who's been taking care of her—or rather, *not* taking care of her? Because she's . . ." His voice rose toward accusation, judgment, anger.

"Wait. It's not what you think. It was her choice. She's a Christian Scientist, and she just needs proof that she's not pregnant so she can enter one of their hospitals."

"To do what? To die? Because she's going to."

"Yes, I know. She does, too."

"Of all the insane . . . Jesus! Does she know what this is? Does she have any idea that . . ." he sputtered angrily.

I interrupted him. "She knows. It's her faith, and she's not upset."

"I know, I know. That's what I don't get. I did her scan, and she was so calm. And she's so *sick*. We've had four techs and two radiologists check the scan. It's the most advanced case of cancer any of us has seen, and she's *smiling* at us."

"So there's no pregnancy in there at all?"

"Oh, hell no. Just huge tumors everywhere, in all the organs and all the spaces in between them. Do you hear what I'm saying? You can't even see what's what, you know? And it's very upsetting."

I sighed and pressed my fingertips to my eyelids. "I know. I'm so sorry it's upset all of you. I don't feel very good about it either. Just send her back and mail me the report as usual, okay?"

"Yeah, but with surgery and modern medicine, she might have lived."

"Yes, I know. Thanks."

I dropped my head into my hands. I had held a shred of hope, praying I was wrong, that there was some logical, treatable explanation for her condition. Now that tiny hope evaporated. Truly, she would die.

A few minutes later Patricia returned, and I handed her the letter written on my letterhead. For her, it was so simple. She just wanted a piece of paper to allow her to enter a place where she would be treated with love and compassion while she made the final and most important journey of her life. A letter, just a few lines long. The bare minimum had been asked of me, and the bare minimum was what I provided. A single piece of paper that said, "Visual, bimanual, and ultrasound examinations all confirm the following: Patricia Adams is not pregnant. If you require more information, please contact me at the above address."

I hugged her as she left my office. She smiled and stretched out a thin hand to touch my cheek. Again, it felt like a blessing, a moment of grace.

"Thank you so much. You've been kind," she said.

"I wish you well," I answered, struggling with the lump in my throat.

"I'll be fine."

"Yes. I know you will," I nodded, and I turned back to the waiting room where two women wrestled with noisy toddlers fighting over a colorful pull-toy.

Ten days later my phone rang in the evening just as I poured rice into boiling water.

"Mrs. Vincent? This is Tim Adams."

Tim Adams, Tim Adams. I searched my brain, but I just couldn't place him.

"I'm sorry, what did you say your name was?"

"Tim. Tim Adams. Patricia Adams was my wife."

Ah, Patricia Adams. The belly, the skin, the tumors. Her peace.

"Okay, yes." I took a deep breath. "I remember Patricia very well."

"She passed on a few days ago."

I sat down hard and fast. "Oh, I'm so sorry."

"Thank you. And thank you for helping her."

"I only wish I could have been more help. I wish . . ." What did I wish? I had wished for something different from what she had chosen to wish for. I sucked in my breath as I realized her wish had been granted.

"Well, Patricia's fine now. But there's something you can do for me."

"Of course. Do you need more documentation? Are there legal problems?"

"No, no, nothing like that. It's quite simple, I'm sure. Close to the end, her mind wandered, and she talked about some flowers. During a lucid moment, she told me she'd seen flowers at your office. I want to plant some in her memory, but she couldn't remember what they were called."

My chest heaved with a sob, and I covered the receiver so he wouldn't hear me. She was still God's perfect child in his eyes, and I heard no sadness in his voice. He sounded as much at peace as she had been on that morning ten days ago. I mustn't burden him with my tears for what might have been. This was my grief, not his.

"Hello?" he said into my silence. "Mrs. Vincent?"

I took a breath and steadied my voice. "Bougainvillea," I said, in a whisper. "Purple and magenta bougainvillea."

~ *Labor's Not So Bad*

"Just take it moment by moment, Judy, and when a contraction's over, let it go. It's gone forever. Try to stay in the present."

I'd expressed the same philosophy thousands of times over the years, helping women stay grounded. Helping them keep from feeling overwhelmed by the relentlessness of childbirth.

But Judy didn't need that coaching. She'd already figured it out. During her uncomplicated, twelve-hour labor with her first child, she'd spent long hours in the shower. This time around, the big bathtub appealed to her. Before I finished speaking, her eyelids flickered, and she slid lower in the tub, tuning out the world. She reclined like a pregnant maharani in the cramped bathroom of the alternative birth center. I sat on the toilet lid, and Bonnie sat on the edge of the tub.

The three of us had spent considerable time in Greece, and we talked about the incredible blue of the sky, the books of Nikos Kazantzakis, and sunsets behind the Acropolis. We recalled the clicking of worry beads, the rows of octopus drying on clotheslines, the taste of *ouzo,* and where we'd found the best *baklava.* Every few minutes we stopped talking and watched Judy close her eyes, rocking beneath the warm water. Then she sat up and said, ". . . and did you take the donkey ride on Santorini or did you walk?"

I shook my head and smiled, marveling at her composure. Long years ago when I first started teaching childbirth classes, I often tried to predict how individual women would handle labor. Within a couple of years, I weaned myself of the fruitless practice. The impossibility of predicting what kind of labor a woman would have was only half of the reality check. Given the unpredictability of labor, one must tack the unpredictability of a woman's response onto it.

I once watched a tense and prim woman dressed in a tailored suit sit through a series of six evening childbirth classes. She clutched her navy leather purse in her lap, crossed her legs at the ankles, and neither varied her expression nor spoke a word. I pegged her for a quick cesarean based on what appeared to be her total inability to relax.

I happened to be on duty when she entered the hospital in labor. I was nearly as astonished as her husband, who had clearly never seen this hidden side of her personality, when she pulled the pins from her long blond hair, peeled off every scrap of clothing, and threw herself naked onto the bed. With hair streaming like wet seaweed across her sweat-drenched face, shoulders, and chest, she rocked and rolled through a tumultuous labor that left her, breathless and triumphant, with a baby in her arms in six hours flat.

Acknowledging that there are too many unknowns, too many variables, to make the art of prediction any more accurate than throwing a dart toward an unseen target in a dark pub, I gave up trying.

I began suggesting that women write up their ideal birth in as much detail as they wished. Then I encouraged them to hold a little New Age ceremony—and burn it to ashes. That written scenario might be as close as they would ever come to their dream birth. Women can't possibly know if they'll have a wham-bam-thank-you-ma'am six-hour labor or a grueling forty-hour affair with relentless back pain. The long menu of unknowns facing each woman at the end of her pregnancy makes planning seem ludicrous.

But luck and anatomy predestined Judy to have easy labors. And she also knew with rare intuition how to go from moment to moment during the contractions—how to let go and return to the present when they ended.

Her husband, David, stuck his head into the bathroom and said, "Honey, do you need me to rub your back, or help you with your breathing?"

"No, David, no thanks, I'm fine." Her voice trailed away as she sank down till just her face, nipples, and bellybutton showed above the water. David watched, fidgeting with his watchband and shifting from one foot to the other. "Well, just let me know. I brought lots of stuff. Juice, tennis balls, Scrabble, a mandala, sour candy."

Judy smiled at him and waved him out of the room, saying, "No, I'm fine."

He backed out, pulling the door shut behind him, but not before I saw relief flood his face. Bonnie and Judy saw it, too, and Judy chuckled and said, "Poor guy, he's out of his depth."

"Well, you can't blame him," said Bonnie. "Many men feel pretty awkward around laboring women. I wonder if we really did men a favor when husband-coached childbirth came into vogue. It's a lot to ask of your average guy."

I remembered my husband's comment after Skylar's birth: "I was so glad all those women were there to take care of you. I could never quite get the hang of how I was supposed to 'coach' you the previous times, when I've never had a baby. It was such a relief not to have that pressure so I could just be there for you, however you wanted to use me."

During the years when I taught natural childbirth classes, I always encouraged couples to pick a woman to come along as a second support person. And I cautioned the men not to take it as a personal rejection if the laboring mom turned toward the woman near the end.

Celeste, a mother of four, explained her feelings: "As soon as I started humming my labor song, I wanted my sister close by. Her voice was on the same pitch as my song, her movements mirrored my own, and soon I felt like her heart and mine were beating in harmony. Randy's a great guy, but everything's different with a man—his voice, his energy, the feel of his body. That difference is part of what makes sex between a man and a woman so good—but in childbirth, I want what only another woman can give me, the softer touch, the gentler rhythm. That's part of why I use a midwife."

David peered through the steam several more times to check on Judy's progress, but mostly he stayed in the labor room rummaging among the bags and baskets they'd brought to the hospital. He hauled out his camera and toyed with angles and focal length. Prowling the room with his light meter, he muttered about exposure and f-stops.

So it was just us ladies in the bathroom, which soon felt like a Women Only spa. Eventually Judy stopped talking altogether. Bonnie and I continued our conversation, voices soft in the mist.

We paused whenever we noticed Judy sink beneath the water. Pink circles appeared on her freckled cheeks, and then we saw a telltale shred of bloody mucus float from her body. Like a red ribbon trailing through the water, it was the herald of late labor, the sign of the last bit of cervix melting away. Bonnie and I exchanged a glance and stood up together.

Why can't it always be this simple? I didn't even need to examine Judy to know that birth was imminent. She opened her eyes and saw us standing above her.

"It's time," she whispered.

"I know," I whispered back, helping her to her feet.

With a transfixed expression, as if she were balancing on a tightrope where the merest zephyr could topple her, she stepped from the tub. Glancing down, I saw the lips of her vagina begin to separate. The labor had been so graceful, and it looked as if the baby would emerge the same way.

Bonnie took Judy's hands and backed up, leading her out the door. I followed behind cupping the fuzzyheaded baby's scalp, now bulging as big as a billiard ball. With Bonnie in front and me hunching along behind, we made our way toward the bed, just eight steps away. Judy waddled along with her legs apart like a toddler who needs a diaper change.

"Wait. My camera," said David as he saw our strange parade. Whirling in a circle, he searched for his misplaced camera.

The head surged again, now as big as a tennis ball. Judy took another tiny step.

"David, it's here," I said. Still one step from the bed, the rest of the head slid into my palm. Judy made not a sound, just put one bare foot on the metal footstool and one knee up on the mattress. I heard David twisting a lens into place.

Judy placed her hands with precise care, palms down on the folded bedspread, as if it mattered somehow. The baby's top shoulder slid beneath the pubic bone. Judy still had one foot on the footstool. David still had his back to us, advancing the new film to the first frame, muttering, "Yeah, here we go."

I cradled the shiny, wet body with my hand and felt the other shoulder swing past the perineum as Judy's tissue stretched with the elasticity of bubble gum.

"Um, David, the baby," said Bonnie.

"Wait a sec, I'm nearly ready," he said. He aimed the camera at the window and then toward the darkest corner. "If I bounce a spot off that wall, it'll be perfect."

The baby's belly, hips, and legs came out, sliding onto my extended arm like a sausage moving along a conveyor belt.

Pushing the baby forward between Judy's legs, I murmured, "Take her."

Judy grasped a waving arm and pulled the baby further onto the bed, right beneath her damp and dewy face. "Ooo, look at you," she crooned, using a corner of the bedspread to wipe mucus from her daughter's cheek.

The baby didn't seem to know she'd been born. She stretched and arched her back, wiggling her bony little chicken hips. She opened her eyes. Judy placed her pinkie in the baby's palm, and the tiny fist closed around it. Judy smiled and kissed a powder-puff cheek.

When David turned around with his camera in front of his face, it was all over.

"But . . ."

Judy lifted her other leg onto the bed and curled onto her side, nose-to-nose with her second daughter. Bonnie and I dealt with cord-cutting, placenta-delivering, baby-wrapping, and propping David up till some color returned to his face. A couple of minutes later the placenta slid out, and David snapped off three shots of it from various angles. As I plopped the placenta in a blue plastic basin, he aimed and clicked the camera once more.

Later, as she completed Judy's chart, Bonnie shook her head in awe. "That was the most effortless birth I've ever seen. How did you do that?"

Judy looked up from her nursing baby and said, "Labor's not so bad, you know," and she must have seen our incredulous glances, because she added, "Well, except for the contractions, of course." She waved her hand in the air as if to erase something so inconsequential as "the contractions."

We stared at her for a minute, and then Bonnie burst out laughing. "Oh, 'the contractions!' Pffhht."

"Really, you guys," said Judy. "Each one is just a minute of pain, and then it's gone. You go from one to the next, and that way it's not so bad. Oh, I can't explain."

I laughed and reassured her. "No, you're absolutely right. It's just that so few people figure that out. I never could. Even though I've talked the talk for years, I still can't walk the walk the way you just did."

"Well, really, I don't mind labor at all. What do you think, David, shall we have one more? It might be a boy, you know."

"Yeah, sure, what the hell," said David, who had set his camera aside to cuddle up next to her. He reached his arm across her to stroke the baby's velvety cap of fine, dark hair. "Let's go for it in a year or so. I mean, anyone who can have babies so quietly that I miss the whole thing, even though I'm standing right in the same room, probably ought to go into production. But I swear to God, Judy, I'm not going to take my eyes off you. The next time, I'm leaving my camera at home."

~ *Goose Abuse*

Phyllis made the best vegetable soup I'd ever tasted. I spooned broth into my mouth, wondering how someone who could make something this good could have such a negative outlook on life. From the bedroom came her shrill voice, complaining to her husband.

"Nick, it doesn't help when you press there. You can never find the right spot. Why are you so stupid?"

Having delivered her first child just eighteen months earlier, I should have known what to expect during her second labor—I had hoped things would be different. But as I scooped chunks of potato and rounds of carrots from my bowl, I realized my prayers to the Birth Goddess for an easy second birth for Phyllis had gone unanswered.

Soon I would have to go back to her. I ran through my bag of tricks. I'd already used so many. Acupressure, massage, chanting. Reflexology was worth a try, but I knew I was scraping bottom, and she adamantly refused to consider moving to the hospital for pain medication.

"I'm going to die! I want to die. But I'm afraid I *won't* die. It'll just go on forever," she yelled. Taking a deep breath, I squared my shoulders and reentered the small bedroom.

She had her husband in a headlock, backed against the wall. I smiled at her as a contraction ended and brushed hair from her sweaty forehead. She pushed my hand away. When her friend, Cynthia, offered a glass of water, Phyllis threw it to the floor.

The next time she sat down, I pressed my thumbs into the pad of tissue below her big toes, massaging the tops of her feet at the same time. I said, "Breathe down through the pain, right into it and past it, out the other side. Yes, that's right, all the way down to your feet." I felt her toes relax for a few heartbeats, but then she recoiled and kicked my leg, knocking me against Nick's knees.

"Nothing works for me. I knew it would be just as bad as last time. Why me? Why doesn't anything go easy for me? God, why aren't you trying to help me?"

I stood up as she leapt to her feet. She yanked Cynthia forward and draped herself across her friend's back. Another contraction began, but as her husband and I pressed on two tried-and-true acupressure points, she whined, "No, not like that. Don't touch me at all. Just leave me alone."

We moved back and glanced at each other. Her husband sighed as she shrieked, "Don't go away! Why are you leaving? Can't you at least try to help?" He moved toward her, and she turned aside. Pressing my fingertips to my eyes, I sighed and leaned against the wall, thinking of better days.

Women who labor with negativity drag everyone down with them. I frequently joked to my pregnant moms that the only thing I requested of them, besides good chocolate and Peet's coffee, was that they keep me entertained. People always laughed, but really, I was only half-joking. Long ago I recognized that a woman's ability to maintain her sense of humor is the best predictor of a positive birth experience, even if there are difficulties. Fortunately, most women who choose home birth are well prepared to handle the pain and have an upbeat sense of the absurdity of this thing we call labor. But Phyllis had a different attitude. I was not entertained.

During the next hour, she shrieked through her contractions in high-pitched tones of tension and panic. I have no problem with noisy women in labor. In fact, I encourage them. But there's good noise and there's not-so-good noise. Shrieks and shrill screams increase fear and pain, where low-pitched roars, moans, groans, and yells release tension.

I said, "Phyllis, try to get your voice lower. Put the sound into the back of your throat. Try it with me. Ahh, ahh, ahh, see if you can—"

"EEEEeee! Shut up. Nothing's working, nobody's helping me. None of you are any good. Yeoww!" she shrieked, in a range high enough to make her dog howl in sympathy.

Cynthia and I went to the kitchen for more soup. We didn't speak. We leaned over the steaming broth and listened to the litany of complaints from across the hall as we stared toward the distant skyline. I returned to the bedroom, but I knew my line of credit on patience was about to run out.

I suggested that Phyllis sit down instead of acting like a frantic child playing musical chairs. She yelled, "I can't sit down. It'll hurt more. I'm so tired. I need to lie down. Where are the pillows. Nick, did you take the pillows again?"

If I'd known hypnosis, I'd have suggested it, but I suspected it would have met with the same response as all my other offers of help: angry refusal, rejection, and abuse.

"How 'bout a shower?"

"No, no, no, it hurts my back to stand still. Don't you understand? Can't you make it better?" She leaned against her husband for five minutes as he stroked her back, and then she smacked at him, whining, "Don't get so close. I can hear you breathing."

Hundreds of times over the years, I've willingly spent long hours nose to nose with a laboring woman having a difficult time, helping her surf the waves of pain. In more than thirty years of caring for women in labor, I have rarely been at a loss for some way to comfort a woman. But Phyllis had created a no-win situation.

Her rounded shoulders hunched even further forward as she whined and kvetched through another hour. Looking at the tight slash of her mouth and the deep frown lines made me sorry for her joyless outlook. She demanded help but refused it. I felt drained.

For the first time in my career, I found myself completely frustrated with a woman's refusal to cooperate on any level with me or with her body. I had lots of special little tricks up my sleeve, but she dismissed them all. I felt rejected and useless, a failure. I couldn't seem to come up with a single technique to make this labor go more smoothly. To make matters worse, at four centimeters of dilation, she was barely into mid-labor. Both Phyllis's friend and her husband behaved like saints in the face of her steady abuse, but I was losing it.

On the edge of total meltdown, I knew I had to take a break, even at the risk of damaging my reputation. With fists clenched in the pockets of my jacket, I gathered my courage and said, "Phyllis, I need to spend some alone time. I'm running out of ways to help you, and I'm feeling really frustrated with our inability to work together. I hope if I get some distance for half an hour or so, I'll come back with some new ideas."

I babbled on, astounded that I was saying these things aloud to a paying client. I filled the charged space between us with words, afraid of what she might say if I gave her a chance. If this got out into the community, this monologue of mine, what would the repercussions be? I felt sure no other midwife had ever before done this. But I feared if I didn't calm down, I might say things I'd live to sorely regret. Truly desperate, I plowed ahead with my speech. "Perhaps while I'm gone, you can see this labor in a different light. Right now it's really difficult for all of us, especially for you. And I need to pull back for a while."

In surly silence, she leveled a glare at me and snarled, "What if the baby comes while you're gone?"

"I'll be ten minutes away. Page me." I looked at Nick and Cynthia. They nodded. Nick heaved a deep breath and exhaled with force.

I left.

It was a beautiful December afternoon, but I barely noticed the decorated Christmas trees visible through many bay windows. Gripping the steering wheel so hard that for days afterward I picked pieces of black plastic from beneath my fingernails, I tried to calm the tightness in my stomach so I could focus on the narrow road. I swerved around the curves toward Lake Anza, parked, yanked my clunky purse off the seat, and stomped across the grass.

Lake Anza, home to many ducks and several geese, sits at the center of Tilden Park on the ridge above the Berkeley hills. In one spot, a low stone ledge keeps toddlers from falling into the water. With mothers in tow, several little kids crowded the area, feeding the already-fat ducks.

As I walked toward the lake, I kicked at candy wrappers and torn potato chip bags, mumbling to myself like a bag lady—and suddenly a huge goose obstructed my progress. Perhaps he mistrusted my threatening manner. He lowered his head, spread his wings, and came at me, leading with his snapping, clattering, yellow beak. It had a bony hump at the top, right between his eyes.

Filled with righteous fury, I didn't break my stride. Instead, I swung my purse at him, knocked him out of my way, and stormed on by, swearing softly like a madwoman.

About twenty steps farther, I heard this insane honking and turned to find him running toward me again. He flapped his wings and clacked his beak, honking and weaving his head from side to side, looking for the best angle of attack. I'd heard of geese used like guard dogs, and it crossed my mind that this aggressive gander must be the alpha male of the flock. As he came close I dodged, looked him in the eye with a mean glint in my own, and swung my purse a second time, connecting with his hefty body hard enough to divert him. He squawked once and moved away, lurching along in a stiff-legged, macho goose-waddle with his wings still spread. I heard him muttering to himself as he rounded the wall.

I reached the lake and sat on the ledge with my back to the water, stared up at the trees and the clear sky above me, took a few deep breaths . . . and there he was again! He was up on the wall and heading my way fast, head lowered and neck stretched toward me. He was silent this time—and full of deadly purpose.

I stood up and took an offensive stance, fists clenched, feet apart, chin thrust forward, and I shrieked, "Okay, Brother Goose, I'm warning you, you've picked the wrong lady at the wrong time. Leave me the fuck alone!"

This attracted the undivided attention of all the nearby mothers of small children. But he, stupid goose, didn't listen. He kept coming.

So I took two or three steps back, got a running start, and, using the side of my foot à la Women's World Cup soccer player, I kicked him, beak over tail feathers, about fifteen feet above the lake.

I couldn't believe how heavy he was. Nor could I believe how far he traveled—or how hard I must have kicked him. The sound of my foot on impact with his midsection was part whumph and part thummmp, hollow but heavy, like an under-inflated volleyball landing on the sidewalk after being dropped from a third-floor window. The impact vibrated all the way up my leg into my hips, and continued right up my body like a vibrating tuning fork. It gathered all the anger and tension I'd been holding and sent it up to my head. It all rattled around in there for a moment or two and then burst out in a stupendous, tingling rush of laughter.

As I staggered to regain my balance, I watched, a joyous grin on my face, as the astonished goose floundered, fluttered, and flapped through the air in a high arc, squawking loudly as he landed with a splash. Very surprised, he quickly began rearranging his feathers into a semblance of dignity, trying to look as if the whole affair had been just a prank of his own creation.

All the mothers herded their children to the far end of the lake.

I felt rather silly, but overwhelming my embarrassment was a renewed sense of power, of being back in control. As soon as the goose landed and glanced back at me with something that looked like respect, I felt great. Kicking the goose had cleared out the bad energy, but, even more important, it knocked some sense into my head. Phyllis was paying me for one thing: to safely deliver her baby. The way she chose to deal with her labor was none of my business and shouldn't be my problem.

What *was* my problem was that I took her rejection of my best efforts to ease her distress as a personal failure. As soon as I realized this, the problem vanished. Within a few minutes I skipped back across the lawn and drove along the ridge, muttering, "I think I can, I think I can," out loud in my car.

Affirmations. I had one more technique left to try.

As soon as I opened the front door, I knew nothing had changed. Phyllis pounded her fists on the wall and cursed at her friend. I held her shoulders and looked into her eyes. "Try this, Phyllis," I said. "Say it with me. 'I can do this, I can do this.'"

"I can do . . . No, no, no, I can't, I'm just no good at this. I can't do it. Oh,

I must be your worst patient ever," and she spun away and pulled at her hair.

But I felt calm. My shoulders weren't tense. As she pressed her forehead against the doorframe, I spoke into her ear. "Phyllis, your baby will be born in a few more hours. If you need any help, just let me know. I'll be close by."

And I went into the kitchen and started copying the soup recipe onto a file card. Phyllis's continuous stream of negative comments rolled off me like water off a goose's back. Four hours later she pushed her second little girl into the world. I tucked her daughter in beside her. The baby began nursing contentedly, and Phyllis smiled at last.

So did I.

I put the recipe for that dynamite vegetable soup into my purse and drove down from the hills. As I passed Lake Anza and spotted a flock of geese on the grass, I rolled down my window and shouted, "No hard feelings?" I honked my horn, and I think one of the geese honked back. The big one with an orange hump on his beak.

I knew my clients well by the end of their pregnancies. Each prenatal visit lasted half an hour, and after the five minutes it took to measure a belly, take a blood pressure, and listen to a baby's heartbeat, my client and I could settle down for twenty-five minutes of girl talk. Dads usually came to some of the visits, but occasionally I didn't meet the baby's father till labor actually started. Now and then, a particular pairing surprised me.

Although I blinked maybe twice, I think I adequately covered my astonishment when lithe and graceful Angelique, a radiant Hare Krishna devotee, introduced me to her partner. I smiled as I shook the paint-stained, gnarled hand of Joe, a sixty-five-year-old street artist.

Hannah, a six-foot-tall Jewish woman with a Ph.D. in astrophysics, gazed with devotion at her husband, a five-foot-six-inch Irish Catholic auto mechanic, and I marveled at their mutual attraction.

There's just no accounting for people's tastes, and I like to believe I celebrate these differences. The unusual types of people I met were one of the most interesting aspects of my job. But when I attended Mara's birth, the behavior of her young husband, Nicky, made me uneasy.

Nicky, a man—no, a boy really—with the features of a Greek god, seemed to be hitting on me. Me, a middle-aged woman thirty years his senior. Under other circumstances, I might have been amused or even flattered, but this was downright outrageous. His wife labored on a futon three feet away, and his stepdaughter sat in my lap.

With dark, softly curling hair framing his pouty, almost girlish face, Nicky strutted like the prancing drum major of his own parade. Bare-chested and barefoot, he looked like Adonis with an attitude, and he trailed one fingertip across the back of my neck as he passed behind me. His drawstring pants, so sheer I knew he wore nothing beneath them, hung far enough below his navel to make me nervous.

Mara, this man-child's wife, groaned in labor in their funky apartment, and I sat on the floor beside her with five-year-old Natasha leaning against me. I played This Little Piggy Went to Market with her toes, trying to ignore Nicky.

Impossible. Like a magnificent butterfly searching for the best flower on which to display its splendor, Nicky flitted around the room. He rubbed his thigh against my shoulder each time he passed.

Fate had blessed Mara with Gaelic beauty: long legs, full breasts, black hair, and creamy skin. But her thick-lashed, sapphire eyes wore blinders when it came to picking men. Natasha's father, a commercial artist twenty-five years older than Mara, had been a handsome rake demanding adoration from a steady procession of lissome young women. For her second attempt at parenting, she chose Nicky, a boy sixteen years younger than she, a kid who wanted me to lie on the birth certificate so it would appear he was at least twenty.

At thirty-five, Mara earned a marginal living as an artist and a costume designer. She had sublet her spare bedroom to Nicky eighteen months earlier, right after his parents kicked him out. During a prenatal office visit, she tried to explain her attraction.

"I needed the money, and besides, he agreed to pose for free, and Lord, what a body." Dreamy-eyed, she toyed with her hair as she continued. "He'd only been living with me three days before we were shacked up. Wait till you see him, Peggy. He's gorgeous. You'll just love him."

Gorgeous? Yes. But I didn't love him.

With Mara struggling through strong contractions, I tried to direct his attention to his wife. "Nicky, Mara's got a lot of back pain. Why don't you massage her, right here at the top of her sacrum? You're strong, you can push harder than I can, I'm sure."

"I'd rather not," he murmured, spinning away. "My art requires me to stand for long periods of time. I might injure my back if I bend over too long."

I seethed. Mara labored on as I rubbed her back. She didn't see his gauzy thigh just touching me as he slithered past. She didn't notice his heavy-lidded glances.

The modest apartment felt overwhelmed by Nicky's monstrous sculptures in plaster, paper, wood, and concrete. Spatters of paint in psychedelic colors dominated not just his work but also the walls, floor, and ceiling of the large living room.

"Come see my masterpiece," he'd said during a prenatal home visit a month earlier. He dragged me into the master bedroom to view a ten-by-six-foot plaster, three-dimensional painting hanging on the wall. With an odd and enigmatic smile on his face, he waited for my reaction. I stared at the enormous construction of repetitious castings of some odd shape that meandered across the surface. The entire piece vibrated with hot tropical colors: pinks, purples, citron, and chartreuse.

I tried to think of something nice to say while Nicky stared at me like a malicious Pan, but I just didn't get it. I twisted my head this way and that, trying to make sense of the piece. Finally I mumbled the kind of blather that people say when the meaning of artwork escapes them. "Very nice. You certainly have a talent. You must be very proud of this piece."

He curled his lip and looked at me as if I were as dense as mahogany.

Now I sat in that same bedroom with Nicky vamping around, posturing and preening. After refusing to rub Mara's back, he sashayed to the small kitchen, and I heard him rattling crockery. When he returned, he posed in the doorway with one hip cocked higher than the other, the thin cotton pants dipping even farther below his hipbones as he sipped a cup of tea. He hadn't offered to make me a cup, and I looked at his mug with resentment.

"God, it reeks in here," he said, wrinkling his nose. "Does birth always smell this foul? I'm going out for some fresh air."

I didn't discourage him, and the charged tension flowed out of the room as he left. Mara relaxed and began progressing more quickly. We both felt calmer with Nicky gone. Even Natasha seemed lighter, freer. She bounced out of my lap and skipped around the bedroom, finally coming to rest beside her mother. She lay down on her tummy and propped her delicate little chin in her hands, staring at her mom. Mara reached out and coiled her daughter's spectacular black curls around her fingers. She pulled one out to its full length and watched it bounce back into place. When a contraction came, Natasha didn't mind that Mara slid her whole hand into the masses of curls and grabbed a handful, drawing her closer. Throughout the pain, Mara breathed with her nose buried in the clouds of curly hair. Natasha smiled a coy little smile at me.

It was nice. Just us girls.

I went to make myself a cup of tea. Outside on the narrow balcony, Nicky stood in a sunbeam, smoking a joint. Now backlit by the sun, his near nakedness was even more obvious, and his genitals were spectacularly visible. Perhaps aware of the stares from tenants in other apartments across the U-shaped courtyard, he posed like an artist's model.

I looked toward the bedroom where Mara lay. Behind her hung the enormous wall sculpture. Suddenly I saw the familiar shape behind the wild colors. I looked at Nicky again, moving a few steps to one side to get a better angle, then back toward the artwork. Uh-huh, I was right, and I started to laugh.

The sculpture displayed multiple castings of his genitals in various stages of arousal. The individual "packages" had been randomly mounted on the background and set at various angles, making the identification more difficult than if they'd been arranged in the proper direction. I remembered my comment from the home visit: "You must be very proud of this piece." I giggled aloud.

"What's so funny?" asked Nicky when he came inside.

I waved my hand in the air. "Nothing, nothing."

Less than half an hour later Mara began pushing. "Nicky," cried Mara, stretching her hand toward him, but he didn't reply. Natasha knelt behind her mother and stroked the hair off her forehead.

As I moved to her side, I glanced at Nicky and caught him in an unguarded moment, a fleeting second when dark clouds of self-doubt raced across his arrogant face. He stood against the wall hugging his arms to his chest, staring at Mara writhing on the floor as if she were a nest of snakes. He saw my glance and tried to mask his expression. But I'd seen it. Nicky was terrified. He'd probably never in his life been around something as elemental as childbirth. He looked like he might bolt at any moment. Mara wanted Nicky to catch their baby, but he didn't seem to be in any shape to manage it.

"Nicky, do you still want to catch?" I asked him.

"Well, but I might mess up and hurt the kid or Mara."

"I'll help you," I assured him. "It's a chance most people never get, and I'll have my hands on top of yours the whole time."

"Aw, jeez, I dunno," he mumbled, but he edged closer. Finally he crouched beside me and just then the dark-haired baby slid into view. "Is that . . . is that its hair?" he whispered, and I nodded.

He slipped between Mara's feet as I moved aside. I knelt behind his nearly nude young body with my hands on top of his, and I felt his spine trembling as he leaned forward to catch the slippery infant. As Nicky's hands received the baby's body, the newborn flung his arms wide in a gesture well known to TV evangelists. The baby screamed.

Then Nicky cried. He couldn't manage the scissors to cut the cord, so I took care of that and wrapped the baby in a warm blanket while Nicky cried on and on. He cried in the touching way of a child who makes no effort to cover his face or wipe his tears. He cried when he saw his son take his first breath. He cried when he looked at his bloody hands that had just caught his child. He cried like the boy he still was. Mara stretched out both of her arms and gathered in Nicky on her right and the swaddled baby on her left. Nicky lay with his head on Mara's shoulder, blinking into his son's scrunched up little face. Looking at each other across Mara's motherly chest, both of them cried. Natasha looked at me, rolled her eyes, and heaved a melodramatic sigh.

I patted Nicky's back, handed him a tissue to blow his nose, and caught Mara's eye. She shrugged and gave me a wry smile.

A boy. A man. A father. Nicky, between worlds.

I feared their marriage would survive about as long as the thin cotton pants he wore, but I could no longer be angry with him. He was a kid, the same age as my eldest. Egotistical, insecure, confused, and just nineteen.

I left a couple of hours later. As I gathered my supplies, Nicky scrambled to help me. He shook his curls out of his eyes and pulled his pants higher, retying the drawstring.

"Here, let me carry those for you," he mumbled like a Boy Scout trolling for a merit badge. Refusing to let me carry anything, he staggered down the dingy stairs of the creaky old building and loaded my supplies into the VW. He scrambled to open my door, but before I could slide behind the wheel he wrapped me in a hug.

"God, thanks. Thank you. That was wonderful," and his eyes filled with tears again. "I just had no idea. I mean, I never knew . . . well, anyway, thanks a lot."

I'm often awed to see birth work its transforming alchemy on those privileged to attend, but rarely have I seen such a dramatic change as in Nicky. I squeezed his arm and said, "It's pretty amazing, isn't it?"

He just nodded, but as I started the engine, he grasped the doorframe. "About earlier. Well, I'm sorry. I didn't mean anything."

"I know. I appreciate your telling me, though. I'll see you tomorrow," I said.

When I looked back through the rear view mirror, he was standing barefoot on the gritty sidewalk, hands dangling at his sides, the pants snug around his waist.

Then he turned and headed upstairs, back into a room where he would try to figure out what it means to be a father, before he'd even gotten the hang of what it means to be an adult.

It's Just So Interesting

Naked, Julie hunched forward on the toilet, wiggling her toes at top speed. Rocking like an autistic, head-banging child, she white-knuckled the plastic seat with both hands as she howled toward the ceiling. For the past hour, she'd sounded like a wild jungle beast instead of her usual, pragmatic, corporate self.

She and Mark had planned a home birth as affirmation of their belief that hospitals, doctors, and drugs are rarely necessary. But Mark had never seen Julie behave this way. He balanced on the edge of the bathtub, staring with desperate eyes at his usually demure and elegant partner. He kept up a dogged and loving monologue.

"You're fine, Julie, everything's going just fine, keep breathing, keep relaxing, keep open to whatever happens. You're doing so well, keep it up, just stay grounded, stay focused . . ."

"Yowee!" shrieked Julie, rocking and roaring. Slick with sweat, she drowned out her husband's earnest voice. "Yowee, zowie, wowie."

Margaret came up beside me, handed me a mug of tea, and leaned against the doorframe. I knelt on the cold tiled floor, smiling into Julie's contorted face. When she had trouble pushing in bed, I had suggested moving to the toilet, thinking she might find it more natural to push there. It worked. Julie had hopped onto the pushing highway, and her baby had seen the exit sign and shifted into high gear.

Mark looked frantic, gulping for air like a fish flopping on a dock. He searched for just the right words to convert Julie back into his ladylike wife of ten years.

"I love you, I love you so much, and you're doing so well. Just stay relaxed, and soon you'll have our baby, our very own little baby."

"Yi-yi-yi, zowie, zow-zow!"

Mark reached toward Julie and then paused, glancing at me. When I nodded, he touched her shoulder, a tentative touch, as if he were reaching across a vast space to connect with something bigger than he'd ever faced before. Gently he said, "Julie, don't be afraid."

She jerked her gaze from the ceiling light and stared at him like she'd never seen him before. Spewing spit with each word, she screamed, "I'm *not* afraid! It's just so . . . so . . . so *INTERESTING!*"

I fell against the wall, laughing.

Mark finally got it that Julie wasn't suffering. All the noisy caterwauling was just her way of coping. He sagged with relief, slipping backwards and nearly falling into the tub. Margaret, choking with laughter, pulled him up while I took a peek between Julie's thighs. The baby's head bulged at the opening.

"We've gotta get her out of here," I said between our laughter and her bellows. They both tried to help me lift her off the toilet, but Julie had the best of us. She clung to the rim of the seat as if it were a life raft. Sucked into the raging ocean of her labor, far beyond the reach of our words, Julie became a pushing machine with only one purpose: Get the baby out.

Although it certainly makes the cleanup afterwards simple and isn't as unsanitary as people fear, I never actually *plan* to do a delivery on the toilet. However, other than the infant's surprise when it hits the cold water, there's no reason to avoid it. I just keep the head above water, then fish the flapping baby between the mother's legs and up over the edge. It's not graceful, but it works.

So Julie's baby plopped into the toilet. As I scooped the dog-paddling infant over the edge, Julie sat up straight and silent like a Victorian at a tea party. She watched me with close concentration while Mark wept beside her.

"Oh Mark, look," she purred, hugging him as she gazed at their little girl. I wrapped the outraged infant in a bath towel and put her into Julie's arms while Margaret scooted downstairs to get warm blankets from the oven. "Is that the end?" Julie asked me, back to her ladylike self. She patted a strand of black hair behind her ear.

"Well, there's still the placenta, but it often takes ten minutes to come out. We can probably make it back to the bedroom."

In the same even voice and without breaking eye contact, she said, "I believe that just came out, also. Would you care to check?"

I peeked into the bloody toilet bowl. There was the placenta, floating around at the end of its umbilical leash. "Jeez, Julie," I muttered as I hauled it out.

"Maybe you should pack a fishing net in the future," laughed Margaret.

"Are we finished now?" Julie asked.

I nodded, and we toddled back to the bedroom.

An hour later, while Margaret helped Julie with breastfeeding, I went downstairs to rustle up some lunch for everyone. As I reheated a pot of clam chowder, I gazed out the window, and I pondered.

"Interesting," Julie had said. She described the pain of childbirth as "interesting."

I marvel at the tremendous leap of faith taken by women like Julie who choose home birth for their first babies. Medication for pain is not an option in a home birth, yet these first-timers, clueless as to what labor pains will actually feel like, willingly create a scenario that won't allow them a choice in pain management. They just say, "I know I can do this. I don't know how. I just know I can."

Usually they're dumbfounded at the intensity of the experience, at the raw primal nature of the pain, the relentless rhythm of it, their inability to call time out. They talk about a trapped feeling, being overwhelmed by the previously unknown power within their bodies. Yet in all my years of doing home births, I never once took a woman to the hospital because of unmanageable pain. Not once. And time after time I had the honor and privilege of looking into the astonished faces of first-time moms as I laid slippery newborns in their arms. They gazed back at me, awed by the intensity of this thing called childbirth, this rite of passage they had just completed. Having made that journey, having tapped depths of strength they never knew they possessed, they crossed a line and never looked back. Right before my eyes, they left girlhood far behind as they stepped with both feet into womanhood, into the world of Women Who Have Given Birth.

Standing at the stove, stirring the soup and looking at the iris and primroses in Julie's spring garden, I remembered Sarah, one of my first home births when I was a brand new midwife. Sarah coped with an exhausting labor that spanned two nights and three days. Near the end of the ordeal, she eyed my array of supply boxes and asked, "Are you absolutely sure you don't have something for pain over there?"

When I promised I really wasn't holding out on her, she sighed and said, "Okay, forget I asked. It's not worth a trip to the hospital," and she never mentioned drugs again.

The soft, splupping sound of the simmering chowder pulled me from my reverie. I filled four bowls, sliced a loaf of French bread, put everything on a tray, and carried it upstairs to Mark and Margaret, and to Julie, the woman who had said that labor was "interesting."

In all my years of being with birthing women, that was a first.

Of course when Julie found herself pregnant again three years later, she and Mark planned another home birth. One night, three weeks before her due date, my phone rang, and Mark said, "Uh, Peggy? Julie's acting peculiar. She's had a few contractions, but now she won't talk to me. She's crawling around the floor in a circle, swinging her head back and forth, chuffing like a steam engine. I don't have a clue what's going on."

I did. Julie's second baby had found the exit sign much faster than its sister had.

I gunned my car across town and left it in a handicapped slot near their condominium. I ran across neat lawns, around hedges, past iris and prim-roses—another spring birth—and up their front walk. Twisting the doorknob and finding it unlocked, I burst into the bedroom seconds later.

Julie lay on the bed crooning to a tiny infant wrapped in a flowered pil-lowcase. Mark, in briefs and a torn T-shirt, hunkered against the far wall with his head in his hands. He lifted his face at my noisy entrance. Staring at me, he remained crouched on the carpet, pale and hollow-eyed.

". . . so fast," he murmured.

Julie looked like an investment banker with windblown hair, completely back to normal. Pulling the pillowcase aside, I found the baby still attached to the placenta, so I dealt with that and rewrapped the infant. Except for being cold and small, she seemed fine, peering at her new world with curious eyes.

I tossed a towel to Mark. He dropped it between his knees.

". . . barely got her onto the bed," he muttered.

He hadn't thought to warm the receiving blankets, so I put four in the clothes dryer. "What's with the pillow case?" I asked as we waited for the blan-kets to heat up.

"Pillow case?" said Julie, plucking at it. "I didn't even notice. I guess it's the first thing Mark found when I yelled at him to get something to dry her off. He ran to the linen closet and brought me this."

A few minutes later, I wrapped the baby in two cozy blankets and then rolled her in aluminum foil to keep the heat in. She looked like a take-out burrito. Slightly premature, she stared at me from a pinched and foxy little face.

At last I turned my full attention to Mark, still on the floor and gazing now at the ceiling. A smear of blood decorated his right cheek.

"So Mark, how you doin' down there?"

"Oh, man," he sighed, shaking his head.

"Not what any of us expected, was it?"

"Man oh man," he repeated, turning his eyes toward me at last.

"Came a little fast, huh?"

"Yeah, I just . . . it was so . . ." His voice trailed away.

"How was it, delivering your own baby?"

"So . . . *interesting*. Yes, just very *interesting*."

~ Okay, Okay, Okay

Certified midwives practice under protocols that define the scope of their practice. They also have their own personal limits based on such things as comfort zone, belief system, and backup arrangements. I know a midwife who refuses to care for any woman who has had an abortion. Another won't accept smokers, and some refuse obese women or those with histories of substance abuse.

My own boundaries were rather broad. For planned hospital births, I accepted nearly everyone. For home births, I set a few restrictions. Trying to stay within a fifteen-mile radius of Alta Bates, I told clients, "I don't cross bridges." Medically speaking, I ruled out home births for women with previous cesareans or severe anemia. In one special case, I insisted that a 450-pound mother of ten deliver in the hospital, knowing that, in case of an emergency, moving her would be difficult.

But with a clientele ranging in age from nineteen to the mid-forties, I never considered age limitations. Then Naeema phoned me.

"Hi, Peggy? Um, you're the midwife?"

"Yes, I'm a midwife," I answered. With her high, sing-songy voice, she sounded about twelve.

"Um, well, see, I need a midwife 'cause I'm going to have a baby? I need a woman to deliver me? Because I'm Muslim?" She had the Valley Girl habit of turning a statement into a question with that rising inflection at the end of her sentences.

"How old are you?" I blurted.

"Like, I just turned sixteen on October fifth?"

She *was* a child, the exact age of my daughter Jill, less one day. I tried to wrap my mind around Jill married and pregnant but failed utterly. Boys, red roses, driver's ed classes, and Madonna's *Material Girl* occupied her thoughts, not choosing a midwife.

"And, um, my husband's mother, you know, Janice? She, like, gave me your name? So, can I be your patient? Is that okay?"

What the heck, I thought. Years of hospital experience had taught me that teenagers usually do well in pregnancy, even on a diet of Cokes and hamburgers. If she developed complications, I could transfer her to my backup doctor's female partner.

"Okay," I said, and I smiled as I heard her shriek.

"Oh, totally bitchin'!" she whooped. "Charlie—he's my husband—he's a senior? Oh, Charlie'll be so happy."

Two weeks later, Bonnie and I heard giggling outside the open windows of the office—girlish squeals followed by running footsteps. A young man's deep voice, rough with laughter and affection, joined in, and then came the splashing, slapping sound of water hitting the asphalt driveway. We peeked out the window and saw two strikingly beautiful biracial teenagers having a water fight with the hose.

The rowdy sounds grew louder as the waiting room door burst open. The kids gasped for breath as they entered the quiet room, and they clamped their hands over their mouths like naughty schoolchildren stifling forbidden laughter.

Naeema and Charlie had arrived. Drenched from head to foot, Naeema wrung water from her shirttails and retied her headscarf. Charlie's loose sweatpants and T-shirt clung to him, and his shoes squelched so badly he took them off before stepping onto the pale gray carpet. Their giggles kept popping to the surface like champagne bubbles, infecting several women in the waiting room with contagious laughter.

Bonnie and I laughed along with them as I peeled the wet shirt from Naeema's skin to listen for the baby's heartbeat. Shy and modest, she pulled her shirt down wherever I tried to pull it up, revealing only a bare inch or two of belly at a time. She blushed through her café-au-lait skin and finally gave up the struggle to stay covered when Charlie said, "Naeema, you're so beautiful. I love your little round belly, and your skin is so perfect. You should be proud. Show them your tummy, honey."

Charlie couldn't keep his eyes or his hands off his lovely young wife. He put his face close to hers and whispered sweet nothings, stroking her cheek as I rolled the shirt back to expose her abdomen.

At five feet, eleven inches, Naeema wore size six jeans, zipped up, in the fourth month of pregnancy. Her legs started high and went on forever. In keeping with her Muslim upbringing, she wore a white scarf pulled forward and tied under her chin. The loose, long-sleeved shirt, meant to discreetly cover all but her hands, now clung immodestly to her body.

This understated attire served only to direct more attention to the most arresting pale green eyes I'd ever seen. Her shy, Bambi glance and the stillness of her posture would have made her look regal had she not been acting like a giddy teenager.

A couple of months later, Naeema phoned again.

"Um, me and Charlie wondered if, like, is it okay if Janice—that's Charlie's mom, you know, and we live with her—if Janice, like, comes to the next prenatal visit?"

"Sure," I replied. My daughter talked the same way, so Naeema's roundabout sentences with all the twitchy, unnecessary words sounded familiar to me.

Janice entered the exam room halfway through Naeema's next visit, and I blinked as I recognized her. She had taken childbirth classes from me eighteen years earlier while pregnant with Charlie, and we often ran into each other at Peet's Coffee or Monterey Market. "I thought Naeema told you," she said, seeing my surprised look.

"No, she just said 'Charlie's mother, Janice.' I didn't make the connection."

"Well, it's me. But I'm not sure I've done you any favors. Wait till you hear what these two are cooking up." She leveled a look at Charlie, who looked at Naeema, who looked out the window.

"Charlie?" I said. I'd learned he was usually easier to engage in conversation than his shy wife. "What's going on?"

"Uh, me and Naeema, we want to have the baby at home."

"See what I mean?" said Janice, folding her arms.

"That's interesting," I hedged. "Who planted that little seed?"

"Just me," said Naeema, for once speaking without encouragement. "I have nine brothers and sisters, and my mom, like, she had a bunch of them at home? I was with her for the last four. I think she, you know, kinda wanted to scare me into not messin' around and getting pregnant? But it didn't scare me at all, even though she yelled and screamed and told me how it's the awfulest pain a woman can have."

"How did that make you feel?"

Charlie had his arm around her. Janice stared at the ceiling.

"Well, she always talked about, like, the agony of it, but, see, I've known my mother my whole life, and I think I handle pain a lot better'n she does. I can't imagine going into a hospital for something as simple as having a baby."

"What did Janice tell you about childbirth?" I asked.

"Hmmpf," grumped Janice, behind me. "I said the wrong thing."

"You told her labor was horrible, too?" I asked, very surprised.

"No, just the opposite. I tried to counter all the scary stuff her mom's been feeding her and told her my labor was a breeze, even though I was forty-four when I had Charlie. It began after lunch and was over before dinner, and I never gave drugs a thought. It was just dumb luck, but I didn't want Naeema to hear only bad stories. Only I didn't count on her wanting a home birth. She's barely sixteen. What does she know?"

I looked at these two kids. Charlie's thick-lashed, melted chocolate eyes and Naeema's of LifeSaver green, both pleading. I looked at Janice, supportive but doubtful. I thought of my daughter, knowing that she, too, would want to have her babies at home.

"Let's say I'll consider it. Okay?"

Charlie and Naeema grinned and slapped hands in a high-five.

Janice looked at me as if I'd lost my mind.

Naeema breezed through the rest of her pregnancy. With her long, lean torso, she hid the pregnancy inside and never looked more than six months along. Even Janice had to admit that Naeema combined marriage, pregnancy, and high school like a pro.

"It's either a case of 'ignorance is bliss,' or 'a little knowledge is a dangerous thing,' but she's doing great," Janice said when we bumped into each other in the bread section of Berkeley Bowl, a local grocery store that used to be a bowling alley. "She's even given up Cokes."

"Great," I said, "and you live just ten minutes from the hospital. I don't see that we've sacrificed either safety or sanity by letting them try it at home. If she changes her mind or runs into problems, we can zip right over to the hospital."

"Yeah, I feel better about it now than I did that day you said okay so fast."

"God, Janice, how did you feel when Charlie told you he'd gotten his fifteen-year-old girlfriend pregnant?" I asked, changing the subject.

Her answer surprised me. "Oh, it wasn't like that at all. They were married six months before she got pregnant."

I almost dropped my bag of bagels.

"Yeah, and he said he couldn't figure out how it had happened, since they 'used birth control almost every time.'" She rolled her eyes.

"Oh, lordy."

"They met when Naeema was a freshman and Charlie a junior. Her mom found out she was meeting him around Berkeley and hit the roof. She read her the riot act about her Muslim responsibilities, about modesty and morality.

She said, 'You can get married, but dating is out of the question.' So next thing we all know, Charlie converts to Islam, and two months later they're married.

"At first I was pretty upset, but I had Charlie so late in life I figured I wouldn't live to enjoy my grandchildren. Well, that's sure changed, and I'm a little embarrassed to say I'm actually sorta pleased at how things turned out. But they're awfully young."

Toward the end of Naeema's pregnancy, Charlie, who attended every visit with her, said, "There's something we'd like to ask you. See, Naeema wants me to deliver the baby," he said, batting his eyelashes at me. "Would that be okay?"

In for a shilling, in for a pound, I figured. "Okay."

I visited their home the next week, and while Janice stood in the hallway with her jaw hanging down, I used a life-sized baby doll to show her eighteen-year-old son how to deliver a baby. Naeema, her waist-length curly hair uncovered within her own home, sat quietly at Charlie's side, stroking his shoulder.

The following Tuesday, Naeema's three girlfriends stopped at her house as they always did, and the four of them walked the rest of the way to school together. Charlie's classes started later, but he and Naeema walked home together as usual and fixed dinner for themselves and Janice.

An hour later, her labor started, but Naeema didn't tell anyone. She did some homework and went to bed. As soon as she heard Charlie breathing deeply, she got up and started walking to bring the contractions on faster. He awakened at five A.M. when she stumbled and nearly fell on top of him. Charlie woke Janice and called Naeema's mother. Janice took one look at Naeema and called me.

"Well, Peggy, I can hear her in the other room telling Charlie it's too soon to call you, but she's active. They're about three minutes apart. She's real quiet, but it's making her toes curl, and she twists one foot around her other ankle and kinda dances, right? And I've heard these teenagers go really fast sometimes."

"Be right there," I said, already pulling on sweatpants. I called Bonnie and left.

Janice and Naeema's mother were perched on a piano bench when Bonnie and I arrived. Charlie fixed us strong tea laced with milk and then looked at us four middle-aged women. We had fifteen children among us, and two of us were nurses. He took a deep breath and made what I'm sure was a prepared speech.

"Me and Naeema really appreciate having you here. You've got so much experience, but it's kinda intimidating, and we'd sorta like to work it out for ourselves. You're all nurses and mothers, and, well, it's overwhelming, see? I know you have to check on the baby and Naeema and everything, but we'd really appreciate just kinda being left alone. In private, you know?"

Janice and Naeema's mother looked dumbfounded. Bonnie and I just laughed, wondering if these two would ever stop surprising us.

"Okay, okay, okay," I said, "just let me check her, and then come back every fifteen minutes so I can listen to the baby." The baby's heartbeat sounded great. I checked Naeema and found her seven centimeters dilated. Everything was perfect.

"Go," I said, still laughing. They scampered across the hallway like two kids let out of school for summer vacation, ducked into the dining room, and closed the heavy sliding door.

"Well, if that doesn't beat all," said Janice, shaking her head.

Naeema's mother just stared at the closed door, her mouth slack.

True to their word, they emerged for regular monitoring of the baby's heartbeat. With each contraction, Naeema pressed her head to Charlie's shoulder. He stroked her back and whispered in her ear as she silently, silently breathed through the pain. Indeed, the only way we could tell one had begun was when her right foot started to twine around her left ankle. Occasionally she wrinkled her nose and hiccuped. Her amazing hair flowed loose and spectacular, rippling over her upper body. She took off everything except for a ragged, pink T-shirt, and she smiled shyly as she lifted the bottom of the shirt to blot perspiration from her upper lip.

"So?" asked Charlie, with a lift of his dark eyebrows as I removed the stethoscope.

"Everything's okay," I assured them. "Off you go."

Bonnie put blankets in the oven to warm and cracked open the oxygen tank. I organized my birth supplies near the futon and opened some 4 x 4 gauze squares.

The door slid open again. Naeema fixed her eyes on me as she walked very slowly into the living room. With her fingertips, she held a tiny wad of bloody toilet tissue between her legs. She walked straight across the room, stopped square in front of me, and wrinkled her nose as she said, "You know what? This helluv hurts."

We grownups burst out laughing, and I hugged her bony adolescent shoulders.

"Let me check you, honey. I'm sure it's nearly over."

Sure enough, the baby's head was right inside the opening. She squatted on the futon with her knees practically beside her ears, looking like a contortionist. With Naeema's first push, a quarter-sized patch of baby scalp showed. I whispered instructions in Charlie's ear and marveled as he maneuvered the baby's head free of his young wife's body. He sobbed so hard he could barely see, and I heard Janice and Naeema's mom crying behind me. Bonnie and I grinned, and I saw her eyes fill with tears at the same moment mine did.

With Naeema's next gentle push, a seven-pound baby girl slipped easily into Charlie's bare hands. He lifted the baby to his cheek and whispered a Muslim blessing into her ear. Then he handed the baby to Naeema, wiped his hands, and asked his mom to dial his father's number. Charlie's parents had been divorced for many years but were on good terms, and Charlie maintained a close relationship with his dad.

"Dad, it's Charlie. We had the baby, like two minutes ago. It was helluv icy. It's a girl, and her name's Saalima. Naeema was so brave, just hellabitchin', and I delivered the baby myself 'cause we have this hellafresh midwife who taught me how to do it."

An hour later, Naeema sat nursing the baby with her wet hair wrapped high on her head in a towel. Fresh from her shower, she sipped some cocoa while awestruck Charlie hung at her side.

The doorbell rang, and three high school girls in extension braids and tight jeans appeared. Holding schoolbooks to their chests, they clumped into the room, then came to a dead stop when they saw Naeema nursing her baby. One by one they crept forward, going down on their knees like worshipful devotees.

In a sing-songy, teenage voice, one trilled, "Na-eeee-maaaaa, omigooood, you had the baaaaaby."

Another said, "Naeeeeeeeema! How waaaas it?"

Naeema looked around the room. With a half-smile and a lift of her eyebrow, she seemed to realize she had stepped over a line drawn in the sand. She had joined the club of all the women of the world who have given birth. She lifted her chin high, looked at the schoolgirls kneeling before her, wrinkled her nose, and shrugged as she said, "It was okay."

~ *Is My Mommy Happy?*

With his lips already puckered to blow out the five candles on his birth-day cake, Skylar scowled when my pager beeped. Minutes later I turned the party over to Rog, but the image of my son's gaze stayed with me as I drove to Alta Bates Hospital.

Why do women always go into labor when I have something important planned? I wondered. I've cancelled lunch dates, celebrated Christmas on December twenty-sixth, missed the first day of a family vacation, and arrived late to my own holiday party. But Britta's labor had begun, and I was her mid-wife. Skylar's birthday would have to proceed without me.

At the hospital, one of the nurses said, "Why the long face?"

I shrugged and wrinkled my nose. "I'm missing Skylar's birthday party. I'm just not happy to have someone deliver this afternoon." I reorganized all my facial parts into what I hoped would pass for a smile. "Is that better?"

She laughed. "Yeah, that'll do. Your patient's in Room 7."

So I wore my newly minted happy face down the hall to care for Britta, whom I truly liked and whose bright-as-a-brass-candlestick daughter, Jane, always made me smile. During a sibling preparation class, Jane had cracked me up when she asked, "Which comes first, the baby or the polenta?" By the time I reached Room 7, I was smiling for real.

A lazy hour of labor passed, and I sent Britta onto the roof garden. Her sister, her husband, and Jane accompanied her while the nurse and I watched through a window. About thirty minutes later, Britta opened the glass door to come inside.

Britta's eyes always shine huge and bright, but when she lurched back into the labor room, they glowed like blue lasers, fixed, round, and enor-mous. A popsicle stick protruded from the right corner of her mouth. As it had been there for the last hour, I knew the popsicle itself was long gone.

Her husband, Hugh, guided her toward the bed with his arm around her waist. Little Jane with a Buster Brown haircut came in last, gripping her aunt's hand.

"How ya doin', Britta?" I asked, grinning at her frozen expression.

Britta didn't answer. She just looked at me, eyes even bigger, searchlights. Then she switched the popsicle stick to the left corner of her mouth, like Groucho trading sides with his cigar. She even waggled her eyebrows in a Groucho leer, but it turned into a grimace as she spun around and grabbed Hugh. Chewing with a vengeance on her wooden stogie, she jerked him from side to side by his belt loops.

Always so loquacious, Jane watched in silence, then took my hand and said, "I'm so happy, Peggy," and after a pause, "Is my mommy happy?"

Her aunt hugged her and said, "Hey, Brit, Jane wants to know if you're happy."

Smiling through tight lips at her precocious little girl, Britta said, "Happy enough, but I'll be a lot happier after this baby comes out."

"When's it coming out, Momma? When will you be even happier?"

"Maybe Peggy can tell us, Jane." She flipped the popsicle stick, wiggled her eyebrows again, climbed into bed, and spread her legs for an exam.

Just begging to be broken, the amniotic sac bulged with pressure, the only thing holding the baby back. Britta must have felt as if a beach ball was about to pop inside her.

"How much left?" she asked, those eyes drilling into me, unblinking.

"Hardly anything," I said. "Only a little rim around the edge. Mostly there's just water, water, water, and the baby's head is right behind it."

"How much longer if you break it?"

"You'd probably begin pushing within a contraction or two and have the kid in your arms maybe ten or fifteen minutes later."

"Ten minutes?" squeaked Hugh in a soft Irish lilt. "Oh, sweet Blessed Virgin, she was out on the grass not fifteen minutes ago!"

Another contraction began. With a yell that sent Jane reeling against her aunt's legs, Britta rose upright in the bed like a bomb had gone off beneath her. She hated lying down when the pains came, and she braced herself bolt upright, knees out to the sides and feet tucked together into her crotch. She looked like a bloated swami chanting a mantra. The popsicle stick bounced up and down as she chewed on it and groaned.

When the contraction ended, Britta flopped back and waved her hand at me.

"Aw, Jesus, just break it, Peggy. Let's get the little sucker outta there."

"Break it?" asked Jane in a small voice. She stepped close again and put her dimpled hand on her mother's damp hair. "Is Peggy gonna break you to get our baby out? Are you still happy?"

"Jane honey, I'm not going to break your mom," I explained as the nurse handed me a plastic amnihook. "I'm going to pop the water balloon that's around the baby. It's like opening a birthday present to see what's inside."

Although Jane had seen and handled an amnihook in the sibling preparation class, her eyes widened as the long, blunt crochet hook disappear into her mother's body. She glanced at Britta's face and stood very still as her aunt rubbed her back.

"It's like getting your hair cut," I assured her. "Scissors are sharp, but does it hurt when you get your hair cut?" She shook her head and chewed on her fingernail, so I continued. "A lot of water's gonna come out in a second, Jane. It's okay."

But she still jumped, and so did her aunt, as the water gushed. It arced through the air and splashed down eighteen inches away, soaking my arm and thigh. The nurse pushed some towels between Britta's legs, and I took another one to dry myself as Britta's roar heralded her first push.

I glanced at her, then dropped the towel and lurched sideways. Nearly dislocating my back, I lunged for the bald head that rode the crest of the wave like a surfer headed into shore. The head crowned, then paused for a second while Britta took another breath. Jane covered her ears as Britta hollered to the ceiling, and then I blinked my eyes. When I opened them, the whole baby lay flapping in my hands.

"Whoa, Nelly!" shouted Britta's sister.

Behind me I heard the nurse mutter, "Ten minutes, my ass!"

"Mary Mother of God," whispered Hugh.

"Is my momma happy *now?*" yelled Jane, squealing with excited laughter.

Britta spit out the popsicle stick and yanked Jane into her arms. "Haven't been happier since the day *you* were born, darlin'."

Fifteen minutes after the birth, Britta hopped into the shower and Jane posed with her baby sister while Hugh took pictures. I picked up my purse to leave and shouted a goodbye to Britta. She stuck her head around the sliding glass door and said, "Did I hear the nurse say something about this being Skylar's birthday?"

"Yeah, I think the party will still be going on when I get home."

"Hey, Jane? You want to call Peggy's son and sing "Happy Birthday" to him?"

"Yea!" cheered Jane, plopping the baby onto a pillow and running to a phone.

I dialed the number, my husband answered, and he passed the phone to Skylar.

A huge smile pulled at my cheeks as I listened to Jane's off-key voice sing "Happy Birthday to You." Then she sang it again.

"Why did you sing it twice?" asked Hugh.

Jane looked at him like he'd just crawled out of a hole. "Duh, Dad. Once from me and once from my baby sister. She can't sing yet, you know."

A few minutes later I sat at the big round table in the nurses' station finishing my charting, smiling as I filled in the soulless blanks on the routine form. Length of labor, weight of newborn, mechanism of delivery, estimated gestational age. No space asking if the mother was happy. No space to document miracles.

The nurse who'd seen me walk into the hospital two hours earlier handed me a fresh cup of coffee. "You certainly look happier than when you came in."

"Much happier," I agreed.

PART VI

Devices and desires

*"We have erred and strayed from thy ways like
lost sheep; we have followed too much
the devices and desires of our own hearts."*

A GENERAL CONFESSION
BOOK OF COMMON PRAYER, 1928 VERSION

~ *Wrongful Life*

I want a home birth," said Patty. Her blunt-cut brown hair fell forward like a curtain, partly veiling her heavy-lidded eyes. "Will you do it?"

"Patty, I can't. You had a cesarean with your last baby. I can deliver you in the hospital but not at home."

Her voice rose to a whine, like nails on a chalkboard. "Why? Is it risky?"

"Not really," I answered, going on to explain that the fear of catastrophic uterine rupture in a labor following a cesarean is no longer considered valid. But standard midwifery protocols mandate hospital deliveries for all such women. "So I just can't help you, Patty."

She looked like a child who had been told she was too short to go on a carnival ride. "Then I might as well see Dr. Weick. He's a 'preferred provider' on my crappy insurance policy, so there'd be no surcharge, but they won't cover a midwife at all. I'd be willing to pay cash if you'd deliver me at home, but not if I'm going to be in the hospital anyway."

She yanked her purse strap off the back of her chair and flounced out. I exhaled with something like relief. Her intensity, her insistence had made me tense, and I wasn't sorry to see her leave. There was a wariness in her manner, something evasive that I couldn't articulate even to myself. I just didn't quite trust her.

But I understood all too well what she meant about the insurance company. For years I'd tried to become a preferred provider on several insurance plans, but doctors had a monopoly. With the practice of medicine heading steadily toward managed care, midwives more often found themselves being forced into working as employees for physician groups or large health maintenance organizations. As one of only a few midwives with an independent practice, I knew how good I had it, and I hoped I could string it out for many more years.

I rented space from Dr. Weick for my own practice, so when I saw Patty in the waiting room two weeks later, I knew she'd made her decision. Then one afternoon she stuck her head into my room and asked, "Do you have a few minutes?"

I waved her toward a chair and asked, "How's the pregnancy going?"

"So-so. Right now the baby's breech. Dr. Weick says he'll probably turn on his own, but I want to ask you something." She tilted her head, and her hair again hid half her face. "I had rotten luck with both my other births. One horrendous, sixty-hour induced labor eleven years ago and what I believe was an unnecessary cesarean for my other daughter, who's two. I feel both births would have gone better if I'd stayed home longer."

I agreed with her and ended by saying, "As long as everything's normal, I usually counsel women to stay home till they feel as if they're holding up the walls."

She laughed. "So this time I'd like to stay home until I'm really active. Holding the walls up." She laughed again, then turned and drilled me with her eyes. "Do you do labor coaching?"

"No, I'm on call twenty-four hours a day for my own clients, but I'll recommend someone."

"But I want you," she insisted, pouting. "I want a midwife, someone with skills who understands how important this is to me. I had drugs before, and even though I begged for them, I hated it. And I hated myself. I feel like such a failure."

For the first time, I felt she was speaking from her heart. I reached out and put my hand over hers. "Patty, you've got two healthy children. You're not a failure, but I know what you're talking about. Many women feel it's important to their self-image to master childbirth. I do understand, really."

Some of my most fulfilling deliveries were those in which the mom, like Patty, had had terrible previous experiences. To be able to choreograph a satisfying birth, to help the woman over the rough places of labor, to allow her a feeling of control—and ultimately of triumph—always reminded me how grateful I was to be a midwife. Just the previous week, I'd delivered a woman named Lorna who felt she'd been railroaded into a hasty cesarean with her first child. As I delivered her second baby, Lorna squatted on the floor of the birth center. She reached between her legs and pulled her daughter onto her chest, sobbing with transcendent joy. Then she looked at me and said, "This is the first time I've felt whole and complete in two years."

Knowing how important this birth was to Patty, I agreed to her request, as long as she understood that I couldn't promise her anything. I might be with someone else and be unable, therefore, to care for her.

"Yes, yes," Patty muttered, and she waved her hand as if brushing a gauze curtain aside. We settled on a fee, and she signed an agreement that I wrote on the spot.

As she walked out the door, I shook my head. Why had I caved in to her request? Being a labor coach put me in such an awkward position, a position of knowledge but without power, a role of advising but not of acting. She had persuaded me to be her advocate, but a niggling worm of anxiety made me hope I would be unavailable when she called.

Then Patty's baby began flip-flopping from breech one week to headfirst the next, a condition known as an unstable lie. A baby that turns that often can become tangled in its umbilical cord. One afternoon as Patty was leaving the office, I overheard a short exchange between her and Dr. Weick.

"Patty, I want you in the hospital as soon as active labor starts. We need to monitor the baby. Don't stay home too long, okay?"

She continued walking away from him with a sulky expression, and his voice rose. "Okay? Patty?" She gave a desultory wave of her hand and walked out.

He turned, saw me, and pulled me into his office, shutting the door behind him. Exasperated, he leaned against the door and rolled his eyes. "She just won't listen to what she doesn't want to hear."

"What's going on?" I asked.

"She's determined to stay home till the last minute. I can't help but wonder if she's still trying to figure out some way to have a home birth."

"Are you serious?"

"Well, given the way she's been acting, I think it's a distinct possibility. What's your arrangement with her again?" He jammed his hands into the pockets of his pressed jeans and looked at me.

"To send her to the hospital when she's about six or seven centimeters."

"That's too late. You can check to see if it's headfirst at home, but I'd like her in the hospital when she's four. This baby needs to be watched closely."

"And she's not buying it?"

"You got it—and she's really stubborn. Just make sure she understands your role, and send her in as soon as she's active." I nodded.

A few days later, I visited Patty at her home. She met me at the front door, her mouth set in a stubborn line. "I saw you with Joe the other day. Did he talk to you after I left?"

I explained the gist of our conversation. The whole time I spoke, she looked into her lap and slowly shook her head. When I finished, she glanced up, and anger flashed in her eyes. Behind the anger lurked something else, and I remembered Joe's apprehension.

"I think he's overreacting. I want to stay home as long as I can."

"I can't agree to that anymore."

"But I'm hiring you. He's not. You're working for me."

"He's my backup doctor. I won't ignore him."

"What if it's too late to send me to the hospital when you get here? You'll have to deliver me at home." It was a statement, not a question.

"No, I'd call 911 and let them take over."

"Why?" she cried. "You could just say it was too late to transfer me."

"Patty, I know how much you want your dream birth, but it's your baby's well-being we're talking about. Besides, my relationship with Joe is too valuable for me even to consider deceiving him."

"More valuable than my birth experience?" she pleaded.

"Yes, it really is. It represents my ability to help many more women than just you. I'm not going to do it, Patty. Period."

Although she didn't like it one bit, she put a good face on it and smiled as I left. But I no longer trusted her.

A month later, ten days before Patty's due date, I returned home from attending another woman's birth. I pulled on my nightgown and had almost fallen asleep when my phone rang. I groaned inwardly when I heard Patty's voice.

"I'm in very early labor, but there's this bloody show like you get in late labor, so I'm confused. Could you come check me?"

Relief replaced my dismay as I realized she wasn't asking me to come to stay. She lived so close, I figured I would probably be back home within thirty minutes. I pulled on tights and a Polartec jacket, not even changing from my long flannel nightgown. Taking just a few basic supplies, I arrived at Patty's house about seven minutes later.

She'd left the front door unlocked, so I let myself in and climbed a narrow circular stairway. Patty and her husband, Fred, stood in the bathroom doorway gazing in puzzlement at her palm. I gasped when I looked at the goopy stuff in her hand. It resembled a mixture of peanut butter, tar, coffee grounds, and thick pea soup, differing dramatically from common, garden-variety meconium.

Disbelief numbed me, and I knew I wouldn't be going back home any time soon. In the hospital, we call that type of meconium "dead baby mec" because it's the end result of a trauma severe enough to cause total relaxation of the rectal sphincter. It happens at death.

When I found my voice, I said, "Patty, is this what you called bloody show?"

"No, this is different," she said. "What is it?" She scrubbed her hand with a washcloth, but it was sticky as library paste. Smudges still remained when she stopped wiping.

"It's meconium, Patty, really bad meconium. You didn't tell me your water had broken." I heard fear in my own voice, reflecting my unwillingness to believe what I was seeing. For a fleeting moment, I gave into my worst suspicions, believing she'd tricked me into arriving in late, late labor. Then I saw that her confusion equaled my alarm.

"It didn't break. There's only been the mucus until now."

"It must have broken," I said, dropping to my knees to listen for the baby's heartbeat. "It has to break for meconium to come out."

I heard nothing through the stethoscope except Patty's pulse booming at about eighty beats per minute. Nothing else. "There wasn't even a little bit? Maybe some brownish stuff?" I asked, still listening. Silence.

"No, nothing. I didn't even think it was labor, but then there was that chunk of really bloody mucus. I know that can mean late labor, so that's why I called you. What's happening?"

My mouth felt like cotton. "Lie down, Patty, so I can listen better." She scrambled on the bed, and another tablespoon of dark slime seeped out. "Patty, this doesn't look good. I want you to do everything I tell you. Speed is what counts."

"Okay, okay, but what's wrong?" she asked, beginning to whimper.

"I'm not sure yet."

I turned the Doppler this way and that. Nothing. I peeled open a glove wrapper, and Patty automatically spread her knees.

Fred stood at the top of the spiral stairway twisting his hands together and staring at me, his face blank.

"Fred, bring the phone closer, please." He set the phone beside me and backed against the far wall. I couldn't tell if fear or general ineptitude caused his wooden behavior. He moved like a toy soldier.

My fingers quickly found Patty's cervix. In spite of the fact that she'd said she wasn't in labor, she was already five centimeters dilated, and when I felt the baby's hair, my last shred of doubt about the broken bag disappeared.

I feared a prolapsed umbilical cord. I suspected the baby's head pressed against the cord, cutting off circulation so severely that it had already killed him. I swung my fingers everywhere in the silver dollar–sized opening, but I felt only a strand of mucus as narrow as a cocktail straw, as flat as a piece of beach grass. I swept it aside—but it recoiled, snapping back like a loose rubber band. I held my breath.

Carefully, carefully, I slipped my finger beneath it again . . . and it didn't shred apart as mucus would have. I had my diagnosis. Umbilical cords are usually as thick as my thumb, and my heart plummeted as I realized my finger was looped through the smallest, narrowest, most flaccid prolapsed cord I'd encountered in twenty-seven years of OB nursing. And not a single drop of blood flowed through it. It had been drained dry for uncounted minutes, perhaps hours.

Fearing it was too late to make a difference, I pushed the baby's head up to relieve the pressure and said, "Patty, turn over onto all fours and put your butt high in the air. Fred, call 911 to come, and then wait for them at the curb."

"What? What's wrong?" Patty begged, rolling over.

"It's a prolapsed cord. Do you understand that?"

"Yes, it can kill babies," she whispered. "Is mine okay?"

"No, he's in severe distress, Patty. I can't hear the heartbeat at all. We have to get to the hospital right away."

"Oh, God," she keened. "What should I do? Help me."

I stared at Fred. He still held the phone to his ear, and his face looked as flat as pond water. He felt my look and turned, saying, "911 put me on hold."

"Merciful Jesus," I muttered.

Then my heart leaped. The baby's head moved. I snatched the Doppler and pressed it deep into Patty's flesh, just above her pubic hair, and I heard the baby's pulse through the speaker.

But slow. Oh my God, so slow. So irregular I couldn't count it, but I guessed about thirty or forty beats a minute. Much too slow.

"Is that slow one me or the baby?" asked Patty, her voice quavering.

"The slow one's the baby, but at least he's alive."

Patty exhaled her pent-up breath in a ragged sob and then cried quietly, fighting for control.

Fred finally spoke to the 911 operator. He hung up and scrambled down the stairs to await the ambulance. I calculated. Urban neighborhood, but no traffic in the middle of the night, and Alta Bates just over a mile away. I guessed we'd be at the hospital in about fifteen minutes. Maybe a little longer to negotiate the stairway.

I dialed Dr. Weick's answering service. "Hi, this is an emergency. I'm a midwife at a patient's home. She's got a prolapsed cord, and Joe Weick's my backup doctor. I need to speak to him immediately."

Answering service operators can be maddening, but I got lucky. "I'm dialing, honey. I'll stay on the line till he answers. Good luck."

"Bless you," I breathed, as the phone rang.

"Hello," came Joe's voice, thick with sleep.

As I spoke, sleep vanished from his voice. "Do you have a cord pulse?"

"No, it's the most flaccid cord I've ever felt. But his head moved a minute ago, and I heard a weak, erratic heartbeat once through the Doppler."

"I'll meet you at Alta Bates for a cesarean, if the baby's still alive. Are you coming by car?"

"No, by ambulance. There're these weird stairs . . ."

He cut me off. "I'll see you at the hospital."

Patty and I waited in the dark, expecting to hear the siren any minute. To elicit a potentially life-saving pain response from the baby, I scratched his scalp now and then. Once more he jerked away, tossing his head like a circus pony, but otherwise he remained motionless. I heard the heartbeat only once more, even slower.

Where was the ambulance? I glanced at the clock. Eight minutes had passed. I strained my ears. Nothing. "What's keeping them?" bleated Patty.

"I don't know," I muttered.

I called 911 again. In a bland voice, the operator said, "They'd just left when your call came in. I sent another crew from further away, but they'll be there any minute."

I wanted to scream.

Another five minutes passed, and then I cocked my ear. Yes, siren, far away, drawing closer. Loud now, right on the street, right out front. But then . . . quieter, farther away. They'd passed us. "What the hell?" I shouted.

Fred crept up the stairs. Abject with apology, he mumbled, "They didn't even slow down. They crossed Broadway, and went up the hill on the other side."

"Were you standing by the curb?"

"Well, no, I just stood in the door and sort of waved."

Imposing in neither physical presence nor affect, Fred had been easily overlooked by the speeding ambulance driver. But still, I thought, on a street with clear house numbers, they shouldn't have blown right by. I exhaled loudly and said, "Well, they'll figure it out soon enough, I guess," but when another two minutes passed, I gave up. "Let's get outta here. Can you crawl downstairs, Patty?"

But then we heard the heavy thrumming of the ambulance engine, and this time it stopped right out front. Fred ran to let them in, and moments later two men clattered up the stairs.

"Thank God," Patty and I sighed together.

"Okay, folks, what's going on?" said a man with a loud, gruff voice.

"A baby with a prolapsed cord, severe fetal distress," I said. "Third baby, one previous cesarean. Five centimeters, infrequent contractions, no health problems, ten days before term. They're waiting to do a cesarean at Alta Bates. Let's go."

"Who are you?" he said.

"Peggy Vincent. I'm a midwife and . . ."

"Midwife?"

"Yes, I'm a licensed midwife, and . . ."

"Could I see your license?"

"What?"

"Your license. Could I see it?"

"There's a baby with a prolapsed cord here, and you want to see my license?"

"Yeah, I need to know who I'm dealing with, see?"

"God almighty." I exhaled and tried to unclench my jaw. "It's downstairs in my purse by the front door."

I twisted a little so I could see him. Reddish hair, a florid complexion, beer belly like an overweight high school football player gone to seed. Maybe twenty-five or thirty, small blue eyes above puffy cheeks. I squinted to see his name badge. Larry something.

Behind him stood a skinny guy with limp hair like Fred's. No machismo at all. He opened the collapsible stretcher, eyed the tight curves of the stairway, then bent to one of the supply boxes and removed a thermometer.

"I called 911 for a quick, safe trip to the hospital. This is taking too long. Do that stuff en route. You guys missed the house on the first pass, and they're waiting for us at the hospital."

The skinny guy mumbled, "I couldn't read the house number, and I had to drive to the top of the hill to turn around."

Larry interrupted him and spoke to Patty. "Your name, ma'am?" he asked, apparently giving up on my license.

"My baby could die," yelled Patty. "Just get me to the hospital."

"We've got our routines. Things'll go more smoothly if y'all will just cooperate."

"Her name is Patty Wilson," I said. "Hurry."

Fred hugged himself and looked down at the oscillating lights on the untended ambulance. They flashed red-blue-red-blue-red-blue on the bedroom walls.

I took a deep breath and tried to think my way out of this impasse. Fred disappeared into the wallpaper, and I had no power over this blustering Larry. I knew that to him I was just a middle-aged woman in a nightgown kneeling on the floor. He didn't trust me, he didn't like me, and he seemed determined to exert his authority over me.

The other fellow crept forward like a cat hugging the walls and slipped a thermometer in Patty's mouth. She spit it out.

"I'm not sick," Patty screamed. "It's my baby! Get me to the hospital."

"Please, please don't waste time here," I begged, checking his badge. "Wilbur, this is a prolapsed cord. Do you guys know what that is?"

"Of course we know what it is," sighed Larry, rolling his eyes. "We're just waiting for the firemen to arrive." He spoke with exaggerated patience, as if speaking to an imbecile. "There are only two of us. We need more people to get her down that crazy-assed stairway, and it'd be real helpful if we could get some information while we wait." He stepped closer and hitched his tight pants over his gut, lifting his chin in a gesture of defiance.

"There are four of us, not two," I insisted. "There are two of you, there's her husband, and there's me. Let's just pick her up and go."

Fred and Wilbur came closer, but Larry stopped them with a look. "We're gonna do this safely or not at all."

I'd had it. "Patty, come on. I'll help you down the stairs. Fred can drive us."

Patty had both hands on the floor when I sensed Larry moving closer. He stretched out his beefy arm and shoved me back. My hand nearly jerked from Patty's body as I struggled to regain my balance. "Hold it, lady. If I have any more sass from you, believe me, I'll have you arrested for obstructing my job. Everybody just do as I say, y'hear?"

I froze. He towered above me, all 250+ pounds of him. I felt the heat of his rage and feared he might actually strike me. I was powerless.

"Patty, the sooner we make him happy, the sooner we can get out of here."

"That's better," Larry purred.

He had half a page of questions answered when at last we heard the fire truck. The whole house trembled as it stopped out front, adding another flashing red light to the room. One knock, and they entered.

Larry hollered, "Up here."

Two men in full fireman gear came up the stairs. Then they stood looking at the stretcher and the stairway, and I listened as they talked among themselves.

"We can't strap her onto the stretcher that way."

"I don't think that stretcher'd make it around those curves."

"What's the other woman doing?"

"I'm a licensed midwife," I shouted, "and I'm holding the baby's head off a prolapsed cord."

"Well, we can't get the stretcher down unless she lets go." They had their backs to Patty and me.

I trembled, close to exploding again. Fred sighed, Patty wept, and I shouted. Then I saw Fred glance toward the stairway. Another fireman appeared, a guy of about fifty with a weathered face, laugh lines, and the poise of a natural leader. I guessed he might be the captain of the fire engine crew and had been waiting outside with the truck.

"What's the holdup?" he asked.

Larry talked fast. "The stretcher . . . these stairs . . . this midwife person . . ."

"There's no way this stretcher's gonna make it down that stairway," said the captain. "Any jackass can see that. Just pick her up."

"Yes!" I shouted as they all jumped to obey. Rickety and unstable as we were, we moved in one fluid wave down the stairway. Fred woke his step-daughter and hurried her and his sleeping toddler to a neighbor's house.

The EMTs lifted Patty through the ambulance's double doors and locked the stretcher in place along the left side. With my hand still inside her vagina, I scrambled onto the stretcher beside her. Larry climbed in back, and Fred sat in front beside Wilbur, who flipped on the siren and pulled away from the curb. I caught a glimpse of the shocked faces of curious neighbors in bathrobes, their features illuminated by the garish ambulance lights.

"They're expecting us at Alta Bates Hospital," I reminded Wilbur. He nodded.

As we approached the main street, I shifted my weight in anticipation of a right turn. When Wilbur veered left instead, I was thrown off balance and nearly yanked Patty off the stretcher as I scrambled for footing. "You're going the wrong way!" I yelled.

"He knows where he's going," snarled Larry.

"Impossible. Alta Bates is in Berkeley, and Berkeley is now directly behind us!"

"Um, sir, she's right," mumbled Fred. "Alta Bates Hospital is the other way."

"I'm goin' to Alta Bates. I only know one way to get there," said Wilbur.

"Christ, you've just added a mile-and-a-half to the trip," I groaned as Wilbur took the equivalent of the long way around a circle, more than dou-bling the time the one-mile trip should have taken.

At last we arrived at the hospital. Leaving Fred with a compassionate nurse who led him away, we rolled through the double doors of the OR. The response of the staff said it all. "Where in God's name have you been?" they shouted.

"I'll explain later," I said, glowering at the retreating EMTs.

"Do you have a cord pulse?" asked Dr. Weick, his voice crackling.

"No, I've never felt one. Just an occasional erratic heartbeat, and the baby's head moved a couple of times."

"Let me check her." He examined Patty. When he removed his hand, he looked at the telltale meconium and raised his eyebrows to me.

"That's how it looked when I got to her house," I said sadly.

He listened for a heartbeat. He listened everywhere, then shook his head.

The operating room door opened, and the head neonatologist, Dr. Matthew Fall, pushed a portable ultrasound scanner into the room. "Have you got a pulse?" he asked.

"Just an occasional heart beat that hasn't been heard for the last twenty minutes," said Dr. Weick. He then turned to Patty and took her hand. "Patty, your baby didn't make it. He was probably pretty far gone by the time Peggy got there. It's no one's fault. I don't know what you could have done differently." He paused and smoothed back her hair, a poignant gesture. "I don't see any reason to subject you to a cesarean."

Tears trickled from Patty's eyes. She bit her lips and nodded, wordless.

I turned aside to wipe my own tears and saw the neonatologist plug in the ultrasound machine. He squirted gel onto the probe and approached Patty. Dr. Weick stared at him, but Dr. Fall didn't meet his eyes. He placed the scanner on Patty's belly and flipped on the machine. Why was he insisting on this, I wondered.

Dr. Weick continued talking to Patty. "We'll move you to one of the regular rooms and induce labor, because your contractions seem to have stopped. Is that right, Peggy?"

"Yes," I mumbled, my eyes fixed on the flickering sonogram screen. "I've only felt two since I've been with her."

The neonatologist easily found the baby's head . . . then the curved spine . . . the chest . . . the heart. The heart that wasn't beating. We all stared at it. Nothing.

I expected Dr. Fall to step back, but he continued holding the scanner against her skin, continued to stare at the motionless heart. And then it contracted. Once.

Then, after a long pause . . . once more.

In an emotionless voice, he said, "There's heart motion. Let's cut."

What? a voice within me screamed. What are you thinking?

No one moved. Patty's eyes traveled between Dr. Weick and the neonatologist. Dr. Weick frowned at Dr. Fall and said, "Matt, what would we be accomplishing? Don't you think . . ."

Dr. Fall barked, "Come on, let's get started. There's a heartbeat. You all saw it."

In the hospital hierarchy, he outranked Dr. Weick, who pressed his lips together in resignation. Everyone moved to begin the surgery, but no sense of hope propelled the staff—just rapid, mechanical obedience to orders.

I wanted to run to Patty and tell her to refuse surgery, but it wasn't my place. It wasn't my right, my job. Besides, how do you tell a woman to stop a doctor from trying to save her baby's life? How do you tell her to deny her own hopeful heart? How do you explain the profound consequences of oxygen lack to someone who just heard her baby's heartbeat, a sound that signifies life?

So, under general anesthesia, Patty had a cesarean. In a few minutes, Dr. Weick lifted a flaccid little boy from her body, and a nurse transferred him to the resuscitation table. Led by Dr. Fall, a team of three specialists went to work on the baby with the precision and skill of a military drill team.

I looked at the clock. 3:04 A.M.

"Have they got a pulse?" asked Dr. Weick. His voice sounded sad and resigned.

I caught the eye of the resuscitation nurse. "No pulse," she said.

Other than the whoosh of the oxygen bag, the occasional terse request for drugs to stimulate the heart and lungs, and the clang of an instrument tossed into a basin, no sound penetrated the room's cold silence except the soft, almost continuous murmur of the neonatal nurse. "No pulse. No pulse." My eyes met Joe's above our surgical masks. His looked haunted, and I knew mine did too.

3:12 A.M. Just two more minutes, and then they'd stop trying. The longer it went on, the more certain was brain damage if the baby survived.

"No pulse. Still no pulse."

3:14 A.M. The ten-minute cutoff point ticked past.

But they continued. Still Dr. Fall forced air into the baby's lungs with the bag and mask. Still he performed cardiac compression. Still he ordered drugs and fluids to be administered through an IV line. The nurse looked at me, frowned, and gave a helpless shrug. I wanted to scream, Stop!

A few minutes later, the baby's heart began beating. An occasional beat at first, then closer together. Then a countable pulse. Moments later they rushed him to intensive care and attached him to life support.

Patty and Fred named him Luke.

For the next few days, while the doctors subjected the baby to every possible test to determine brain function, Luke's parents prayed, but they didn't know what to pray for. Life or death? Some sign to give them joy that Luke still lived? Or a swift and loving release from the torture his life might become?

The doctors finally declared Luke brain dead, and Patty and Fred tearfully signed papers to discontinue life support. It would finally end as I had expected it to end from the moment I'd seen the meconium in Patty's upstairs bathroom. I just wished Patty hadn't had major surgery and that Luke hadn't been subjected to days of constant testing.

The next morning, while his parents held him for the first time, Luke's nurse disconnected the IV, the monitors, and the respirator so he could die peacefully in his mother's arms. Patty's tears dripped onto her son's head. She kissed his eyes that would never gaze into her own. She fondled the soft shell-folds of delicate ears that would never hear her voice. She traced with her fingertip the curves of his lips that would never nurse from her aching breasts. Fred sat quietly beside them holding Luke's bare foot between his two hands, feeling the softness of his son's plump little heel.

Patty spoke to the nurse through quiet tears. "How much longer?"

"Not long. Maybe ten or fifteen minutes," she replied, her voice soft with compassion.

But she was wrong. Luke survived.

When his heart still beat twelve hours later, and his lungs still drew in air, the pediatrician inserted a feeding tube, and his parents began to face the reality of life with a profoundly disabled child.

Two days later, Dr. Weick and I happened upon Patty in the lobby. Anger crackled from her every glance, all of it directed at the ambulance attendants and the neonatologist who had insisted on performing the cesarean.

"Somebody should pay for this," she said. "Luke's death would have been sad enough, but his life will be even sadder. Blind, deaf, paralyzed, spastic. What kind of life is that?" She jabbed the elevator button and rode up to the nursery.

As Joe and I left the hospital, he shook his head. "How tragic. And it'll end up in court. That baby will need lifelong care. Who's your lawyer?"

"My lawyer? Why would I need a lawyer? I didn't do anything wrong."

He stared at me. "Haven't you notified your insurance carrier?"

"No, I never gave it a thought. Luke was probably brain dead by the time I got to her house, but if he'd ever had a chance, the EMTs blew it with their delays. I don't honestly think it made any difference, but I'm sure you and I don't have anything to worry about."

He studied me for a moment before saying, "Peggy, you've been in hospitals long enough to know that guilt has nothing to do with most OB lawsuits. Lawyers follow the money, and you're insured for big bucks. Call your carrier."

"Patty would never sue us," I insisted. "How could she?"

"I've known her longer than you have. Patty's grieving now. She's suffered terribly, and with some people, that brings out the worst side of their personality."

"But she'd never sue us, Joe. She wouldn't have a case."

"She doesn't need a case. She's got a damaged baby, and that's all she needs."

"But . . ."

He gripped my arm. "Get a lawyer. Today." He walked away but stopped and turned back. "Today," he repeated.

I spent the next few hours on the phone with the American College of Nurse Midwives, my malpractice carrier, and a San Francisco law firm. Then I sat down to type my recollection of the events surrounding Luke's birth while it was fresh in my mind.

Two weeks later, Patty and Fred buckled their deaf, probably blind, and profoundly retarded infant into a car seat and drove him to a full-time residential facility that cares for children like Luke. Then they went shopping for a personal injury lawyer.

My insurance company referred me to Peter Carr, a medical malpractice defense attorney. Several months later I went to his office to meet with the Wilson's lawyer and the ambulance company's defense lawyer. I would give my deposition as a witness. While we waited for them to arrive, Peter brought me up to date.

"Initially the Wilsons wanted to sue Dr. Fall for wrongful life," he began.

"Wrongful life?" I interrupted. "That's quite a term."

"Patty argued that he shouldn't have ordered the cesarean, let alone continued the resuscitation for so long. But her lawyer refused to take the case on those terms. He said no jury would condemn a physician for trying to save a life. So she sued the ambulance company."

"Well, those guys were incompetent," I said, "but I'm not convinced it would have made much difference."

"Don't offer that opinion. Just answer their questions."

A few minutes later, two other lawyers walked in together, laughing loudly. The ambulance company's lawyer, a short, crinkly-eyed guy in a flapping sports jacket, bounced on his toes and greeted me as though I were his new tennis partner. The Wilsons' lawyer stood erect in a buttoned navy suit with a regimental striped tie. He smoothed back his graying hair and smiled, showing white teeth. It looked like a smile he practiced each morning in his bathroom mirror.

I didn't trust them, but I knew I'd done everything according to standard procedure. Looking over my notes, I could find no flaw in my actions, not one spot where a lawyer or medical expert could say I should have acted differently. So as we waited for the stenographer, I felt calm. I knew my facts. I folded my hands and listened to the repartee of the three expensively dressed lawyers. I marveled that these men who might someday be tearing each other apart in front of a jury obviously had many years of friendship behind them.

"I had to make reservations at Chez Panisse a month in advance."

"What's our starting time on the golf course this Saturday?"

"Johnny-boy, when are you going to show us the new boat?"

The recorder arrived, efficient-looking in a pale blue silk suit. Fingers with professionally manicured nails click-click-clicked at the keys as the two lawyers questioned me.

The deposition began in jocose friendliness, as if we'd all shared teething biscuits in nursery school. But soon the questioning focused on the nature of my intended role, the scope of my practice, my professional relationship with Dr. Weick, and the details of the scene with the ambulance attendants. The lawyers sat forward like alert terriers, eyeing each other and watching me. They became adversaries, but they played it like a subliminal game, the surface as still as a lily pond to the casual observer.

My lawyer sat back and watched. He tapped a pencil eraser on the polished tabletop, occasionally making notes on a yellow legal pad. "Don't answer that," he said once, when Patty's lawyer asked my opinion of the baby's condition on my arrival.

When the stenographer finally turned off her machine, the lawyers stood up. Their adversarial mood of alley cats in a standoff vanished. By the time I shook their hands, picked up my papers, and turned to leave, they were acting like littermates.

The next week I returned to review and sign my deposition. Peter folded his hands and said, "There's no money in dead baby cases."

"What?" Had I heard him correctly?

"It's too bad, of course, that the baby lived, but since he did, well, now there's big money at stake. Dead babies aren't worth much, just a one-time settlement, but when a baby needs financial support for life, the stakes go up. Way up. You did well in the deposition," he continued, "and you'll do fine in court, if it comes to that." He shifted in his chair, looked out the window, and paused before continuing. "I feel confident the Wilsons have no interest in suing you at this point."

"Well, God, I hope not! Why would they?"

"I'm getting to that," he said, holding up his hand. "As I said, at this point I'm sure they'll only call you as a witness. Their lawyer is interested in preserving you as a friendly witness against the ambulance company, but be careful. You should know that the ambulance company carries limited liability, only $100,000. That amount, less legal fees, won't begin to cover Luke's expenses. I suspect the Wilsons will go after the big bucks."

"Big bucks? You mean, deep pocket?"

"Yes, it refers to whoever carries the most insurance."

"Mmm-hmm, deep pocket," I said, feeling my mouth set into a grim half-smile. "I've heard that term for years."

"Yes, it means the lawsuit follows the money trail, naming everyone until it finally taps the sources with the greatest coverage. You're insured for a million, and so is Dr. Weick, so you're both in the line of fire. But for now, you can rest easy. The Wilsons aren't interested in naming you or Dr. Weick in the case, at least not yet."

I left his spacious top-floor office feeling as if I ought to look overhead to see if a black cloud followed me. "Not yet." Had I heard him right?

As it turned out, I needed to wait only six months to find out.

～ Cut Me!

Patty Wilson's disastrous delivery and tragic outcome haunted me as I delivered healthy babies in the weeks following Luke's birth, but Joe Weick and I rarely talked about it. The memories were too painful. Powerless to affect the outcome, I think we both hoped the threat of being named in the lawsuit would go away if we pretended to ignore it.

"A lawsuit is the only way parents of these brain-damaged kids can get enough money to care for them," my lawyer had said.

"All doctors should contribute to a state fund dedicated to supporting kids like Luke, where there's been no malpractice. But the lawyers would squash that idea because they want their piece of the pie," Joe had said in the days after Patty's delivery.

"How could they sue you?" Margaret and Bonnie asked me when I voiced my fears. "You did everything right."

I explained, "It seems being right isn't enough. Being unlucky is apparently all it takes to be sued."

"Patty would never sue you," Margaret insisted, but without my protecting cushion of innocence and ignorance, I was no longer so sure. The possibility hung over me like a storm cloud, and my mind reeled with the enormity of it.

Everyone seemed to be keeping an eye on those distant dark clouds, wondering if they'd erupt into a downpour or blow over. Sandi and Lindy, my closest midwife friends, knew all the details, as did my assistants. Because of the high profile issues involved and the amount of insurance carried by Alta Bates, administrators examined the hospital's liability. Even the nurses who had assisted at the cesarean scrambled to check their personal insurance policies.

But, other than occasional comments that rumbled like distant thunder, there was very little talk. I said to Rog one evening, "It seems as if everyone's practicing magical thinking, like if we don't mention it, it doesn't exist." I'd told my children about Luke's birth, but they were fourteen and sixteen at the time, teenagers with their own lives. When nothing more happened in the following weeks, I knew they believed the storm had blown out to sea.

A month after Patty and Fred put Luke into a home with other severely handicapped children, Margaret and I drove to the suburbs to care for Erica. I'd met her seven years earlier when Dr. Rider, the control freak, had reluctantly entered Alta Bates's birth center to deliver her second baby. In the intervening years, Erica and her husband, Jordan, had traded crunchy-granola Berkeley for the monochromatic suburbs for the same reason many did: the good schools.

Erica had said she'd have her next baby at home—but only if I could be there. Now I'd been at her house for the past four hours, and her wish was about to be granted. I tossed my exam glove into the wastebasket while Margaret checked the baby's heartbeat. Stretching, I stood with my back to the bed, staring out the patio door. Brittle with drought-shriveled grass, identical backyards stretched up and down the block. Every yard the same size, each with a swing set out back and a Volvo, BMW, or SUV out front. Everything about this birth seemed as predictable as the Weber grill on each patio. The baby's heartbeat—we knew it was a boy—had chugged along steadily for four hours. Erica was eight centimeters, and I'd just broken her bag of water to nudge her into the final phase of labor.

Erica's quick wit and flip humor had always entertained me, and I wondered how she was adjusting to the suburbs, if she felt bored by the sameness. I'd always known about the suburban dress code, but every time I drove through the tunnel and into the 'burbs, I forgot to switch my Birkenstocks or Tevas for something less Berkeleyish until it was too late.

I figured Erica was strong enough to stand up not only to the dress code but also to what appeared to be a lawn, car, and house code, as well. I felt equally sure that I wouldn't have been so successful. All those maroon Volvos precision-parked in double driveways gave me the willies. My beat-up VW bug looked like a baby whale stranded in a herd of sleek seals.

I sipped my iced tea and looked again at the peaceful lineup of backyards. Does anything exciting ever happen here?

Margaret looked puzzled. "I can't hear the baby's heartbeat," she said in a voice that meant she felt certain everything was fine, but for some odd reason, right at that moment she just couldn't find it. She frowned, twisting the Doppler this way and that.

Startled out of my reverie, I stared at her, feeling my chest tighten. Vivid images of Patty's labor flipped before my eyes like flash cards, and I knew Margaret was thinking the same thing. Another prolapsed cord? At such moments, I wonder what possessed me to be a midwife. Why not a lawyer, or better yet, an accountant? A job where a budget out of balance would be the worst thing that could happen.

I knelt beside Erica. "He sounded perfect a minute ago," I said, my voice flat with artificial composure. "Check again."

She aimed the probe everywhere, then shook her head and handed me the Doppler. Jordan sat up straight and stared at me. Silent. Frowning a little.

That's so weird, I thought. I just felt the baby's big head filling the whole space within a little rim of cervix. If it's a cord, it's hidden, occult.

I listened. Ka-whoosh, ka-whoosh, ka-whoosh. But that was Erica's pulse. Slow, loud, and throbbing. I wanted to hear the faster, dancing heartbeat of a healthy baby who ought to be jitterbugging into the world in about half an hour. This third child shouldn't be giving us any trouble, especially since Erica had already zoomed into late labor, nearly fully dilated. She lay on her back looking at us, mild concern furrowing her brow. With her long, graceful arms and legs, wide smile, and big brown eyes, Erica resembled an Italian movie star from the fifties. A very pregnant Sophia Loren with short hair.

I listened everywhere, but I couldn't find the baby's quick, clickety-clack pulse either. My own heart rate soared as I opened another glove and examined her.

Just the head, nothing else. No loop of umbilical cord. But still no heartbeat. Disbelief nearly drowned me. I pushed the head up, poking it, trying to elicit a response, but mostly trying to nudge it off what I knew had to be a hidden piece of umbilical cord. It had to be there somewhere.

I gave another shove to the head, and, pocketa-pocketa-pocketa, his heartbeat bounced from the speaker. We all heard it, and Erica smiled. "Whew, I was worried for a moment. Thank goodness he's okay."

But I didn't feel so confident, and Margaret sat very still beside me, eyes wide. An all-too-classic script played out in my mind. You break the bag of water, you lose the heartbeat. You push the head up, the heartbeat comes back. The next scene in the worst-case scenario calls for the heartbeat to fade away again as the head settles back into the pelvis with the next contraction. Then we'd have a diagnosis: occult prolapse of the umbilical cord, meaning the cord is invisible, hidden, but the baby's blood supply is cut off or at least impeded.

Most midwives spend their entire careers without ever encountering this phenomenon, one of the true Code Blue emergencies of obstetrics. The umbilical cord works like a scuba diver's air hose; if something pinches it off, the diver will die unless he rises to the surface immediately. But it's usually breech babies who are at risk for prolapsed cords, and since midwives rarely deliver breeches, we seldom have to deal with this emergency.

But those reassuring odds didn't apply to me. I'd encountered prolapsed cords twice before at home births. Both times the baby had been headfirst, and one had been Luke.

Erica jerked as another contraction began, much stronger than the previous ones. With my fingers still inside, I felt more of her cervix melt away as the baby's head plunged into her vagina.

"Gone again," said Margaret, looking frightened.

I pushed hard on the head. Erica looked at me in shocked disbelief, her raised brow and wide eyes asking why I seemed to be working at cross-purposes with her efforts. Jordan stood up, and I heard his breathing quicken.

"It's back again, a little slow, about 90. Okay, it's picking up now, really fast, over 180. Steady now." Margaret chewed her lip. She knew.

If I could find the cord, I might be able to correct the situation. I explained things to Jordan and Erica briefly and said, "This is going to hurt, but it's important. Your baby's in trouble, and I'm going to try to fix it."

Erica nodded vigorously and said, "Sure. It's just pain. That won't kill me. Go ahead." She grabbed Jordan's hand and brought it to her mouth, pressing his knuckles against her bared teeth. Her breathing hissed in and out as I forced my fingers all the way up beside the baby's head. Carefully I probed the circumference, checking every quadrant.

Then I found it, just the edge. A smooth, looping arc that felt almost like the top of the baby's ear. But it had a slow and throbbing pulse. As I felt along its length, my finger slipped into the loop. It lay alongside the baby's temple and jaw, getting squeezed each time his hard head crushed the cord against Erica's pelvic bones.

"Hold on, Erica. Here goes," I said. Pressing my fingertips together, I pushed the loop up, up, up, trying to get it beyond the head, into the baby's neck or chest area. My whole hand squeezed alongside the head. I knew how painful it must be, but Erica just pulled Jordan's hand over her eyes and sustained one long continuous moan, tossing her head from side to side until I finished. Otherwise, she remained motionless.

I thought I'd done it. For about two minutes I couldn't feel the cord at all. Margaret smiled broadly, tapping her finger and nodding in rhythm to the bouncy, healthy heartbeat we could all hear through the Doppler's speaker.

Then the entire loop slipped past my fingers, past the head, and down into Erica's vagina, almost to the opening. The baby's pulse plunged. 50 . . . 40 . . . 30.

"Okay, we've got a big problem here," I said, jumping up. "Erica, flip onto all fours, stick your butt in the air, and stay that way. Jordan, there are several hospitals out here. Which is closest?"

"John Muir," he whispered, pale as smoke.

"Great," I spun around and punched three numbers into the phone. "We need to get there right away. Erica needs an emergency cesarean."

Then I saw Margaret staring at me open-mouthed, her face rigid. "What?" I mouthed, as the phone rang in my ear.

"You're not calling 911, are you?" she said under her breath. "I mean, after what happened with Patty?"

"No! God, no. I called Information, 411, for John Muir's number."

Margaret slumped with relief.

I twisted the cord around my fingers, wishing we were in Berkeley instead of way out in the suburbs. Erica's voice jerked me from my reverie when she said, "Can't you do the cesarean here?" I spun around. Was she joking at a time like this? No, she wasn't.

The operator answered.

"John Muir Hospital, labor and delivery . . . Thanks." I jotted the number on a torn glove wrapper.

"Just cut me," insisted Erica. "Do it now. I mean it."

"No! God, Erica, no. You need anesthesia and IV's and . . ."

"I'll hold still, I swear. You know how. You've seen hundreds. Just cut me."

"*NO!*" I shouted, and I turned my back. "Jordan," I said, grabbing her statue-like husband and twisting him to face me. "Carry her to the car upside down like she is." He didn't move and I shook him a little. "Jordan! Right now. What kind of car do you have?"

"Um, a Volvo wagon."

"Great! Put her in the wayback. I've got to make a quick phone call, but I'll be out there before the next contraction."

He turned like Frankenstein's monster with stiff limbs and bulging eyes, but he bent, lifted her in his arms, and walked out. Watching him, I knew he'd have carried out the refrigerator, too, if I'd asked.

As I dialed, I shouted, "Margaret, turn off the oven, open the car for Jordan, then push the baby's head up." She dashed off.

Thank God the other kids were with their grandmother. One less thing to think about, I realized, checking items off my mental list.

Please, please, please, I silently chanted while the phone rang. The attitude of whoever picked up the phone could determine the survival of Erica's baby. As a home birth practitioner, I operated on the thinnest margin of acceptance within the medical community. One step out of line, one mile out of my neighborhood, one procedure code out of my parameters, and I opened myself to persecution and vilification. I had experienced both. When far from my home base, I always feared some mother or baby would suffer because of my circumstances. In Berkeley, everybody at the hospital knew me, but out here in the land of strip malls, I might as well have been a tree trimmer for all the credibility I had.

A woman's voice answered on the third ring.

"Hi, you don't know me," I said, willing a composure I didn't feel into my voice. "I'm a licensed midwife with a practice in Berkeley, but I'm in Concord with a woman having her third baby. She has a prolapsed cord with a cephalic presentation, and she's nine centimeters and pushy. We're on our way in by car. *Please!* Please, please, *please* have everything ready for an immediate cesarean when we get there."

"I'll try my best. Good luck to you," she said. I sagged with relief. Whoever she was, clerk, nurse, or volunteer, she didn't know me from Adam's housecat, and she could have turned this day into a living hell.

I grabbed Erica's chart, the Doppler, two sterile gloves, and my purse, dashed out the door, and helped Margaret out of the back of the Volvo. "Go ahead to the ER, Margaret, and prepare them for us," I said as I crawled in beside Erica.

Jordan peeled rubber like a fifteen year old on a joy ride as he turned right and headed for the back roads. I squirted KY jelly onto a glove and plunged my whole hand into Erica. With her bottom showing above the car windows, she was perfectly visible to everyone in the cars we passed, but she didn't care. Neither did I.

"Hurry, hurry," she begged Jordan and then screamed as another contraction ripped into her. I felt like screaming myself as the contraction ground my fingers to mush. As hard as her uterus tried to push the baby down, I tried just as hard to push him up, to keep the pressure off the cord. Quickly my fingers went numb, then my hand and wrist. By the time I saw the hospital in the distance, it felt like the wringer on my grandmother's old-fashioned washing machine had chewed up my arm.

Jordan swerved onto the main drag a block before the hospital and slammed on the brakes. At eight A.M., the peak of morning rush hour, four solid lanes of cars stopped us. We needed to make a left turn to reach the emergency room. About eight cars idled ahead of us at a red light. Boxed in,

Jordan morphed into James Bond. He flipped on the emergency blinkers, flashed his headlights, blew the horn, and lurched onto the median strip. Jordan smashed an entire half a block of flowers and low shrubs as he roared to the end of the divider. I glimpsed the astonished faces of bug-eyed drivers to our right as we blasted past them. Their jaws dropped, but not a single driver honked as we streaked by, gallumphed off the curb, and turned left against the light, taking the corner on two wheels.

Margaret was arguing with an orderly outside the emergency room doorway, and she flung her arm in our direction as we stopped beside her. The orderly's face drained to the hue of skimmed milk when he saw Erica's rear end with my arm disappearing inside, both of us writhing in pain. He ran inside, reappearing in ten seconds with a stretcher and two nurses.

Somehow they moved Erica and me onto the stretcher as if we were welded together. She hunched onto her knees with her chest and head on the sheet, and I knelt behind her. Margaret threw a sheet over Erica and ran alongside the gurney. An ER nurse zoomed us at high speed through the corridors, into an elevator, down a hallway—and then we zipped around another corner and turned into a labor room.

"No!" I yelled. "No, no, not a labor room. The operating room. They're expecting us." A crowd of people in green OR scrub suits ran our way. Something in my tone, and perhaps the stampeding reception committee, convinced the nurse that maybe I knew what I was talking about. She did a 180 in the middle of the hall, flew back the way we'd come, rounded another corner and slammed to a standstill in the operating room.

Then the hoard of professionals surrounded us and shifted Erica to the operating table, me still attached by my numb arm. Numb, that is, except for the tip of my middle finger.

A pulse. I still felt the baby's erratic pulse in that loop of umbilical cord. 60, 100, zero, 50.

Questions. Everyone talking at once. Clattering basins. Shouting. People everywhere. The squeak of an IV pole. Green sheets. More questions.

"Hold it!" shouted the obstetrician, taking charge. "What's her name?"

Before I could answer, Erica spoke for herself in a way that none of us will ever forget. "My name's Erica Slade," she responded, as rapidly as machine gun fire. "I was born April 15, 1960, and this is my third baby. I'm a week overdue, and my blood type is A-positive. Cut me. Save my baby. I don't need drugs or gas. I swear I won't move. Just cut me right now. Hurry."

Silence. People exchanged glances. The anesthesiologist leaned toward me and whispered, "Where'd you find her? She's fantastic!"

"Aaaah," I groaned. Erica's contraction chewed my hand.

"Erica, we'll operate as soon as possible, but we need more information."

"Okay. My due date was June fifteenth, it's a boy, I weigh 152 pounds, uh, I had a tetanus shot five years ago, I think. Um, I'm 5'6" and I'm not anemic, I, I, what else do you want to know? Please, just cut me." She was still upside-down with her face pressed into the stretcher, talking to the sheet.

The doctor placed his hand on my shoulder and asked, "Is she completely dilated?"

"Yes," I said. "And pushing."

"Do you have a fetal pulse?"

"Yes. Very erratic, but the baby's head is moving."

"Great! Let's go," he said, and everyone went into high gear.

"Yes, hurry, hurry, hurry," chanted Erica. "Just cut me."

The anesthesiologist bent to her ear and said, "We're hurrying as fast as we can, honey. We'll get your little baby outta there in a few minutes, but I need to start an IV first."

Pressing her nose and forehead into the stretcher, her bottom sticking high into the air, Erica wordlessly thrust both arms straight out in front of her, offering them to whoever could get an IV line in place the fastest. She couldn't have chosen a more poignant gesture of total cooperation, a mute plea for speed. I caught a nurse's glance and saw tears fill her eyes.

As he taped the needle in place and allowed fluids to rush into Erica's body, the anesthesiologist again looked at me in awe. "Do you think we could clone her? There's gotta be a market for women with her kind of guts!"

Then four people flipped Erica onto her back, and she was drugged, anesthetized, intubated, and cut. Finally, cut. A scrub nurse threw a drape over Erica, burying me, too. I rested my head on her sweaty thigh as the instruments came closer to my fingers. I whimpered, "Don't forget me. I'm in here. My fingers are right beside the baby's head."

Somewhere on the other side of the drape, they muttered, "Yeah, yeah, yeah, we know," and they continued slicing and dabbing, pushing and cutting. Fighting the fear that my fingers might be amputated at any moment, I twisted my toes inside my shoes and held my breath, waiting for the bite of the scalpel. They got closer and closer. I felt them millimeters away, only a few layers of tissue between us . . . and then the surgeon's fingers touched mine as he said, "Okay, we've got him. You can come out."

I slumped as my arm slithered from Erica's body. Someone helped me to my feet, and I cradled my limp right hand like a dead kitten.

Looking over my shoulder, I saw them lift a pale baby from Erica's abdomen and lower him onto the resuscitation cart. A pediatrician, the anesthesiologist, and a nursery nurse crowded around his limp body. Visions of Luke rushed back. Blind with the pain of circulation returning to my arm, I listened for some sound of life from the child, remembering that lightning can indeed strike the same tree twice.

Finally I heard a gurgle. Then a cough. Another fifteen seconds of silence. Then another cough followed by a weak cry that got stronger and louder and more insistent until it was the loudest sound in the room.

"All right!" said the obstetrician. "That's what we like to hear." He had no idea how wonderful that cry sounded to me. Margaret and I, still in our street clothes in the sterile operating room, fell into each other's arms and wept.

An hour later, drowsy Erica lay in the recovery room with her son in her arms. Stroking his cheek to make him turn toward her breast, she whispered, "It was pretty scary for you, wasn't it, little guy? I was plenty scared myself. Uh-huh, that's one morning none of us will forget."

I watched as he began to nurse. I touched his hand. He grabbed my finger in a reflex grip, and I thought about all those accountants in cubicles, working over their computer spreadsheets. I didn't envy them a bit.

~ *You'd Better Sit Down*

At noon one day in June 1988, my lawyer called.

"Peggy. It's Peter Carr. You'd better sit down."

I felt as if he'd punched me in the stomach, and I sat down. "They're suing me?" Just saying the words took my breath away.

"Yes, both you and Dr. Weick have been named."

The room whirled, and I heard nothing except a ringing in my ears. Midwives are almost never sued, I told myself. Good care, good outcomes, but most of all, good relationships with our patients accounted for the scarcity of lawsuits against us. That's why our insurance premiums were so low.

Eight months had passed since Luke's birth. During various depositions, I'd listened as Patty's lawyer described the baby's condition. Deaf, visually impaired, and profoundly retarded, he could express himself only by screaming. His shrieks echoed through the house nonstop when Patty and Fred brought him home for a visit. The doctors had told them to expect nothing more, not ever.

"Why?" I whispered into the phone. "On what grounds are they suing me?"

"They've only listed 'unprofessional conduct,'" he said, "but Patty's claiming Dr. Weick didn't explain the risks involved when a baby changes position so often."

"Oh, that's bullshit. I heard him that day in the office, trying to get her to listen. She just ignored him and walked out."

"Well, you'll certainly have an opportunity to share that information. Can you come in next week for another deposition?"

"Of course," I said. I had previously been careful not to portray Patty in a negative light, but it would be a relief to speak unguardedly at last, now that I had recovered from the initial shock of actually being sued.

So, for what I hoped would be my final testimony before we began preparing for trial, I headed for the plush San Francisco office building. But as the afternoon progressed, I found it was just more of the same: lawyers twisting speech, pouncing on every turn of phrase, asking the same questions with different slants. Each query seemed an attempt to catch me in a moment of monumental boredom, a slip, a contradiction. I was prevented from elaborating or offering relevant information.

Three hours later, Peter sighed and said, "Well, that went pretty well," but I went home depressed. Now I understood what he'd meant by "Dead babies aren't worth much." If Luke had died, Patty and Fred might have sued the ambulance company, but that would have been the end of it. Because he had survived but needed constant care, everyone circled around a pot of gold.

However, I never lost a moment's sleep. I felt no guilt, no self-doubt, and was certain a trial would exonerate me. But I had no idea the process would drag on for two-and-a-half more years. Nor could I even begin to suspect the final outcome.

PART VII

The measure of my days

~ *Guardian Angel*

H ello? Peggy?" whispered a soft child's voice over the phone. "This is Grace."

"Grace?" I prompted. I didn't know anyone named Grace.

I heard whispering in the background. "Uh, you're Peggy? The midwife?"

"Mmm-hmm."

"Well, you delivered me."

I heard her draw a deep breath, and the rest came out all at once. "I'm ten years old this month, and my mom and dad wanted me to say thanks for helping me get born and everything. We live in Albany, and I take piano lessons, and I help my mom cook dinner. My dad works for, umm, yeah, he works for an elevator company. And my mom teaches nursery school. Bye. Thanks again."

The receiver buzzed in my ear. She had hung up ... and I had no idea who she was.

I pulled out my birth log and thumbed the stained pages back to August, ten years ago. Running my finger down the rows, I looked for a baby named Grace. When I found it, I followed the blue-ruled lines back to the mother's name on the left side of the page.

My eyes filled with tears. Elizabeth and Guido. I remembered everything.

"Ah, my guardian angel!" Guido's relieved shout had boomed out as I pushed through their front door. Mariachi music blared from the neighboring apartment unit.

Not more than six feet from the door, Guido sprawled on the floor, leaning against the couch. Elizabeth hunched between his thighs, naked except for a pair of fuzzy purple socks and a pink plaid ribbon in her hair. Guido peered around her head as he saw me lurch in, banging my gearboxes against the doorframe. When my eyes adjusted to the dim light, I understood his relief. The baby trembled on the Brink of Born, as I often told women who asked, "How much longer?"

I dropped to my knees and stretched out my hands, pondering for the umpteenth time how much additional stress this baby would add to Elizabeth and Guido's already tenuous existence. The simple fact of their survival surprised those who'd known them longest, and the realization that they'd set up housekeeping as a straight and hardworking couple pushed at the boundaries of the miraculous.

But a baby added to the mix? I worried.

During Elizabeth's prenatal visits, Guido had done most of the talking, bouncing on his toes with coiled energy. "Oh, I dunno why I fell in love with Lizabeth," Guido tried to explain. "It ain't a good idea for a dealer to get personal with his customers, but she was special. Still is," he finished softly, looking at her with dewy-eyed devotion.

Elizabeth explained that ten years earlier, when she went to prison following her third drug-related arrest, Guido visited her with pockets full of change. They stood by the vending machines, holding hands and staring at each other while he spent all his money.

"Sheesh, fresh fruit she wanted. Fruit, fruit, fruit."

"No, Guido, you bought me potato chips, too, and remember when I went on that Reese's peanut butter cup binge?"

"Yeah, yeah, but that was the exception. Mostly fruit."

He came every visiting day. They sat at the picnic benches in the hardscrabble prison yard while she told him about the Buddhist nun who taught meditation twice a week. She talked about knitting and poetry classes, and how she'd finally learned to swim in the prison pool. As they planned their life together after her release, she asked him to look for an apartment near a swimming pool and a Buddhist temple.

"A what? A Buddhist temple? Swimming pool? You some crazy broad, y'know?"

"I mean it, Guido. It's important." But three weeks before her release, Guido was arrested for drug trafficking and eventually went to prison.

Elizabeth moved into a local YWCA and immersed herself in Zen Buddhism. She became a vegetarian, gave up alcohol, read books on yoga, and meditated daily at San Francisco's Zen center. She landed a job in a bookstore in North Beach, and for the first time in twelve years, she earned an honest living. She even opened a savings account.

At one of Elizabeth's prenatal visits, Guido shifted from one foot to the other, eager to talk while Elizabeth weighed herself and checked her urine.

"She came all the time when I was inside, you know? I could count on her. The other guys were so jealous. When I got out on parole six years later, me blinking in the light with only a paper bag and a lot of dreams to my name, God, there she was with that gorgeous smile. So fresh and pretty. I couldn't wait to get my hands on her."

"Guido!" But she threw her arms around his neck and kissed him.

"Yeah, but you know all that Buddhist shit? It never stuck with me."

Indeed, Elizabeth never managed to convince Guido that Zen Buddhism could be his salvation, as it had been hers. I sensed Guido figured Elizabeth herself was his deliverance. She had strength for both of them, and in spite of the odds, they stayed straight. Guido worked in construction, she had her job in the bookstore, and somehow they managed to keep from backsliding into their old lifestyle.

Then, at forty-two, Elizabeth missed her period. The pregnancy test came back positive. It had happened a couple of other times in her life, and she'd had abortions, knowing she was in no condition to raise a child, or even to place one for adoption.

"No, no, too many drugs in my body," she said. "I wouldn't wish that on any child. Not on any adoptive parents, either. I still think I did the right thing, those other times." She looked out the window with a wistful stare.

But now she suffered agonies of ambivalence. Her social worker, her sister, Guido, and his parole officer all urged her to schedule an abortion. She and Guido still grappled for a fragile foothold on the tenuous slopes of propriety, and everyone who knew them feared the stress of adding a child to their lives would send them tumbling back into crime.

Torn with self-doubt, Elizabeth nonetheless harbored a shred of hope. She sought guidance from the Zen priest, she wrote to her mother for the first time in five years, and she prayed.

"Children are our teachers," said the priest.

"Babies are messengers from God," her mother replied, enclosing twenty dollars.

But Elizabeth, listening to her heart, still wondered and worried.

Months later as she sat talking to me with both hands stroking her belly, I asked how she'd finally reached her decision. She told me that one day as she meditated, a white light appeared, and a clear voice told her that the embryonic soul she carried within her was an angel of grace, a little girl, an affirmation of life and love.

"I will bow to something bigger than I am," she'd whispered aloud. "I will say yes to the future."

From then on she stood as strong and tall as a sequoia. Despite Guido's dismay, she remained adamant in her decision to give birth to a new life.

"Oh, God," said Guido later, running his hands through his dark hair. "Oh, God, Peggy, I was scared. I thought maybe she was on drugs again, you know, her brain fried for good. Such a crazy choice. But she just looked at me and wouldn't say nuthin'. She put her arms around me, and I didn't have no choice, did I? I mean, if I wanted to stay with her—and I did—it looked like we was gonna have a kid. But I was so scared."

The added obligations terrified him. One evening Guido railed against their financial situation and the fearful additional responsibility they were about to accept. "I can walk out this door right now and come back in an hour with more money than I earn in a whole month in construction," he shouted.

"We're not raising our child on dirty money, Guido. If you do this, I'm leaving."

Guido stayed home, and they clung to each other through the long hours till dawn. The next day, Elizabeth began prenatal care with me, planning a home birth as further affirmation of her decision.

At forty-two, and never having given birth before, Elizabeth expected her labor to be arduous, maybe even complicated. With single-minded fanaticism, she devoted herself to the preparation of both mind and body. She ate yogurt, brown rice, and organic produce. She practiced yoga daily. By the end of the pregnancy she could swim a mile without resting. I loaned her books on pregnancy, nutrition, exercise, and childcare. She gobbled them up like M&Ms. And she meditated twice a day, kneeling on a Japanese *zafu* and staring at the calm face of Buddha on her bedroom altar.

As the months passed, Guido calmed down, at least a little. He still thrashed in bed at night and had frequent panic attacks, moments when he hyperventilated and broke into a clammy sweat. But his eyes softened whenever he looked at Elizabeth. His breathing quieted when she put her hand on his cheek. The tense lines around his mouth relaxed when he gazed at her rounded shape. He came to every prenatal appointment.

"Oh, Mother of God, just look at her, will you? Ain't she somethin'? You ever seen anything so beautiful?" he said, as she lay bare-bellied on the exam table. With callused fingers, he touched the moving baby parts through her stretched skin, and his eyes grew round with awe. "I can't believe how much I love her belly. I've always preferred skinny women with big tits . . ."

"Guido!"

". . . and Elizabeth was skinny, but she never had much in the tit department."

"My God, Guido," but she giggled.

"But now I'm a pig in shit. This is great. I got a skinny lady with big tits and this insane pumpkin belly stickin' out the middle that I'm madly in love with. God, I'm the luckiest man alive."

Strong as Elizabeth was, I knew she feared labor and had made her decision to have a home birth partly because of her terror of the easy availability of drugs in the hospital. "What if it's more painful than I can bear?" she asked during one visit. "I've been clean for more than eight years, but not a day goes by that I don't crave drugs. I'm afraid if I'm in the hospital, they'll offer me narcotics, and I think I'd take something, and, well, I'd be a junkie again."

But contemplating childbirth without the option of pain relief made her eyes go blank with fear.

Guido, however, never doubted she'd give birth at home with ease. "Aww, whaddaya talkin' about, woman? Holy St. Joseph, you're strong as an ox, I'm tellin' ya. You gonna spit this bambino out like wet soap. Trust me, I know you better'n anybody, right?" She nodded, still scared, and he continued, "Just relax, it's gonna be a piece a pink Italian wedding cake."

From the moment labor awakened her just before dawn, the pains piled on sharper and closer than she'd expected. Then, at eight A.M., midway through breakfast, Elizabeth's bag of water broke.

"Oh, my God, Guido, the baby's coming. Right now!"

Not a calm man under the best of circumstances, Guido totally lost his composure when he saw Elizabeth strip off her clothes and flop naked to the living room floor. He ran around in circles. He jerked open the front door and looked up and down the balcony, came back inside . . . and changed his shirt. Then he put a pot of water on to boil, threw a stack of old newspapers into the living room, emptied the wastebaskets, and brought Elizabeth a cup of tea and a cold washcloth she hadn't asked for.

She screamed at him to call me. He couldn't find my phone number.

"It's on the wall beside the telephone," she gasped, pressing her hand to her crotch.

"Which phone?" he hollered as he raced toward their bedroom.

"Guido, we only have one phone. In the kitchen!"

So when my phone rang, Guido sounded a little excited. At least he spoke

English and not Italian. In a voice full of the rhythms and inflections of Don Corleone, he rasped, "Ah, Peggy, itsa comin'! Elizabeth's having the baby really, really fast. There's water all over the place, and some blood even. Lotsa blood, you know? And she's gruntin' like the sow in my mama's back yard in Sicily. You gotta come quick, quick, 'cause I dunno what the fuck I'm doin' here."

Before I got out the door, he phoned again. "Peggy, hurry! It's really comin', I'm a-tellin' ya. Just listen," and I could hear her in the background.

"Call 911, Guido, and tell Elizabeth to yell and blow and try to keep from pushing. I'm on my way." I grabbed my equipment and dashed to my car.

Fuming at traffic, I swore aloud and barely acknowledged stop signs as I hurried to the part of Richmond best known for its high crime rate. When I finally jerked to a halt in front of their apartment, I glanced up and down the block. No ambulance in sight. Probably Guido had been too distracted to call.

With California in the fifth year of an epic drought, I'd long ago stopped expecting green grass in narrow curbside strips. But here, in addition to bare dirt and the stubble of dry weeds, I saw crushed beer cans, broken glass, and a used condom. I kicked a syringe into the gutter, marveling again that the neighborhood ambience of crack houses, smoky bars, and doorways reeking of urine hadn't sucked them back into their past lives. Somehow, Guido and Elizabeth had stayed above their dismal surroundings.

The rusty railings screamed in protest as my boxes banged against them. The apartment door stood ajar. I kicked it open, lunged inside, and saw the whites of Guido's eyes. Then he spread his arms in a grandiose Italian welcome and shouted, "Ah, my guardian angel!"

I dropped my supplies and knelt between Elizabeth's legs. Just one push and a single scream lay between the baby and the world. With Elizabeth's next contraction, I caught her baby in my bare hands.

It was, indeed, a girl. They named her Grace.

Ten years ago seemed like yesterday as I snatched up the phone and dialed *69. Elizabeth answered on the first ring, and I wondered if she'd been waiting to see if I'd call back.

"Elizabeth? It's Peggy."

"Oh, I didn't know if you'd remember us."

"Trust me, Elizabeth. I remember you perfectly."

We talked for nearly half an hour. It hadn't been easy, Elizabeth admitted, but as she filled me in on their ten years of struggle, I heard triumph and pride in her voice. In order to be free to care for their daughter, Elizabeth had worked at a series of part-time jobs, mostly in the childcare industry. Guido had a union job with an elevator maintenance company, full benefits, and a month of annual paid vacation. They had visited Italy the previous summer, and Grace met thirty-five of her cousins while Elizabeth learned to make homemade pizza, Sicilian style, from one of Guido's seven sisters.

Grace played the piano in the background, a familiar aria from *La Traviata*.

During Elizabeth's pregnancy, I'd been hopeful but not optimistic about their chances of forging a future together, but they'd done it, done the improbable.

Guido had called me his guardian angel, and I'd felt like one that morning as I held their crying baby in my hands, looking down at their smiling faces while water and blood pooled around my knees.

But now, ten years later, I blinked through a mist of tears as I listened to their child playing the piano. And I knew the truth. They surely did have a guardian angel, but it wasn't me.

It was Grace.

~ *Allah's Blessing*

I always glowed with pleasure when a former client asked me to midwife her through yet another birth because, of course, it was a vote of confidence, but also because I'd get a peek at the older children, the ones whose births I'd attended in years past.

Perhaps the tiny baby I'd last seen as a six week old, just practicing his new trick of smiling, would now be a coy two year old peeping from behind his mother's leg. The toddler who had watched her brother's birth from grandma's lap would be bringing *papier maché* dragons home from kindergarten. Many of "my babies" are now riding bikes, playing competitive soccer, choosing high schools, flirting, learning to drive, attending prom night, and going off to college. Maybe even marrying.

But rarely did I witness the maturing of the parents themselves from teenagers to community leaders. Charlie and Naeema gave me that chance.

I marveled at this teenaged couple. In the eighteen months since I'd delivered their first child, Charlie had grown from boy to man. He now dressed in loose cotton pants instead of tattered blue jeans, and his Def Lepperd T-shirts had given way to conservative long-sleeved tops. He'd lost the loose-limbed movements of a high schooler, walking now with the confidence of a young man. He took his conversion to Islam seriously, studied the Koran, brushed his teeth before praying the requisite number of times daily . . . and he'd changed his name to Hameed.

But I had trouble remembering.

"Peggy? It's Hameed. I think it's happening really fast."

"Hameed?"

"Yeah, Naeema's been in the shower the last half hour, but now she's hiding in a corner and won't talk to me."

"Oh, Char . . . Hameed! I'm on my way."

Thank God they live only ten minutes away, I thought. As I sped toward their house near Albany High, I coasted through stop signs and barely curtsied at red lights.

Naeema and Hameed were the exact ages of Jill and Colin, seventeen and nineteen, but there the similarity ended. Jill grabbed a bagel and ran to tennis lessons after school while Naeema grabbed her toddler and headed for the prenatal clinic. Colin and Hameed skateboarded together a few times after Naeema's first birth, but those days were part of Hameed's past. He now shouldered more obligations than people twice his age. While Colin surfed through his sophomore year of college in Santa Barbara, Hameed carried a full schedule in a community college. Four afternoons a week he worked at a camera store, and on the weekends he sold Muslim prayer beads from a booth at a flea market. But they still lived in the bungalow with Janice, Hameed's mother.

I felt like a Sherpa on Everest as I lugged all my gear up the old wooden steps. I made so much noise crashing my boxes against each other that I felt certain someone would open the door immediately. No one did. The dark windows stared at me, and a noisy electronic hum came from within.

I knocked hard. Nothing. The droning noise varied in pitch and volume, loud in the otherwise quiet night air. They probably couldn't hear me, I thought, so I turned the handle and barged in. Once inside, I could tell the noise was a vacuum cleaner, probably Janice tidying up at the back of the cottage.

I sniffed. Mexican food. Chilies, salsa, fried corn tortillas. Maybe the spicy salsa had triggered Naeema's labor.

The room to the left of the entryway had been the living room, but Hameed and Naeema now used it as a large studio apartment for themselves and their daughter, Saalima. From the far corner of the big room, a dim light glowed.

I slipped off my clogs and crept through darkness toward the single point of light. After stumbling on a child's toy, I felt my way around a desk, letting the light lead me on. It came from a tiny Christmas tree bulb in a closet. In the weak beam, I finally made out the shape of a naked woman in the corner of the living room, down near the floor. A naked woman with no face.

I couldn't understand her position. It looked like the front of her body but the back of her head, the way an owl can do a 180 with its neck, but I'd never seen a human do that. As I bent over to figure out how this creature was put together, Hameed leaped from the darkness with a yelp.

"Wah! Oh, it's you." He lurched upright, clutching his hand to his chest.

"Agh! God, don't do that to me, Hameed!" I wailed, heart pounding. We shouted at each other, straining to communicate above the loudest vacuum cleaner I'd ever heard.

"Naeema," I yelled, for it had to be her, this naked, owl-woman sitting so still on a futon. "I need some light. Can I open that closet door a bit more?"

I received the barest of nods.

Magic. With the door opened about a foot, things made sense. Glistening with lotion, Naeema's sleek body sparkled. The bones of her shoulders, little knobs under her satiny skin, stood out in the shadows, and the slats of thin ribs marked the upper edge of her pregnant belly. She drew one knee up under her chin, and her waist-length hair cascaded over her face. Slowly and rhythmically, she pulled a wide-toothed comb through her crinkly hair, releasing the flowery aroma of chamomile shampoo. Hidden inside the tent of hair, she combed it over her knee. Over and over, she reached the bottom of one section and then started again at the top, lost in mindless repetitions, calm in the eye of the hurricane of birth.

The vacuum cleaner rasped on and on. It sounded as though it had sucked up nails, safety pins, pine needles, and maybe a drawer full of knives, forks, and spoons.

I hollered into the mass of hair, "Naeema, is the baby coming right now?"

She nodded and kept combing.

Hameed cleared debris from the desk with a single sweep of his forearm. Pens, paper, schoolbooks, baby toys, a stapler, file cards, and a coffee cup crashed to the floor. He yanked open a cardboard box and began unloading birth supplies onto the desk. Pulling out a pie pan, he set it beside me with a few other things, some washcloths, a flashlight—Yes! I thought, a flashlight!—a pile of blue Chux, and some baby blankets wrapped in aluminum foil.

"Did your bag of water break?" I asked Naeema, taking a wild guess where her ear might be. One quick nod, then a contraction started. Her behavior didn't change, but I saw her round, taut belly tighten, shining in the low light beneath the curtain of her hair. And I saw the rolling lurch at the top that heralds pushing. A tiny gasp came from behind the curtain, but the comb never stopped.

"May I check you?"

Her head bobbed twice, quickly. I examined her and, no surprise, found a hard little head with lots and lots of curly hair hovering half an inch inside. Still Naeema combed and combed.

Then she leaned forward and clutched my arm. Her green eyes peered between strands of wet hair as she said, "T ... uh ..." She took a deep breath and combed furiously for a few seconds, gathering energy to try again.

"Naeema, what?" I urged, knowing there wasn't much time.

She took another deep breath and said, "Tell ..." I leaned closer, but a contraction halted her. I stroked her long, adolescent back while she hunched into a push, gripping the comb tightly as her belly heaved.

"Hameed," I shouted, "it's time." He'd delivered Saalima, and I knew he wanted to do the same with this baby. He wiggled past Naeema's knees and wedged his muscular body in front of her.

Jammed into the corner, I wondered again at the primal need of women to find a close, dark, protected space in which to safely bring forth their babies. Time after time, I watched laboring women reject the prepared pile of Chux in the middle of a king-size bed, preferring instead the crowded slot between bed and wall, the space between toilet and bathtub, or even the shoe-strewn floor of a bedroom closet. Naeema had the entire room at her disposal, but we were confined by walls, futon, and door into three square feet of space.

Naeema said, "Tell . . . J," but again a contraction caught her. "Agh! Umph!"

Hameed's eyes, shiny as coffee beans, glowed with adoration.

The lips of her vagina separated, and an inch of baby hair appeared. Not much longer, I knew. She groaned again, and I felt a tightening in her body, a shift of balance. She made not a sigh, but when I glanced between her legs, most of the head slid out on its own without her even pushing, as a bead of water slips down the side of a crystal glass.

"Hameed, it's coming," I hollered, for he still stared at her face.

He looked down and his hands shot forward. "Yikes!" he blurted.

He supported the surprisingly large head with a confidence that came from having done it once before and therefore considering himself an expert. Being just nineteen might have had an influence, too.

Naeema finally stopped combing her hair. She leaned back, flopping her knees out in the boneless manner of a yogi. Flinging her hair back, she locked her eyes onto mine. I could almost feel the heat from her gaze as she hissed in and out, tossing her head in rhythm with her noisy gasps.

"You're okay, Naeema. It's overwhelming, especially since it's so fast, but it's almost over. Just keep sighing. The baby will come right into Hameed's hands."

"What should I do?" He sniffed back his tears, sounding like a teenager again.

"Put the palm of your hand over the head so it comes slowly. We don't want it to pop out too fast. Okay, here comes another one. Naeema, just keep breathing. Hameed, let the baby's head push your hand away, oozing out like lava. Perfect. Feel better, Naeema?"

Her face relaxed, and she leaned forward to look over her belly at the curly hair of her second child.

Keeping his hands on the baby, Hameed wiped his tears with his shoulder. I grabbed a 4 x 4 gauze square, wiped his eyes, and started to toss the gauze aside.

"Blow," he mumbled, and I held it for him while he blew his nose. I wanted to hug him to my chest as if he were my own.

"Hameed, try to get one shoulder out at a time. Oop, here we go again. See her belly curl over? Press the head down, a little more." I spoke just inches from his ear so he could hear me above the omnipresent vacuum cleaner. "This is a bigger baby than your first. We need room for the top shoulder. Mmm, press harder."

But it wasn't moving. I put my hands over his and pressed in a way that should have brought the top shoulder into sight. Still nothing.

"Hey, Naeema, I said you wouldn't have to push, but I lied," I yelled. "Push once for me, long and hard. Really bear down. This is a *big* puppy."

With my hands pressing steadily on the baby's head and with a heroic push from Naeema, the shoulder slipped free. I removed my hands.

"We're on the home stretch, now. Lift the baby's head up, Hameed. It'll come out, that's good, just grab it with both hands and lift upwards."

But the body, born to the chest, just didn't budge. And the vacuum cleaner roared on. In such a small house, I figured she must have been vacuuming the walls and ceiling at this point. There couldn't be that much floor space.

"Lordy!" I hollered. "Naeema, jeez, push again. Forget puppy. You've got a big-bellied moose in there."

As Naeema gave an enormous grunt, amniotic fluid splashed onto Hameed's pants. A huge baby girl flopped out like a salmon landing on the deck of a fishing boat.

"Tell Janice . . ." roared Naeema, but Hameed held his hand up, and she stopped.

Hameed gulped and sputtered through his tears and put his mouth next to the wailing baby's ear. His duty as a Muslim father demanded that Allah's name be the first words his baby heard.

"*La ilaha illa Allah.*" There is no God but God.

Then Naeema bellowed, "TellJanicetoturnoffthatvacuumit'sdrivingme-crazy!"

Laughing, Hameed ran down the hall. Finally the house fell silent. Hameed reappeared at the door with an astonished Janice in tow.

"Charlie, for heaven's sake, it's already over? I didn't even know she was in labor. Why didn't you come get me?" She shook her head in amazement.

"No time, Ma. I hollered, but you couldn't hear me, and I couldn't leave her, and it went so fast, and Peggy came, and well, anyway, it's another girl."

As I packed to leave a couple of hours later, I thought again of the special family this couple had created, bound by youth, love, and their common faith. But I wondered about that Islamic blessing being the first thing this baby girl had heard. Personally, I felt absolutely certain that she'd heard the vacuum cleaner loud and clear, but I decided not to argue the point.

End of the Drought

Seven years into a severe drought, California lawns withered to hard dirt. Children passed through toddlerhood never knowing the joy of running through a sprinkler on a hot afternoon. Of necessity, we had all become drought experts.

I stood in the shower, just so. At my feet, a bucket collected rinse water flowing off my body; I'd flush the toilet with it later. Brushing my teeth with two measured ounces of precious water, I listened to the washing machine's rinse water flowing into a barrel. That water would irrigate our precious apricot tree. Everything else had died long ago.

Water. I couldn't imagine California ever again having enough. So as I toweled dry, I savored my first errand, a visit to the marina where Megan and George, wayfaring young adventurers, lived on an old sailboat.

When I met them for the first time, Megan wore yellow gumboots and smelled like fish. Her red cheeks looked like a fond auntie had pinched them too hard, red hair sprouted beneath her black knitted cap, and her seven-month-pregnant belly stretched a stained fisherman's sweater to its limits.

"We sailed into harrrbor just two days agoo," she explained in a thick Scottish brogue. "Me and George are goona stay in Berkeley till the wee bairn coomes."

For Megan, that was a long speech. She hid behind her cloud of hair and left most of the talking to George, a laid-back, lanky bloke from Yorkshire, as dark as she was fair.

"Aye," said George, "I bought me boat, the *Kestrel,* up in Canada. That's where we met. Megan was working in a cannery nearby and she said she'd love to help me sail round the world."

I'll bet she did, I thought to myself. And I'll bet all the fish made googly eyes at the mere sight of him. He could probably just scoop them up with a little net.

As I recorded Megan's medical history, I realized that, except for a visit to a shaman in the San Juan Islands, I was the first professional she'd seen in her pregnancy. Megan spoke again, "And the ould man said it'd be a wee healthy bairn."

After parking at the marina that morning, I stepped into a watery world of boats, ropes, and fish. A gull swooped by with a french fry in its beak. George waited at the locked gate to let me in. Beside him, two construction workers tinkered with metal pipes and rolls of fencing. The hinged gate squeaked loudly on my left when George pushed it open. As we began the long walk to Slot 17, I guessed the dark, wooden sailboat at the end, the one with red and green trim, would be the *Kestrel*. Riding low in the water, it looked like a Viking ship, something from a medieval fairy tale.

We headed down the pier, but after twenty paces I found myself staggering. "This is pretty weird, George. Why am I dizzy?"

He strode along like the surefooted sailor he was. "Ah, it's quite common. The pier itself is actually floatin', jest like the boats. Yeh need sea legs."

Toddling like a cautious penguin, I reached a set of rickety wooden steps on the slice of dock between his old sailboat and their neighbor's streamlined cabin cruiser. Megan with her flyaway hair popped above the railing like a jack-in-the-box clown, and she steadied me as I stepped over the high sides and into the boat.

Down a few stairs, I entered the low-ceilinged cabin where clutter accumulated by these two packrats overflowed from the cupboards and shelves lining every inch of space. Megan boiled water for tea on a little Bunsen burner. The mug of Earl Grey smelled slightly of fish as I lifted it to my lips.

"Do you guys fish all the time?" I asked.

George said, "Aye, fishin' supports us. The boat herself's fished for a hundred years."

Smells like it, I thought, but within half an hour I no longer noticed.

I took Megan's blood pressure, measured her belly, felt the big baby punching inside, all knees and elbows, and we talked about the contractions she'd been having. Megan still had three weeks to go, but contractions came so frequently that George said he'd almost called me a few nights earlier. I did a vaginal exam and found her cervix already open to the size of a lima bean— about two centimeters—soft and stretchy, all thinned out.

"You're ready, Megan," I said. "I can't imagine you'll last three more weeks."

"Ah, yeh really think me bairn'll cooome soon, then?" she asked, and I nodded. We chatted a bit more as I snooped around the fascinating old boat. Then I drank my fishy tea and headed home to water the apricot tree.

As the week went by, I continued measuring my tooth brushing water, but the weatherman swore rain was heading our way at last. At dinner, my husband and I flipped the TV to the weather channel, watching the swirling patterns on the meteorological map as a huge storm in Canada turned south and began its relentless progress down the West Coast. On Tuesday, the sky turned the color of soot. On Wednesday, strangers waiting for the subway discussed how much rain to expect as wind blew their coats open. On Thursday afternoon a light rain fell, and the air tingled with the burnt smell of wet dust on cement.

Maybe the drought really would end. Maybe California lawns would turn green and the reservoirs once more fill with water. Maybe.

On Friday, the full force of the storm reached the Bay Area. Sheets of frigid rain slammed straight down. The world turned monochromatic, a chameleon adjusting to the gray tones of sky, rain, and sidewalk. Children coming home from school in rain slickers looked like splashes of yellow paint in an old black-and-white movie.

At three in the afternoon, the lights went out. At four, George called. Megan's bag of water had broken. By eight, her labor began to speed up. I notified Bonnie and loaded my car.

Jill stared at me. "You're not going out in this weather, are you?" When I nodded, she turned to the window and hugged her arms to her ribs.

"I'll be okay, honey. I don't think there will be much traffic. I mean, only midwives and cops will be on the road on a night like this." But as I headed out the door, I could see I hadn't convinced her. Her anxious face in the living room window was the last thing I saw as I pulled away from the curb.

The world around me was as dark as the bottom of a mine, but the freeway blazed with flashing lights from police cars, ambulances, and fire trucks. Traffic jams caused by the lack of stoplights snarled traffic flow even more. With accidents everywhere, it looked like a war zone. A trip usually requiring fifteen minutes stretched to nearly an hour.

Squinting past my windshield wipers, I spied the marina's off ramp and started across the narrow causeway. Gripping the steering wheel, I finally turned into the parking lot. The asphalt surface had flooded beneath two inches of water, and the narrow entryway could just as easily have been a boat-launching ramp leading straight into ten feet of angry, inky, oily bay.

With three boxes of supplies, a canvas bag, my purse, an umbrella, and a flashlight, I knew I'd never get everything onto the boat in one trip. I picked up the tackle box holding my most essential equipment, grabbed the flashlight, popped open the umbrella, and stepped into the storm.

Before I'd taken ten steps, rain flooded my boots, and wind blew my umbrella inside out. My narrow flashlight beam, more suited for repairing vaginal lacerations than for lighting my way toward a boat during the storm of the decade, illuminated four feet ahead of me as I inched toward the gate. George had said he'd rig the gate with tape to keep it unlocked. I pushed at it, but it didn't budge. Oh, no, George forgot, I moaned inwardly. Double-checking, I realized I was looking at the hinged side, not the latch. Confused, I thought back to my last visit, sure the squeaky hinge had been on my left.

I shone the light at the sign above the gate. Yes, this was the right place. Sidestepping an iridescent puddle of oil and fish muck, I checked the other edge.

Bless George, there was the tape wound around the latch. I pushed it open and stepped onto the dock. The gate bumped my shoulder as it swung shut. I stepped aside to avoid it but realized something was wrong. Something subtle about the glistening dock. Or was it . . . water?

My foot came down onto nothingness. I dropped everything behind me and, as I fell toward the bay, I grabbed the swinging gate. I crumpled to the dock, hanging half over the edge with my boot in the roiling water. My flashlight rolled away, and, trembling, I snatched it back from the edge.

I had come within half a heartbeat of walking into San Francisco Bay.

As I huddled in the rain waiting for courage to return, I wondered how I could have been so certain the gate opened the other way. Soaked to the skin and frightened, I finally stood and inched through the darkness, aiming my flashlight like a blind man using his white-tipped cane—sweep, sweep, scan, scan. Centering myself, I concentrated on the planks stretching in front of me and tottered straight ahead as if the dock were a tightrope. It was a straight shot, and it was ten or twelve feet wide, but it writhed like an angry snake. The pitching boats banged into pilings, rigging groaned, and metal fittings screeched. I felt as if I'd stepped from a spaceship into an alien world.

Finally, the *Kestrel* loomed from the darkness. Weak lights flickered below-deck, and a storm lantern swung from the mast. The wooden sailboat banging against the dock suddenly looked like the safest haven I could imagine. But there were those pesky little steps again. No way was I going to climb them without help. Catch hold of this bouncing boat and step over the sides in the dark? With the wet, the wind, and the fish oil?

"Uh-uh, no way," I said aloud. I'd had enough excitement for one night, and I hadn't even gotten aboard yet. Using my umbrella, I banged an SOS in Morse code on the side of the boat. Bang-bang-bang. BANG . . . BANG . . . BANG. Bang-bang-bang.

Looking like Darth Vader rising from the gloom, George emerged in a hooded slicker and helped me over the side, pointing me toward the steps down to the cabin. Then he began hauling fishing nets and heavy boxes onto flapping pieces of plastic.

I went down a couple of steps before I remembered that most of my equipment was still in my car. I turned and grabbed the hem of George's slicker as he swooped past, a specter in the dark. He bent to listen. "I could only carry one box with me. My other stuff's in my car, the VW bug. It's unlocked. I can't deal with that pier again."

He nodded and vaulted over the side.

I watched in amazement as the plastic tarps on the deck rose with the wind, dragging heavy boxes with a grating sound I heard above the storm's roar.

Then a different kind of roar made me turn. In the cabin lit by two oil lamps and many candles, Megan looked like a wild jungle child huddling in the lower bunk. A fuzzy mohair shawl draped her shoulders, and she squatted, leaning forward with her knuckles pressed to the bed. With her hair covering her face and the furry shawl, she resembled a redheaded yeti. Her growls intensified the image.

A drop of freezing water bounced off my nose. I took another step, and a steady trickle ran down the back of my neck. Then I heard it everywhere, dripping and splashing into buckets, onto towels, into cups and pots and pans. But George would have needed all the pots from the kitchenware department of Macy's to collect the rain.

The boat was leaking from above. Seriously and steadily leaking. So that's what George was doing with all the plastic on deck, I thought. Stopping the leaks.

I was examining Megan when George clattered down the steps with the rest of my equipment. "Jaysus, it's bloody thick out there," he shouted, shaking himself like a wet dog. "There's no more'n a gob of spit to stop yeh stepping off the end of the dock. Those fookin' eejits reversed the fookin' gate and didn't put up a railing. I damn near walked into the water."

"That's where I fell, George. Something stopped me just in time."

"Oh, Christ, ya fell? Almost in the water? Oh, bloody hell, I'm glad yer all right. Yeh are all right, aren't ya?" He took a good look at me. "Hell, woman, yer soaked through. Here, get somethin' dry on. Then I'll fix yeh up with a slicker, and ye'll stay warm, ye will." He tossed me enough clothing for four people and pointed toward a narrow door that looked like it led to a broom closet.

I stepped into the world's tiniest bathroom. Bumping elbows and knees against the walls, I stripped to the skin and pulled on clean long johns, oil-stained sweatpants, a pink T-shirt with an arrow pointing down to the word *Baby,* and a thick sweater that smelled of fish. But the feet were a problem. My boots were drenched. Holding two pairs of thick socks, I wiggled out barefoot and asked George what to do.

A man of instant solutions and endless supplies, George opened a bin holding about ten pair of gumboots. He helped me find a pair that fit, then pushed my arms into a slicker and gave me a towel to dry my hair.

Geared up, warm and dry, I looked more like a fisherman than a midwife. Although neither Megan nor George seemed to find anything comical in my attire, I bustled around with a big grin on my face.

Bonnie clattered down the steps a few minutes later, her topsy-turvy umbrella gripped in her hand and rainwater streaming from the end of her knee-length braid.

"Whoosh!" she exclaimed. "What a night. And I nearly fell off the dock."

George muttered oaths as he tossed her a towel and a slicker.

As Megan approached late labor, she pulled George's head into her chest, twisted her fingers in his hair, and yanked his body side to side as the contractions slammed into her. I feared she'd give him whiplash, but he just planted his hands on either side of her and let her sling him around like a boat tossed in a wild storm. She growled deep in her throat, and George matched her sounds, keeping her company. Singing the woman's spontaneous labor song with her was a technique I'd taught for years, but George discovered it on his own. Together they swayed and rocked, growled and moaned.

Then there was a grating noise and loud bumping from above. Rain again poured through the cabin ceiling.

"Aaagh!" shouted George. He wrenched himself away from Megan, pulled the slicker over his head, and dashed up the stairs. "Oh, fook! Bloody fook!" he screamed, disappearing into the blackness. It was fifteen minutes before he reappeared, fifteen minutes during which it sounded as if he was smashing cars with a coal shovel. Gradually the solid curtain of rainwater became just drips again. George and his plastic had triumphed, at least for the moment.

The mattress on the bunk above Megan had so far absorbed the leaks, so fortunately, the space where Megan labored remained dry. But every other surface glistened with moisture. Looking around, I asked George where to put my instruments.

"No problem."

He unfurled an enormous blue and gold, UC Berkeley stadium umbrella, attached a rope to the finial, and tossed the other end over a beam above the table. With the swish of a towel, he created a dry area big enough not just for my instruments but for Bonnie and me as well, our own little island in the middle of the flood. While Megan once again busied herself with George-tossing, Bonnie and I brewed tea, found some stale gingersnaps, took off our slickers, and sat under the umbrella for a cuppa.

Soon Megan's growls changed to grunts, and bloody mucus dripped between her legs. George looked over his shoulder at me, his eyes wide with questions. Is this really okay?

I smiled, checked Megan, and reassured George that everything was normal. Normal, that is, except for the weather and the leaky boat. And Megan was pushing.

I often told women, "Stop thinking and just be. Brains don't know how to have babies; bodies do." But Megan did it naturally. Already trusting her body's superior knowledge, she required very little coaching.

I glanced at the stove. No oven. How would I warm six flannel receiving blankets in a leaking boat on a night as cold as the nose of a ghost?

"George, how can we heat the baby blankets?" I asked without much hope.

"Oh, yeah. See that cupboard next to the loo? There's a hot water bottle in it. Just fill it with hot water, then wrap the blankets round and round, cover the whole lot with foil, and shove 'm into this plastic bag. It'll be brilliant."

Bonnie swung into action, and George was right. It was brilliant.

Megan squatted to push, not rising even to take a break from her cramped position. In less than forty-five minutes, the baby's wet, wrinkled head slipped out. With my hands on top of George's, I steered the process as George caught the baby boy himself. Then Megan reached between her feet and pulled him, wet and bawling, onto her chest.

"Jaysus, he's a red-headed bugger, he is," whispered George. His eyes widened in awe as Bonnie toweled the baby dry, fluffing the strawberry fuzz on his head. She examined the baby and weighed him in at nine and a half pounds. George's thick fingers fumbled with a tiny shirt and diaper pins, and he did a passable job of cramming two pinwheeling, pudgy feet into the legs of an all-in-one fleecy baby outfit. I wrapped the wee bairn in two more heated blankets and a hand-knit shawl thick enough to warm a hypothermic Eskimo.

Megan walked to the bathroom with her seaworthy legs spread only slightly more than usual. When she emerged, she wore clean thermal underwear, a cardigan that hung past her knees, and those yellow gumboots. Adding a slicker, she looked ready to go fishing with the rest of us.

George brewed more tea, and Megan pulled a pan of Rice Krispie squares from a cabinet where they'd stayed dry. She nursed her new baby while the four of us sat beneath the umbrella and had a midnight snack. In the candle-light of the dim cabin, we resembled an old Dutch master's painting as we listened to the storm lashing at the rest of the world.

The baby slept soundly with his fists balled beneath his chin, and Megan's head drooped. Eventually I could find no excuse to prolong my stay.

"I'll help get yer car loaded," said George, "and then I'll walk ye out. Jaysus, when I think what might of happened . . ." He disappeared with my supplies.

I had just kissed the baby's nose when George returned. He helped Bonnie and me over the side of the boat and guided us down the center of the still-pitching dock. Once we reached the relative safety of the swamped parking lot, George put the tackle box into the back seat and hugged me. I was eager to get out of the rain, and he was eager to return to Megan. My little car roared to life; I waved to Bonnie and pulled away.

It was still pouring, but the wind had died down. With almost no traffic at two A.M., I made it home in twenty minutes. As I started up our front walk, an errant blast of wind blew my raincoat hood off and dumped about a quart of water down my neck. I gasped aloud and cursed into the darkness. Soaked again.

Leaving my raincoat, boots, and umbrella on the front porch, I crept upstairs in stocking feet. Remembering Jill's anxious face as I'd left home hours earlier, I scrawled a quick note and slipped it beneath her bedroom door to let her know I'd made it home safely.

In the bathroom I peeled off my borrowed clothing, pulled on a flannel nightie, and brushed my teeth. I stared at the two inches of water in the cup.

Grinning, I filled it to the brim, took a long drink, and poured out the rest. I refilled it and brushed some more. Then I spat, swished, spat again, drank a few more mouthfuls and rinsed the sink with the rest, watching it wash away the residue of my flamboyant, water-wasting, tooth brushing extravaganza. Finally I called it quits, turned out the light, and collapsed into bed.

Rog turned and wrapped me in his warmth. Then he froze mid-cuddle and whispered, "You're wet. And cold. And you smell like fish."

"I'll tell you all about it in the morning," I mumbled. "But I really think this drought is over."

You Can't Be Serious

After my lawyer's phone call telling me Patty and Fred were suing me, I expected swift legal action, but my lawyer urged me to relax and just get on with my life.

"The wheels of the law turn slowly, Peggy. I'll be in touch when you need to know something."

In fact, two-and-a-half years passed with frustrating sluggishness.

Joe Weick, neither a patient man nor one to suffer fools gladly, was incensed by the mere fact of the lawsuit against him. He was married to a midwife, and their last child had been born at home. Joe always put his time, energy, and reputation behind his beliefs, and he was convinced that someone, perhaps Patty's lawyers, had influenced her decision to sue him. This and the ponderous slowness of progress toward any resolution eventually took their toll.

Early in 1990, he made plans to relocate. "I've got to get out of the Bay Area. Californians initiate lawsuits in a knee-jerk reaction to bad luck. Patty's lawyers may be putting words in her mouth, and they actually think they can make a case against us. That's just the last straw." When he moved to Oregon six months later, Bay Area midwives lost one of their most outspoken backers.

With Joe gone, I felt more vulnerable, especially as the possibility of a trial moved closer. It didn't help that I knew I played the pawn in this chess game, destined to move forward slowly and with little power.

Patty's lawyer planned to say I'd been acting under Dr. Weick's direction, so my lawyer needed an explicit explanation about our separate agreements with Patty. Again I went to his office to make it clear that my arrangement with Patty was equivalent to a second job. The fact that her obstetrician was also my backup doctor was coincidental.

"There was nothing secretive about it," I reiterated, "but Patty wasn't officially my patient, nor was I serving as Dr. Weick's agent." I'd said the same thing before in umpteen different ways.

And again, weeks, then months, of silence followed.

Finally, in January 1991, while holiday wreaths still decorated doorways, Peter again called me to his office. This time, however, no other lawyers would be present, just a representative from my insurance company.

"Polly Stroud," she said, standing up as I entered the office. She looked harmless enough. In fact, with her tidy blue suit, silk blouse, and print scarf, she looked like a flight attendant. A dark brown pageboy swinging below her ears and medium-heeled pumps added to the image. But when she failed to meet my eyes as we shook hands, I felt my chest tighten. Intuition pricked at my psyche, and something told me not to trust her.

Peter sat back in his leather swivel chair, fingers steepled beneath his chin as he began talking. "Dr. Weick's malpractice carrier settled out of court two days ago, and the hospital settled last month. Only the lawsuits against you and the ambulance company are outstanding."

"We'd like to offer the Wilsons a quarter of a million," said Ms. Stroud.

I started to speak, but Peter held up his hand. "There are several issues at stake. Luke is three years old now, and this case has dragged on for almost as long."

"And the legal fees keep mounting," interrupted Ms. Stroud, checking her nails.

"Besides," Peter continued, "the insurance company is reluctant to go to trial. A baby with injuries this serious—well, imagine if they parade Luke in front of the jury. Blind. Deaf. Spastic paralysis. Just enough brain stem function to power his heart and lungs, but otherwise he's a vegetable. How would the jury react?"

"It would break their hearts," I said.

"Yes," agreed Peter, "and a sympathetic jury might return with a multi-million dollar award, just out of pity. San Francisco is notorious for juries that give preposterous amounts to plaintiffs."

"But it feels like an admission of guilt," I said. "And I did nothing wrong."

"Settling out of court is simply an insurance company's attempt to cut their losses. It isn't an admission of anything," Peter assured me.

"Well, it sure feels that way," I said.

Ms. Stroud pushed forward a copy of my contract. "We'll never settle without your permission. Your contract makes that clear." She pointed to the pertinent clause.

I scanned it, then said, "Fine, let's take it to court." I leaned back and relaxed for the first time during the meeting.

Both Ms. Stroud and Peter sighed. He tapped a pen against the desktop and stared out the window toward the Golden Gate Bridge. She toyed with her ring.

"You're both making me wonder if there's something else at stake here," I said. "What's up?"

"Nothing's 'up,' Peggy," said Peter. "It's just that the contract also explains what happens if we proceed to trial against the insurance company's advice. If we go to court and lose, and the jury awards the plaintiff, say, two million—or ten million—then the difference between a quarter of a million and ten million comes from your pocket."

"You can't be serious," I gasped, but they nodded. Polly Stroud had the grace to blush as she fiddled with her sheets of paper. I was incredulous—and furious, but I was also trapped. "I don't have a choice, do I? Why bother with that clause about not settling without my consent if they're going to stick me for the difference? Is it the same with Dr. Weick's insurance? Is that why he settled?"

"Yes," said Peter. "It's why people decide not to risk the outcome of a trial, especially in a personal injury case where the stakes can be so high." He pushed a pretyped agreement across the desk toward me as Ms. Stroud spoke.

"Juries don't understand the situation for professionals who are defendants in these cases," she said. "They see a tragic situation and want to throw money at it, regardless of blame. They figure there's plenty of insurance money available and can't comprehend what a person like yourself stands to lose."

I looked at the expanse of polished desk, at the ceiling, at Ms. Stroud's perfect hair, but there was really no point in stalling. I picked up the pen and signed, giving the insurance company permission to offer the Wilsons a quarter of a million dollars.

I felt defeated as I slid the papers back, but I was surprised that I also felt a certain relief. At least it was over. I could put the whole case behind me and continue doing what I loved best: delivering babies.

Polly Stroud stuffed the papers into her briefcase and stood to leave, but she hesitated at the doorway. "How long have you been a midwife?" she asked. For the first time, she looked directly into my eyes.

"Ten years."

She kept staring at me as if there might be something else she wanted to say. I looked back at her, my face deliberately wooden. She just worked for the insurance company. She hadn't written the contract. She seemed nice enough, but I found it impossible to like her. A "kill the messenger" attitude polluted my heart.

Hovering in the doorway, she said, "The company might refuse to renew your policy."

"What?" I said, certain I hadn't heard right. She nodded and gave a half shrug. "No, you can't be serious," I said, and the blood rushed to my face.

"Well, it's a possibility, because of the money they've lost on this case."

She blushed and looked down at her hands, and I wondered if she was speaking out of turn. But I didn't believe her. I know many doctors, good doctors, who've been sued several times. It's rare for an obstetrician to go through a whole career without being sued, and usually the case isn't about placing blame—it's about finding an excuse to give money to someone who has an unfortunate outcome. But regardless of the grounds, the doctor's coverage is almost never discontinued. So why would my carrier do that to me? It made no sense, and I pressed for more information. "That's ridiculous. Why wouldn't they continue my coverage?"

She stood with one foot in the hallway. "I have another appointment," she said, shrugging helplessly. "I just think you might want to explore other options—" and she disappeared, her hurried footsteps echoing down the marble corridor.

I looked at Peter. He sat in his leather chair with his back to the fabulous view. A peregrine falcon landed on the ledge outside the high window and stared in at me, its eyes hooded like Peter's, neither of them blinking.

"Is it true?" I finally asked.

"I've never heard of that, but I've never defended a midwife before."

"How could they ethically do that? I mean, what's the point of insurance if they force you to settle and then refuse to cover you any more because you cost them a quarter of a million? Like, one strike and you're out. That can't be right."

The falcon cocked its head and dove from the ledge, falling like a stone toward its prey, no doubt a hapless pigeon. Peter saw the sudden movement from the corner of his eye. He unfolded from the chair and moved to the window, following the raptor's flight before shifting his gaze back to me.

"I do know they can refuse to sell insurance to an individual 'without showing just cause.'"

"I never realized it was such a one-sided relationship. But I still can't believe it could be true. I mean, Patty wasn't even my patient, for God's sake. I was like a Good Samaritan."

He shook his head. "As a licensed professional, you'd never be judged under the Good Samaritan law. You'd be held to a higher standard."

"But I did everything right."

"So did Dr. Weick, and he just settled out of court," Peter reminded me.

"But no one's threatening to terminate his malpractice insurance."

"That's true. Well, if it happens, apply to another insurance company."

"Peter, there aren't any others. This is the only company in the whole United States that sells malpractice insurance to midwives. I have ten months remaining on my current policy. If they don't renew me, I'll be out of business this time next year."

He looked down and rubbed the back of his neck. Finally, he shook his head and sighed, saying, "Well, let's just hope she's mistaken."

But when I left his office a few minutes later, I knew how the pale-breasted pigeon felt when it saw the shadow of the falcon.

~ I Just Forgot

After the meeting with Peter and Ms. Stroud, I approached doctors and other midwives with my concerns. I even called the American College of Nurse Midwives. Everyone reassured me, saying they'd never heard of discontinuation of malpractice insurance except for repeated instances of gross malpractice, which this clearly was not. My husband said, "That woman just didn't know what she was talking about. I hope they fire her for scaring you like this. Just forget it. It's over."

When Dawn came to me for the birth of her third child, I felt like I'd put the whole affair completely behind me. As I got to know Jim, her second husband, the idea of having him catch the baby began to grow in my mind. It wasn't an original thought, of course, but I'd been too distracted for the previous few weeks to think of it.

While most fathers are content to let the midwife do the catching, some want the first hands that touch the baby to be their own. Most dads wanted me to keep my hands involved in the action, too, but a few were such naturals that I just knelt beside them and told them what to do.

When Gerry delivered Pamela's baby, I whispered instructions in his ear and marveled as my words traveled to his fingertips with the speed of a single thought; his hands could have been my own.

The reactions of these guys always touched me. Their spontaneous responses were so genuine, so original. When Rog delivered our third child, he whispered, "I had no idea his head would be so hard."

Michael stared at his upturned palms and said, "I feel like I shouldn't ever wash my hands again, like I've touched God."

Tony looked down at the wiggling baby boy in his arms and said, "I did it, I watched it, I saw everything, but I still don't believe it."

"No wonder she's crying," commented Kurt, placing his squalling daughter on his wife's belly. "She must have one helluva headache."

Usually the request for the dad to do the catching came from the couple, but occasionally, I was the one to bring it up. And, with Dawn and Jim sitting before me, it seemed a perfect opportunity to suggest that Jim deliver his own first child. Dawn, a composed pro during the births of her two older kids, probably could have done the whole thing herself.

He had jumped at my offer, but as ponytailed Dawn lay on the living room couch with the baby's head beginning to show, I wondered if I'd made a mistake.

Jim had me worried.

I'd anticipated some nervousness from him. Excitement, amazement, boundless enthusiasm, yes. But not catatonia. Usually Mr. Hail Fellow Well Met, a natural host, he now held himself rigid as a clothespin. A muscle twitched along his jaw. He was sweaty and so, so pale. I thought he might come apart at the seams if I touched him, so I kept my eye on him. A very close eye.

Dawn's older children were from a previous marriage. During those births, her mother had watched from the doorway, shaking her head in amazement. "Dawn, you're one of the lucky ones, just made to have babies," she'd marveled. I nodded in agreement.

Dawn lay on a plastic shower curtain with some towels beneath her, and Jim hunched at her side, carefully easing the edges of her perineum around the baby's head. He followed my whispered instructions exactly. Sweat beaded his brow, and his body stilled with concentration. I'd never known him to be at a loss for words, but he hadn't uttered a sound for the last fifteen minutes. He focused on the expanding sphere at his fingertips. It slid out a tiny bit more, then it paused . . . and stopped. The contraction ended and the pale orb began to retreat.

Another pause—and it quickly disappeared from view, as if someone from inside had grabbed the baby by the ankles and jerked upward.

"Whoa, what was that?" Dawn gasped. "What happened?"

"It's okay," I reassured her. "The baby's just backing up for a running start. It'll come barreling down again with the next contraction."

Dawn laughed and relaxed, but Jim stayed still, not even blinking. He zeroed in on his wife's crotch with the intensity of a cat fixated on a mouse hole. If he'd had a tail, the barest tip would have been twitching.

"Jim, you okay?" I asked him. I received one terse nod in reply. I sneaked a peek at his face. Pale, really pale, and he didn't blink.

As another pain began, Dawn grabbed a big breath and lunged into what she sensed would be the last contraction needed to push her baby's head out. She was a machine, efficient and businesslike. It looked like hard work, but for her, it just didn't look all that painful.

As soon as Dawn started pushing again, the baby's head zoomed down to where it had stopped after the last contraction. Jim jumped to place his fingers back where they'd been before.

"Jim, I'm going to touch you, okay? I'm going to touch your shoulders."

A jerk of his head told me he'd heard, but he still twitched when he felt my hands.

Cold, clammy sweat soaked his shirt, and new beads of moisture appeared on his neck. Oh, dear, I thought, this big, macho guy might pitch over like a tree.

I talked right into his ear, keeping my hands on him. "That's it," I whispered. "A little more pressure on top, don't let it turn upward yet. Okay, now rock your hands back and forth. Let some at the top come out, now some at the bottom. Good. Top, and now bottom again. Perfect."

Jim followed my instructions to the letter, doing exactly what I told him, easing the baby out slowly so his wife wouldn't tear. I began to relax a little. Maybe I'd been wrong. Probably just an understandable case of nerves, but I kept my hands on him. Just in case.

Dawn squeezed her child along another few millimeters. At last the widest part of the baby's grapefruit-sized head filled her perineum, teetering on the point of no return.

"Okay, Dawn, stop pushing. Let your breath out. You don't have to push any more. The rest of it will come oozing out, just like toothpaste."

Most of the time, asking a woman to stop pushing at this point is to ask the impossible. It's completely contrary to the message her body is sending her: *Get the baby out.* To say "stop pushing" is like telling someone to do a backward somersault in the middle of a fifty-yard dash. And I don't ask all women to stop at this point. Besides, most of them are so far out in space that I can't even get their attention. But Dawn stayed right with me, very much in her head, eyes open, watching everything. She stopped pushing as soon as I spoke, once again making the impossible look easy. She whooshed out her breath and peered over her belly where the child's head bulged.

I spoke to Jim. "Ease the rest of her perineum back with your fingertips. It's like pushing away layers of slippery onionskin. See, it's just sliding out."

And there! The baby's whole head lay in Jim's right palm. It wasn't that the head came forward, really. It was more that her perineum eased backward, slipping out of the way to leave the head behind. When it happens that way, it's beautiful. Slow and gentle and . . . just magic.

Relaxed and smiling, Dawn focused on the baby. She hoisted herself up on her elbows to see better, and both of her knees flopped aside like a marionette's. I wondered once again what combination of luck, attitude, and anatomy makes childbirth so straightforward for some women.

A baby comes through the birth canal with its head looking over one shoulder. The head twists and turns on the neck to navigate the various curves of the mother's pelvis. But once the head is free, it naturally turns to align with the rest of the body.

Dawn's baby did this. The head turned in Jim's palm, turning to face him. And the baby opened its eyes, blinked twice, puckered up its lips and blew a bubble.

"Agh! Oh! Omigod!" Jim shrieked, and his whole body seemed to come apart beneath my hands. I yelped as he leaped to his feet. He flapped his arms a few times, and then he curled over, grabbed his stomach, and hollered again.

Meanwhile the baby lay with its head sticking out. I supported it with one hand.

"Jimmy, what on earth?" Dawn shouted, looking at her husband in amazement.

"Agh! Ohgodohgodohgod. It's a *baby*. And it opened its eyes. And it *looked* at me. And . . ."

"Well, what did you expect, a German shepherd?" she said.

"But, I mean, *it looked right at me,* and it's *alive*. Like, *really* alive! I mean . . ." and he turned in a full circle. "Whoa, I just forgot, I guess."

"This is a *good* thing, Jim. To be alive is a good thing," I said in a voice meant to be soothing. I slid in beside Dawn and prepared to deliver the rest of this very patient baby.

"No, wait a sec. Whew. That was like something out of a science fiction flick. Okay, yeah, I can do it," he assured me. "I just forgot."

"You sure you're ready?" questioned his wife, the picture of calmness.

"Yeah, yeah, yeah, I'm on top of it." He took a deep breath, wiped his hands on his jeans, and knelt in front of me once again. Moments later the whole baby boy uncurled into his hands like a purple jumbo shrimp, and Jim was laughing and crying and shouting and sobbing and whooping and sniffling and then laughing some more. Back to the Jim that I knew.

Dawn sprawled with her hands behind her head and enjoyed the show. She beamed at her husband with proprietary fondness and said, "Do you believe this guy's for real?"

As I laughed, feeling my eyes brim with tears, I thought about what he'd said: "I just forgot." I knew what he'd forgotten. He'd forgotten it was a baby. Jim had been so absorbed in following my instructions, working to get this large, round, slippery, hard, faceless, unknown Thing out of a tight spot that he'd forgotten a living person with eyelashes, lips, a tongue, and fingernails would emerge. When the baby looked at him and blinked, it scared the bejeezus out of him, as if he'd lifted a fragile pink egg out of an Easter basket, and it had turned into a talking head.

It's not unusual for women to forget there's a purpose to all the work. They get so lost in the process, the pain, and the exhaustion that we frequently hear their gasp of surprised awe, "Oh, a baby!" at the moment of birth. And it's usually the man who looks at the woman in skeptical wonderment, as if to say, "Well, duh!"

But this time the tables were turned. After I cut the cord and delivered the placenta, Dawn and I watched Jim waltz around the living room with his son pressed to his green flannel shirt. He was still crying and laughing, still repeating, "Oh, my God, I just forgot! It's a *baby!*"

~ Soccer Mom

Iknow how the village midwife in olden days must have felt. I'll bet she could hardly get her marketing done without women stopping to greet her. Like her, I bump into someone who knows me almost everywhere I go. My world seems full of smiling women eager to show off their round-faced babies, shy toddlers, bored school-aged children, or embarrassed teenagers. It's wonderful to reconnect and makes me feel blessed for the lives I've touched. But the timing isn't always ideal.

I tried to pretend I didn't notice the woman waving frantically from a car at the far end of the crowded parking lot. I'd come to the athletic field to drop Skylar at soccer practice and had a mile-long list of errands to run. As Skylar struggled to corral three soccer balls in the wayback of our car, a sedan backed in front of me, blocking my way. Two little boys in red and white uniforms slowly untangled their seat belts and wrestled with gear bags.

"You forgot your water bottles," hollered their mother, and they turned back.

I was trapped. "I wonder who that woman is," I mused as she inched closer, jockeying between other cars. "I just don't have time to chat."

"There're a bazillion people here, Mom. How do you know she's waving at you?"

"Just a feeling."

"Did you deliver her babies?" When he was in kindergarten, Skylar believed I'd delivered all the kids in his class. Indeed, I *had* caught four of them, but not all twenty. However, "Did you deliver her babies?" had become his standard question whenever he saw me talking with a stranger.

"Maybe," I answered. I watched the woman edging around swarms of children in bright uniforms, and she signaled vigorously when she drew close enough to make eye contact. She finally pulled alongside as Skylar scampered across the grass.

"Peggy?" She squinted into the sun, shielding her eyes with her hand. In the back seat of her silver Audi, three grimy, sweaty, towheaded boys nudged each other with muddy elbows while sucking on water bottles.

I hate those awkward moments prior to recognition. "Yeah, hi," I said, smiling. She looked familiar, but I couldn't put a name to the face.

"I'm Sarah. You delivered my last little boy at home. He had clubfeet."

My eyes jerked to the boys in the back seat, and I barely heard the rest of her sentence. The child in the middle stared at me. I stared back as every detail of his birth zoomed into focus: the worst clubfeet I'd ever seen, including photographs in orthopedic textbooks.

On one of those glorious Mediterranean-warm days we often have in Berkeley in March, Sarah labored with her third child on the ground floor of her brown-shingled home. Pete, her dermatologist husband, raised the windows to catch the warm breezes and the scent from the wisteria clusters that drooped from a trellis outside their bedroom. A gray cat groomed herself on a redwood picnic table. Sarah's boys played in the back yard with their *au pair*. Squeaky tricycles and shrieks of laughter punctuated Sarah's moaning labor sounds. A neighbor's hammer tap-tap-tapped in the background as he reshingled his garage roof.

"Sss-ah, sss-ah. Oh, oh, oh, oh! Oh, Pete! Aah. Sss-ah. Oh, my God."

The hammering stopped. The neighbor climbed down a ladder and disappeared into his house, reappearing in a few minutes with a bottle of beer. Up the ladder he went, and the tapping resumed.

Sarah lay cradled in Pete's arms and rocked within his embrace as the pains came closer and stronger. Coming right along, I thought.

I turned to the dresser beneath the open window to check my supplies. A cake pan holding 4 x 4 gauze squares, my instruments, blue suction bulb, and a pair of sterile gloves. Oxygen tank cracked open. Blankets in the oven. IV handy, just in case. Yep, everything ready.

"Sss-ah, sss-ah. Oh, Pete, oh, yes. Yes. Yes, ah." Listening to her noises, the tempo and pitch rising on a crescendo and then falling away, getting sharper and more urgent as the last bit of cervix stretched open, I knew it wouldn't be much longer. No need even to examine her. I took a sip of Diet Coke and waited for the first signs of pushing.

Bare-chested, Pete lay beside her, his body glistening with almost as much sweat as hers. Pushing damp hair off her forehead, he crooned into her ear and stroked her shoulder. Sometimes birth is such an intimate affair that I feel like a voyeur. To speak feels like a violation of some sacred and private event. Sarah's labor fit that description. She and Pete formed a complete unit, just the two of them. I moved to the window again to give them space.

Tap-tap-tap went the hammer. Squeak-squeak-squeak went the tricycles. A breeze blew purple wisteria petals into the room, and a few landed on my supplies. I gathered them into a little pile, crushed several between my fingers, and smelled them.

Sarah's voice hit a new pitch, and I turned, jerked from my reverie. Her body arched backward, then curled forward. She grimaced, and her labor song changed.

"Uh. Uh. Oh, Pete, oh! Aagh, umph." She heaved into a silent push. Another one followed right behind the first, and she yelled, called Pete's name, and pushed again. She sounded so urgent, so intense. I wondered how the children and the man roofing his garage would react to these incredible noises. I glanced out the window as I reached for the pan of equipment. The children played at the rear of the property, perhaps herded from earshot by the *au pair*. The neighbor seemed to have abandoned his hammering in favor of working on his tan. He lay on the garage roof with a beer bottle resting on his stomach.

I sat at the foot of the bed, letting Sarah's legs rest on my shoulders. Pete wiped her forehead and held a glass of iced tea to her lips. He kissed her cheek. She smiled and kissed him back.

The baby's head surged to her perineum with the third push, and as the baby stretched her vaginal opening, Sarah yelled, "Oh! Oh, oh, oh, Jeezis! Oh, God, *it's cooooooomiiiiiing!* Oh, thank God."

As the little body emerged, I curled him up and onto Sarah's belly. She reached down and scooped him to her chest. Pete rested his cheek on Sarah's head and stretched out a hand to cradle his son's floppy head.

Then I saw the feet.

Grotesquely curled and twisted so the soles faced each other, both feet folded sharply upward against his shins. The most extreme case of clubfeet I'd ever seen.

I snatched a towel and began drying the baby, keeping his feet covered. Studies have shown parents cope best with infant deformity if they're first introduced to all that's perfect about their child. I held his feet with the towel, pretending I was keeping him from slipping off Sarah's belly. "Oh, he's beautiful," I said. "Look at his adorable nose, and he's sticking his tongue out." I caught his waving hand, and he gripped my finger. "And look at his fingers, so perfect."

"Check out his long fingernails," exclaimed Sarah as she caught his other hand. "I'll bet those sharp nails broke the bag of water and started my labor this morning."

Pete stood up to call the boys. "Hey, kids, come see your new baby brother! His name is Micah."

The guy on the garage roof leaped to his feet. "Yo, Pete," he hollered. "You mean Sarah just had the baby? Right there? At home?"

"Yeah, about five minutes ago."

"*HA*. Oh my God, I'm dying. *Ha-ha-ha-ha!*" He shrieked with laughter.

"I don't know why Mel's so tickled," mused Pete as he returned to the bedside. Then we heard the older boys approaching from the kitchen. I tossed a sheet over Sarah's body and wrapped the baby in a flannel blanket, turning my back to Sarah and Pete as I swaddled him. Seconds later the boys burst into the bedroom with Marianna, the Danish *au pair*.

Chaos and giggles surrounded us for the next five minutes. But the boys quickly tired of the baby, finding him boring since he couldn't sing the Barney theme song, laugh at their bathroom humor, or ride a tricycle. They disappeared, and we heard them clattering in the kitchen, helping Marianna make dinner.

The long, slanted light of late afternoon came through the window. Everything felt so peaceful. I dreaded what I had to do, but I'd stalled long enough. I took a deep breath. Sarah met my eyes with a steady gaze and before I could speak, she said, "Let's check those feet now." I stared at her, speechless. "Yeah, let's check those tootsies," she murmured. She began to unwrap her baby.

Pete heard something odd in the tone of her voice. He turned away from the closet where he'd been searching for his shoes. "Feet?"

"Yeah. I got a quick look before Peggy covered them up. There's definitely something funky about those feet," she said softly, ever so slowly lifting the last fold of blanket. "Oh, brother. Oh, my Lord." She put her hands to her face and shook her head. "It's a blessing we have good medical coverage, because this little fella is really going to need it."

"Jesus," whispered Pete as he drew close and stared. "Oh, my poor son."

"Sarah . . ." I began, ashamed of the secret I'd kept for nearly half an hour.

"No, you did the right thing," Sarah assured me. "But when I noticed how deliberately you kept his legs covered, well, I knew it was bad."

I thought I'd been so discreet, so clever, so casual in my attempts to keep his legs wrapped, and she'd known all along.

But Pete hadn't. He sat down hard on the edge of the bed. He took the baby from Sarah and kissed him on both cheeks, cradled him against his chest, and then he wept. Sarah rolled over and curled around Pete's hips, stroking his back as he cried openly.

Then Pete took a deep breath, and I gave him a Kleenex. He wiped his eyes, blew his nose, sat up straighter, and flipped into doctor mode. He laid Micah on his lap and examined the feet carefully. Although he was a dermatologist, he'd had pediatric training as all doctors must. He tried to unfold and turn the feet into proper alignment, but the bones had long ago fused into their unnatural position. They didn't budge.

Pete passed Micah to Sarah and called their pediatrician. When the receptionist heard Pete identify himself as a doctor, she put him right through.

"Hi, Paul, it's Pete Franklin. Yeah, Sarah had the baby half an hour ago, and they're okay, but the baby's got clubfeet. No, this isn't the kind you can correct with massage and shoes. Here, let me have you talk to the midwife."

The pediatrician had a heard-it-all-before tone to his voice: "There's no cause for alarm. Most of these foot things are positional. We find they resolve with daily massage and proper alignment with firm shoes from infancy."

"Doctor, this one's different. The feet don't move, not with gentle massage, not with firm massage, not with anything. The anklebones are lower than the heel, the toes are up near the knees, and the soles of the feet touch all the time. I've often seen the kind you're talking about. This is different."

Sighing, he agreed to see the baby the following day.

Subdued, but each trying to act upbeat for the sake of the other, Sarah and Pete showered together. Except for his feet, the baby was beautiful, and he certainly wasn't in pain. When I left two hours later, he lay nursing in his mother's arms with his hands clasped beneath his chin, looking like a Sistine Chapel angel.

Thirty-six hours later, I returned for a home visit. Pete and Sarah looked tired. "What did the pediatrician say?" I asked.

"Not much," said Pete. "He just turned around and called an orthopedic surgeon. They want to do the first surgery in three months."

"Whoa, three months," I murmured. We sat in silence, pondering the enormity of surgery on such a young baby.

Someone knocked on the door, and Pete went to answer it.

"Hey, Sarah, it's Mel. Can he come back to see the baby?"

"Sure," hollered Sarah. She settled the drowsy baby on her lap and pulled her bathrobe across her exposed breast.

Barely visible behind an enormous bouquet of lilies, tulips, iris, and daffodils that he carried in front him, Mel came in with a bottle of chilled champagne in the crook of his other arm. He made appropriate baby-admiration noises as he looked into Micah's peaceful face. Mel had a sunburn from his roofing work, but he turned even redder when Pete asked, "Mel, what made you laugh when I told you Sarah had a home birth?"

"Aw, shit, Pete, I was hoping you'd forget all about that." He put the champagne on the dresser and handed the flowers to Sarah. "God, this is embarrassing. I heard those sounds Sarah was making. Of course, I didn't know she was in labor, so what was I supposed to think, huh?"

Pete looked confused, but I knew where he was heading, and so did Sarah. "Oh, lord," she muttered, burying her blushing face in the flowers.

"I mean, all the sighing and moaning and stuff. Jeez, I thought you guys were . . . Well, I just figured you were havin' yourselves a nooner. Only it went on and on and *on,* and I kinda got distracted. I'm lyin' up there on the roof thinkin' to myself, damn, Pete's really something. Yeah, that's my buddy. Pete's *da man!"*

Pete's face matched his friend's sunburn. "Mel, stop!" begged Sarah, laughing.

The two men threw their arms over each other's shoulders and went to the kitchen with the champagne, their loud guffaws echoing down the hallway.

"That is *such* a guy thing," giggled Sarah as the champagne cork popped.

Snuggling her son on her chest, she laid her cheek on his downy head and looked out the window at the dangling wisteria clusters. Dreamy-eyed, she said, "It was sure a great birth, though, wasn't it? Such a blessing we didn't know what would lie ahead."

I completed my exam on both of them. Before heading home, I had a half-glass of champagne and a piece of the lopsided birthday cake Marianna had helped the boys make for their baby brother.

After her six-week postpartum checkup, I didn't see Sarah again till that day in the parking lot. I stared at the blue-eyed boy in the middle of the back seat. Dirty face. Grass-stained knees. And black soccer shoes on his feet.

"Sarah, is that really Micah, that one in the middle with soccer shoes on?"

She looked at him. "Umm-hmm. Can you believe it?" Tears came into her eyes. Mine, too.

Micah looked at his mother and groaned. "Aw, Mom, not again."

We laughed and wiped our eyes. She said, "He's had a zillion operations and wore a cast almost constantly till he turned five. At first they doubted he would walk without braces. Then they said he'd have a really bad limp. I thought, hey, a limp we can live with. He's such a tough little guy, he'd handle a limp. And by that time, Pete and I knew we could handle anything.

"So they took that last cast off, and his legs were so small and shriveled. No muscles, just like jelly. But he got down onto the floor right away, and somehow he crawled. A month later he started walking, and I swear, in three months he was running. The next year, he wanted to be on the soccer team with his brothers."

The oldest boy said, "Yeah, come on, Micah. Show the midwife how you can dribble."

"Aw, Jordan," moaned Micah, but his brothers dragged him from the car and pulled a soccer ball from the wayback. Sarah and I stood side by side watching her three boys, ages seven, nine, and ten, perform soccer drills behind the bleachers. All that straw-colored hair, all three dressed in the green and yellow uniforms, all so close to the same height. They began to merge and blur, and I soon lost track of which was Micah.

Then I realized what I'd been anticipating. The thing I'd expected to see that would help me pick him out. When I turned to Sarah, I saw she'd been watching me, eyes glistening again.

"But, Sarah, Micah isn't . . ."

"Limping?"

I nodded, wordless. The boys dribbled and passed the black and white ball back and forth, streaking away in the other direction.

"No. He's not. He told me he wasn't going to on the day he stood up for the first time. And he was right."

The three little boys, as alike as if they'd been shaped by the same cookie cutter, piled back into their car, and Sarah drove off with a jaunty wave. I glanced at my watch and saw it was far too late to run errands. I pulled a paperback from the glove compartment and sat on the grass beneath a eucalyptus.

Soccer practice ended fifteen minutes later. Skylar came running by and saw me.

"What are you doing?" He's not used to seeing me just sit.

"Reading. Waiting for you." I squinted up at him, backlit by the sun.

"Did that woman talk a really long time? Did you do your shopping?" He wiped his sweaty cheek, leaving a mud stain on his face as we walked toward our car.

"No, I never made it to the store. Say, do you know a kid named Micah?"

"Sure. Was that his mom?" I nodded. "Micah's really good," he continued, throwing his balls into the car. "We played his team last week, and I blocked a couple of his shots on goal, but he's really, really good. Why? Did you deliver him?"

"Yes, I did."

"Cool."

"Yeah. Way cool."

~ Hello from Rosie

Home from college for the summer and working as a valet parking attendant, Colin pocketed a wad of tip money and took a date to a fancy restaurant in our neighborhood. It was the kind of place that serves fetal vegetables with leaves and roots still attached and charges $12 for a "mixed green salad of arugula, mizune, frisé, and baby spinach tossed with a light blend of imported olive oil and a raspberry-infused balsamic vinegar."

The hostess seated them at one of the small tables along a side wall. Rog and I have also dined at this restaurant, and I know the close spacing of the tables can occasionally be irritating. One time, the strong perfume worn by a flamboyant woman eighteen inches from my elbow made my mahi-mahi taste like lilacs.

Colin and his date were discussing a movie they'd seen, one she had liked but that he branded a "chick flick." She had launched into her defense when he whispered, "Wait a sec," and leaned a bit toward the woman on his right. Listening closely, he heard this stranger talking about her two home births more than a decade earlier.

"And my midwife drove a VW bug that backfired like crazy."

"Did the license plate say MITWIFE?" Colin asked her.

The woman stared at him, too stunned to speak.

"Sorry," Colin said, smiling, "but I heard you talking about your home births."

The poor woman blushed crimson and stammered an apology. "I'm so sorry, so embarrassed. These tables are too close together, but still, it's not a topic I should be talking about here. I'm really sorry to have disturbed you."

"No, don't apologize. I think I know your midwife. Was she Peggy Vincent?"

"Yes, but . . ." she trailed off, completely flummoxed.

"She's my mom."

"Your mother? Oh gosh, you're Peggy's son?" She babbled on about the small world syndrome and the six degrees of separation, which seem to shrivel to two degrees when you live in Berkeley, the world's largest village. Finally she slowed down and said, "Wow, tell your mom hello from me."

"Sure, what's your name?"

"Donna Glover, although she probably won't remember me after all these years. But, hey, she'll remember Rosie. Tell her Rosie says hi."

"Rosie, is that your daughter?"

"No, it's my tarantula."

Colin shouted, "A tarantula?"

Several nearby patrons looked alarmed and lifted their feet.

Donna laughed. "Yeah, I had a tarantula named Rosie, and your mom brought your little brother over to visit. When tarantulas grow, they crawl out of their old skins and grow new ones. I kept all of Rosie's old body casts in petri dishes. I called them her baby clothes. Your brother was pretty fascinated."

"I can imagine."

"Oh, my God," Colin's date whispered, as the woman got up to leave.

Colin called me the next morning. "I met a lady in a restaurant last night, and you were her midwife. She says to tell you Rosie says hi."

"Rosie who?"

"Rosie with eight furry legs, Rosie the . . ."

"Rosie the tarantula!" It all came back to me, not just Rosie, but Donna, her stack of petri dishes full of Rosie's baby clothes, the pattern of her bedroom curtains, and the African drums her husband played while she pushed her first child into the world. I also recalled that she had only Dreyer's mocha fudge ice cream and six pounds of Peet's coffee beans in her freezer.

But I thought of my son interacting in that pricey restaurant with a former Berkeley patient of mine. I thought about him discussing home birth with a total stranger and burdening his girlfriend with talk of a tarantula named Rosie. I thought of the times he drove my car with the MITWIFE license plate to school, the occasion when he walked into our guest bedroom where I was teaching a woman how to insert her diaphragm, the looks on his friends' faces as they picked up a random photo album at our house and realized it was full of pictures of women giving birth. I imagined my son's discomfort.

"Honey, I'm really sorry for all the embarrassing stuff I've put you through."

"Hold it, Mom. Would I have spoken to that woman if I were embarrassed?"

"Well . . ."

"Of course not. It made me proud to tell Rosie's mom that you're my mother. What are you thinking? Of course I wasn't embarrassed."

"You weren't?"

"Sheesh, Mom, come on. Bye, I love you."

Well, gee.

A Bitter Pill

As the lupine and poppies of spring bloomed and then gave way to the golden grasses of summer, I dared to hope that Polly Stroud, the insurance rep, had been wrong when she warned that my malpractice policy might not be renewed. The warm days of autumn came, and I heard nothing. Her words floated to the back of my brain where they simmered, repressed but not forgotten. The Wilsons eventually received about three-quarters of a million dollars in settlements, with perhaps a third of it going to pay their lawyers.

I called Dr. Weick in Oregon, and he knew more about the final negotiations than I did. Apparently the defense lawyers had made settlement conditional on the court establishing a trust fund to ensure that the money would be spent only on legitimate expenses for Luke's welfare.

Just before signing off, I asked, "Hey, Joe, you've been sued before, right?"

"Sure, but I've never felt as screwed over as I did in this case. It's left a bad taste in my mouth." We both knew California's reputation for the ease with which people can find lawyers to bring suit against anyone for anything.

I asked if his insurance company had ever threatened to terminate his coverage.

"No, why?"

"Mine might."

"Oh, I don't think so, Peggy. They only lost a quarter of a million, just peanuts."

"I hope you're right."

My insurance needed to be paid by November 30. As mid-November approached, I began looking for the renewal notice. Then Rog brought in the mail on November twentieth, my birthday, and said, "You got a certified letter. I signed for it." He had an odd, tight look on his face.

I froze. "A birthday something?" I asked, crossing my fingers.

"No, it's from your insurance carrier." He didn't hand it to me. He just laid it on the hall table and took me in his arms.

"Oh, God," I said, feeling my heart sink. "Happy birthday, huh?" We held on to each other and contemplated what it meant. Looking at the official envelope on the polished table, we knew that only a miracle could prevent my being out of business in ten days.

I used the first five days to fire off outraged letters and phone calls to the insurance company and to the American College of Nurse Midwives. I spoke with supportive doctors, and none of them had ever heard of such an occurrence. They were all sure it was a mistake—but I knew it was real. A sympathetic woman in the legal department of the ACNM had explained that, with the comparatively small number of midwives and our low insurance premiums, there weren't millions of dollars in the insurance pool to pay out large settlements.

"They probably figure a midwife who's cost them a quarter million on one occasion is more likely to cost them money again," she concluded. "I'm just guessing, but I'll bet I'm right."

When I reached the actuarial department of the insurance company, I was stonewalled. "It's nonnegotiable," the supervisor said. Then he hung up.

So that was that. I had truly become the sacrificial pawn.

Although the hopelessness of my situation sickened me, I flipped into automatic pilot. The next five days flew past in a blur as I scrambled to match each of my fifty pregnant clients with a new midwife or doctor. The most difficult to say goodbye to were women with babies due in the next few weeks. I told those already planning home births that if they'd sign a statement saying they were aware I no longer had doctor backup, insurance, or hospital privileges, I'd still do their deliveries.

This is called "going bare," and it's the way lay midwives have always operated. I had attended midwifery school to avoid exactly the situation in which I now found myself: uninsured and dependent on the good will of my clients.

All my home birth moms signed the statement, including one who asked, "That woman who sued you, do you think she would've, if you hadn't had insurance?"

I shook my head. I felt certain Patty never wanted to sue Joe Weick or me, but she needed money for Luke's care. I suspect the Wilsons never dreamed it would put me out of business.

"So the more insurance you carry, the more likely you are to be sued?" she asked, and I nodded, explaining that the more money professionals are insured for, the higher the malpractice awards. Then the hospitals require their doctors to carry even more insurance, and all that does is encourage more lawsuits with even bigger settlements. It's a nasty spiral with no end in sight.

"But you're the only one who's been penalized, right?"

"Yes," I said, fighting anger and bitterness—and trying not to feel overwhelmed with worry about my future. Rog and the kids knew how sad I was at the abrupt end of my dream occupation, and their compassion often brought tears to my eyes. In so many ways, our family life had revolved around my work, my crazy hours, the sometimes bizarre nature of our dinner table conversations. The whole tone of our existence was bound to change. They tried to reassure me that we'd all do just fine, no matter what, but I worried.

Would the fact that I was one of the rare midwives ever to be sued make it difficult to be hired somewhere else? Would lay people misunderstand the facts of the case and think I had indeed been guilty of malpractice? And I worried about money. Salaried midwives don't earn nearly as much as those in private practice, so I felt concern for my family's welfare, things such as my children's college fees.

Still operating like a robot, I made some phone calls and went job-hunting.

～ Happy Birthday

I had three weeks to acclimate to the changes in my life before beginning my new job. Mourning the loss of my private practice, I wandered through the house, staring out the windows at gray skies and torrents of rain. I didn't know if my mood matched the weather or California's winter commiserated with my grief. For the first time in years, I missed the winters of my Midwestern childhood.

Both Rog and I grew up in states where winter means "weather": snow, frost, sleet, and ice. While we certainly didn't miss frozen pipes, whiteouts, dirty slush, or shoveling the driveway, we cherished fond memories of the softer side of the season. Snow days when kids stayed home and wrote their names on frost-etched windows instead of going to school and writing essays on blue-ruled paper. Ice skating and sipping mugs of hot chocolate afterward as the smell of wet mittens drying by the fire hung in the air.

Skylar once asked if we'd ever cut our own Christmas tree, and Rog said, "Of course, and then a real sleigh pulled it to our car."

"And did you build snowmen every year?" my California child asked.

"Oh my, whole families of them, fat and skinny, short and tall. And snow forts and snow angels."

I told him about breaking off icicles to lick like Popsicles, "but we stored the biggest ones in the freezer till August."

Skylar looked wistful. "It never snows in the Bay Area."

It's true. In winter, we drive three hours to Lake Tahoe to find snow. And when we go, we rent a cabin at a ski resort, take a shuttle bus to the slopes, ski all day, soak our tired legs in a hot tub at night, and that's it. No snowmen, no ice skating, no Christmas tree cutting, and definitely no icicles in August. It's "destination snow," Disneyland style.

"I wish it were snowing instead of raining," I murmured to Rog as I stared out the window. I knew I was depressed and found myself craving the cleansing purity of a pristine winter landscape.

He put his arms around me from behind. "Remember snow days?"

I nodded and leaned against him as he pressed his lips to my hair.

"You need one. Why don't you go visit Sally?"

So I called my college friend and asked if I could pay a quick visit.

"Now? You want to come to Maine in January?"

"Yes, if it's not inconvenient."

"Peggy, no one comes to Maine from California in January. It snows here in January, in case you've forgotten."

I booked my flight.

With my arrival the following week, the snow gods cooperated and delivered an epic blizzard that buried their small, seaside town. Snowdrifts to the tops of cars kept us huddled around the wood-burning stove. Schools closed, and neighborhood kids built snowmen within sight of the beach. I took a very short walk and returned with frozen eyelashes. Thrilled with our winter isolation, I shoveled the steps, brought in more logs, and made hot chocolate.

But Sally and Jim wallowed in the terminal stages of cabin fever. When the plows made it down their street, we followed one into Portland for dinner and a play.

A few flakes were still falling as we negotiated the treacherous brick sidewalks through the old town and stamped snow off our boots inside the entryway of Jim's favorite restaurant. Taking our coats, the maitre d' quickly seated us and offered cocktails.

"Three Cosmopolitans, please," requested Jim, knowing me well, "and is Jonathan here this evening?"

"Yes, yes, I've seated you in his section."

Soon a tall, smiling man with a lean face and hair even redder than Jim's came to our table, bringing Cosmopolitans and menus. Sally said, "Jonathan, this is our friend Peggy. She's visiting from California. The Bay Area, actually."

"No kidding? I used to live in Berkeley, and weather like this makes me wonder why I left. I worked there for five years in a great restaurant, Strawberry Fields. Perhaps you know it."

Kaleidoscopic memories of Strawberry Fields tumbled into place.

"Of course I know it. Were you there when Jerry Johnson was owner and chef?"

"Oh, yes, Jerry and I opened that place. I was his first employee. The world shrinks every day, doesn't it? Did you know Jerry personally?"

"Actually, I delivered Jerry and Melissa's baby in the big flat above the restaurant."

"She's a midwife," explained Jim.

Jonathan stared at me a few moments and then mumbled, "The night the restaurant opened, there was a party . . ."

"Wait a minute," I said, feeling goose bumps on my arms. "If you, I mean, were you at that party? It was the one night Jerry made Melissa promise she wouldn't go into labor, because he'd invited two hundred guests to celebrate his new restaurant. Were you at the opening?"

"That was you? You're the midwife who delivered Melissa's baby during the party?" he shouted. He placed both hands flat on our table, staring at me from inches away. Many eyes turned toward us, and other conversations stopped. "My God, that must've been what, ten years ago?"

"Yep, that was me. And Melissa was noisy. You probably heard her. Every time a contraction started, all talking downstairs just stopped."

"Yeah, yeah, we'd hear her hollering, and everybody would stop, listening to this woman having a baby, like, right above our heads, you know?" Jonathan posed like a waiter holding a tray aloft, one foot off the ground, motionless as in a game of freeze tag. "Then she'd peter out, and we'd all pretend we hadn't heard a thing."

"And upstairs, we'd hear the tinkling glasses, forks scraping on plates, laughter. Another champagne cork would pop, and then a contraction would hit, and . . ."

"And we'd just stop, mid-bite, mid-step, mid-sip, whatever. Time froze. And those sounds she made—just incredible. But then it got quiet, just a groan now and then. We tried to imagine what was happening."

I twirled the stemmed cocktail glass between my fingers, remembering Melissa's labor as if it were yesterday. "Right, she pushed quietly. And the birth went so fast. As soon as the baby . . ."

He stopped me with his hand on my shoulder and looked like he'd been to the mountain and seen the prophet. "Oh, man, I'll never forget the sound of that baby crying," he said. "Not if I live to be a hundred. Just miraculous."

I smiled, remembering. "As soon as the baby cried, Lord, you should have heard the noise from below, up through the floorboards and into the room where the little boy was lying on Melissa's belly. We heard everyone laughing and clapping."

"Some of us were crying. I know I was."

"It was great. We felt like the whole world had spread its arms to welcome that baby. And once Jerry could see that everything was fine, he became a chef and host again."

"Yeah, yeah, I remember. He called downstairs to order food for you guys."

"And fifteen minutes later somebody brought up huge trays and platters of stuff from the party. Champagne, hors d'oeuvres, salmon, caviar, and a whole chocolate mousse cake and fresh Peet's coffee."

"That was me," said Jonathan.

I stared at his grinning, freckled face. "No way."

"Yeah, no lie. I didn't see you, though. I didn't come into the room. Jeez, Melissa was my boss's wife, and she'd just had a kid. I didn't know if she was naked or if there was blood or, well, anyway, I just went to the doorway and handed it to this tiny woman with blood on her skirt."

"That must have been Sandi. She always got bloody," I said.

"Anyway, she showed me the baby, and I went back downstairs and told everybody he had the flattest nose I'd ever seen, except on a boxer who'd lost a big fight."

Sally and Jim hadn't said a thing. Sally's silver earrings glittered in the candlelight as her head swiveled between us like a spectator at a Chinese Ping-Pong game. In fact, every person within earshot in the crowded restaurant stared at us, listening without embarrassment. Several people had pushed their chairs sideways so they could look and listen more easily. A woman wearing gray heirloom pearls rested her elbows on the table and propped her chin on the backs of her clasped hands. She smiled with a dreamy look on her face.

I stood and gave Jonathan a hug, and the woman in pearls began clapping. A few others joined her, and soon about twenty people were applauding with big grins on their faces. So much for reserved New Englanders.

"What did they name the baby?" asked the lady in pearls.

"Let me think," I muttered, pondering. "It was unusual. Um . . . Wolf!"

"Let's drink a toast," she said.

Everyone raised a wineglass. "To Wolf."

The owner scurried over to see what all the commotion was about. "What, what? Is somebody having a birthday?"

"Well, yes," answered Jim. "We *are* celebrating a birthday, in a way."

As everyone laughed, I sat still, absorbing the realization that the joy of a birth done ten years earlier had found me in a Maine blizzard, three thousand miles from Berkeley, where it never snows. And I dared to hope that similar memories would follow me forever.

~ Shift Work

Employee benefits—what a concept. Paid vacation, overtime, retirement fund, sick days, medical insurance, educational leave: I hadn't enjoyed such perks since I quit my nursing job to go to midwifery school in 1980. But in 1992, when I accepted a position as a staff midwife at Kaiser Hospital in Walnut Creek, I knew those benefits came at a price. I would be returning to shift work—and once again following doctors' orders.

With a shudder, I remembered Dr. Clark's callous words, the words that had helped propel me into midwifery school: "Normal birth is a retrospective diagnosis. All births are complicated until proven otherwise."

I knew some Kaiser doctors were certain to share that philosophy, and after twelve years of independence and autonomy, I didn't know how well I'd cope. My own philosophy was the polar opposite: All births are normal until proven otherwise.

But to stay employed, I realized I would need to make concessions. At least I had company as I struggled with the transition. Sandi MacKenzie had recently remarried. She found the wacky hours of a solo midwife incompatible with being a doctor's wife, so she, too, took a job with Kaiser.

We had lunch together in the courtyard on the first day of orientation, reminiscing over the good old days. After we tossed our sandwich wrappings and Diet Coke cans in the trash, she pulled a foil-wrapped package from her backpack and handed it to me. It held two of her signature, chocolate-dipped caramels (see Appendix Six), the same ones she made every Christmas and the ones she'd brought to so many births over the years.

"Is this the spoonful of sugar to help the medicine go down, now that we're shift workers?" I asked, taking one.

Sandi nodded, a little misty-eyed, and we savored her caramels in silence. Then, licking chocolate from our fingertips, we went inside again.

After orientation, I worked two or three twelve-hour shifts a week, alternating between days and nights. Like a factory worker, I faced a new shipment of patients each day. Twice I delivered nine women in the course of my twelve-hour shift—and by morning I could barely remember even one of them. In my old practice, I'd known my clients well. I had known their children and their neighbors, their homes and lifestyles, their belief systems and their dreams. Now, since I never met the Kaiser women during their pregnancies, a stranger stared at me each time I opened the door to a labor room.

Kaiser Permanente, the first and still the largest hospital-based HMO in the country, insures women from every socioeconomic level. A migrant worker might labor next door to an attorney. In the recovery room, a biologist and a bus driver might lie in adjacent gurneys. One day I delivered five women who spoke no English, nor did any two speak the same language. I heard families exclaiming over the newborn in Tagalog, Chinese, Spanish, Hmong, and German.

These women delivered at Kaiser Hospital because that's what their insurance covered. A few showed up at the Walnut Creek facility specifically for its unique midwifery service, not available to the same extent at other Kaiser hospitals. But most came just because it was convenient. We midwives cared for them because they were assigned to us, not because they'd requested us. They didn't care if they got a midwife or a doctor. They usually just wanted drugs, as little pain as possible, and a baby.

"I feel as if I'm working on the Ford assembly line in Detroit," I said one day to Rog. "My only consolation, now that I'm out of business, is that there are so many other nurse midwives to carry on."

During those heady years when Sandi, Lindy, and I had soared around Berkeley on a high-flying kite of confidence, we knew many obstetricians feared and resented our independence, but we felt we had the winds of the future holding us aloft. We never imagined it would end so quickly.

As Sandi and I adjusted to institutional midwifery practice, we read in the ACNM newsletter about a high-profile case in the East. In 1991, a doctor, one of only a handful who attended home births, performed an underwater birth and had somehow allowed the baby to drown. In the resulting lawsuit, CNA Insurance, his insurance carrier, my former carrier, and the same one that insured all certified nurse midwives in the United States, paid a settlement of more than one million dollars.

"Surely this won't affect midwives," Sandi said, but I heard the apprehension in her voice. Then we watched helplessly as CNA withdrew coverage from all certified midwives who attended home births. Another company offered malpractice insurance, but the coverage was too low and the premiums too high to make it worthwhile. Within a few months, home birth by certified nurse midwives across the country all but ceased. Those few who continued to deliver babies at home did it without the protection of insurance.

Then, as if a pebble had been tossed into a pond, the resultant ripples set the lily pads a-jiggling as most nurse midwives took steps to protect their livelihood.

"We're nobodies," said Barbara, a midwife friend in Virginia. "We're small change, and we're at the mercy of the guys with the big guns—the insurance industry, the AMA, and the lawyers." She had decided to close her private practice at the end of the year and take a salaried job with the county hospital.

"But, jeez, Barb. Don't quit. What if all nurse midwives dive under the table?"

"Gotta put food on top of the table," she said sadly.

Agreeing with that sentiment, midwives from Virginia to California, from Montana to Texas, abandoned independent practice and accepted shift work as employees of hospitals, HMOs, or large physician groups.

All studies (see Appendix Three) have supported the excellent outcome of midwifery care, but in spite of that irrefutable evidence, doctors have always argued against independent practice by midwives. I've heard physicians insist that it's fine for a midwife to deliver an anemic, uninsured drug addict, but unsafe for the same midwife to deliver a healthy, fully insured high school teacher. Or, that it's safe for midwives to work for an hourly wage in county hospitals, but unsafe in settings that would allow them to be directly reimbursed by private insurance companies.

I remembered a comment that one of my midwifery school instructors had made years earlier: "Doctors talk about safety, but the real issue has always been competition."

Home births, anathema to many physicians, returned to the hands of non-nurse midwives—that same dedicated group of women who caught babies in women's homes before certified nurse midwives came onto the scene. Obstetricians, hoping to eliminate home birth, succeeded only in eliminating the ability of licensed, insured, certified nurse midwives with ready access to a hospital to be attendants at those births.

It was as if the gains we'd made in that magical decade of the eighties had been erased. Not even a trace of chalk dust remained on the blackboard.

During those glory years, we took midwifery out of the alleys and onto the mainstream highway. We could move a mother smoothly from home to hospital without a break in her care, and with a single phone call we could mobilize an entire labor and delivery department for an emergency cesarean. We knew each others' cars on sight, and when we passed on the freeways at three A.M. with the Bay Bridge lights twinkling to the west, we were proud to be ushering newborns into the world while everyone else slept.

The good days, the best days, were at an end. Some nights after completing a twelve-hour shift at Kaiser, I took my old and tattered birth logbook to bed with me and flipped through the pages, just remembering. . . .

Although I was still catching babies, I knew it might never be the same. Not for me, not for other midwives, not for the millions of birthing women in the future, women who someday would include my own daughter. After watching Sandi give birth to Emilie those long years ago, Jill had said she was going to have twenty-five babies, but only if I could be there to hold her hand. Now, with midwifery so changed, I wondered what her chances would be of finding a competent midwife to help her have even one of those babies at home.

Passing the Torch

I love home births. I love their unexpected diversity. Women react with perfect freedom in the comfort of their own homes, and I learned long ago not to try predicting who would be quiet or noisy, stoical or dramatic. Renée used fourteen rolls of toilet paper during her second labor as she hypnotically wiped invisible spots on the bathroom counter. How could anyone have anticipated that? Josie changed her dress six times during labor, hoping the baby would come faster once she had the right attire. Yellow with chartreuse trim finally worked.

I loved watching Jessica rise on tiptoe with contractions while her toddler sat in my lap and a kitten played with my shoelaces. I loved making brownies with Emily's towheaded sons while she paced on a sunny balcony to hasten her labor. I loved it when Bill crouched on all fours to whisper encouragement into the ear of his laboring wife and didn't miss a beat when his toddler climbed on his back for a horsie ride.

I fed my family with my income from working twenty-four hours a week for Kaiser, a huge hospital machine, but I fed my soul by "going bare" to do two home births a month for women like Alison, a midwife herself, who wanted a home birth for her second baby. And who could resist Lynette, an ER nurse who moonlighted as a belly dancer with a six-foot boa constrictor draped around her shoulders? How about Theresa, five of whose first six children I had delivered? How could I say no to her last two?

And what about the covey of Alta Bates nurses with whom I had worked for so many years? When they began having children, they asked me to deliver them at home. In hard labor, Cherie's comment when her bag of water broke revealed her delivery room training: "Is the amniotic fluid clear? How does the fetal heart sound?" Lynn repeated endlessly, "Wait, you guys, wait a minute," as her labor galloped away with her. Rita's son scared me to death when he marched into the bedroom blowing a trumpet just minutes after his sister was born. Holly cracked us up when she said, "Only seven centimeters? Oh, now I'm starting to whine, and I hate whiners." Lois thought she'd have to go to the hospital to have labor induced and was rendered speechless when I told her she was nine centimeters and we weren't going anywhere, thank you very much. Marion crab-walked backwards halfway into her closet right before her baby came out. My own Skylar was ten when Cindy generously invited him to her second home birth. Skylar stood up in the hush after the birth and began clapping slowly, saying, "Way to go, Cindy!" Then everyone joined in.

These nurses and others like them had made my life easy. They smoothed the way when I hospitalized patients with complications, and they made the births of those who planned hospital deliveries as homey as possible within the tiled walls of Alta Bates Hospital. I *had* to say yes to these women, not just for them, but for myself. I needed them as much as they needed me.

At Kaiser, nearly all uncomplicated women were assigned to a midwife upon admission. I never met them till they came through the doors of Labor and Delivery. Most of them had no real interest in experiencing the raw passion of childbirth with a midwife to guide them.

"This is an obstetrical factory," I said to my husband. "I check these women, order an epidural so they won't feel pain, deliver them, and move on to the next room. I'll never see them again."

Driving east through the tunnel to suburban Walnut Creek twice a week was a far cry from tootling around Berkeley and Oakland in my backfiring VW bug at all hours. I can't travel anywhere without reawakening memories. Driving to Monterey Foods market, I pass the rose-covered cottage where Sirpa lived when I delivered her second baby. Heading to Berkeley Bowl for artichokes and arugula, I see the pastel Victorian owned by Kathleen and Wolfgang and realize I delivered three different women in that house. I often knew when growing families moved away and could tip off others who were house hunting. I should have received a commission for all the sales and rentals I arranged.

When I hike up the hill at the top of my street, I pass the house where everyone wore crowns of tinsel stars while Carolynn smiled throughout a long and arduous labor in a cozy, candlelit bedroom. The closest she ever came to a complaint was "Murgatroyd," when I told her it was still too soon to push. In the same house two years later, she managed most of the delivery of a second daughter all by herself while standing upright at the foot of the bed. Three months later, Carolynn kept three huge and overly protective dogs under control while her friend Charlotte gave birth to Abbey.

Each time I stop at my neighborhood gas station, I pass a tiny apartment in Oakland's flatlands where Anne and Hank lived. Born at Alta Bates, their baby girls were the first set of twins I delivered. The second baby literally floated into the world in an intact bag of water, floated out so effortlessly that even Anne didn't know what had happened. The girls were so identical that every morning for the next four months, Anne re-inked a blue Magic Marker dot at the nape of the firstborn's neck.

My private practice was like being a midwife in a rural village. While no one ever tried to pay me with a sack of potatoes, food often was an integral part of the experience. I remember Pamela's sushi extravaganza after Maggie's birth, Acme Bakery's rye raisin buns at Roseanne's, Rachele's raspberry tart with crème anglaise, and the yummy oatmeal Patrick fixed after Ellen delivered their fourth daughter. Lois and Bert hosted a bay cruise on the S. S. *Hornblower* with a banquet for their entire birth crew, and Vani, who described her labor in halting English as "too many contractions," dished up the hottest curry I've ever eaten. Julie's husband kept me awake with Peet's Garuda Blend coffee, and I've drunk it ever since. I can't eat an onion bagel, take a garden tour, cook cassoulet, watch my children juggle, or hear songs from *Mary Poppins* without memories coming alive.

So when Naeema, the young woman who was barely sixteen when I delivered her first child, became pregnant with her fourth, I never considered saying no. Her labor started just as I completed a busy night shift at Kaiser.

"I'll be there in forty-five minutes," I assured her. I changed out of my scrubs quickly, remembering how fast she'd birthed her second baby, combing her hair the whole time. I zoomed along San Pablo Dam Road and into a working-class neighborhood in Richmond. But I needn't have hurried. Naeema's fourth baby was a lazy one. An hour later, I was still sitting on the carpet of their bare living room, dozing off more than once and jerking awake moments later.

Right before their third daughter's birth eighteen months earlier, she and Hameed moved to an apartment next to the *masjed,* the Muslim temple that had become the focus of their lives. Naeema had adopted *hijab,* the fully robed costume of devout Muslim women, including a veil covering everything except her eyes. The frisky, young sixteen year old I'd met six years earlier had matured into a Muslim matron.

"Don't those robes feel claustrophobic?" I'd asked earlier in her pregnancy. "You grew up right on the Berkeley border wearing blue jeans, and until a few years ago you hung out on Telegraph and Solano drinking mochas. This is quite a change."

Smoothing the folds of her robe over her knees, she'd said, "No, I feel safer like this. I see how guys on the street act with girls wearing shorts or those poor-boy tops. Since I started wearing *hijab* with the veil, they act respectful. They blush and mumble and call me ma'am. Ma'am! Imagine."

Looking at her slim body and those knockout eyes, I could understand that, without the protective robes, she'd be the target of lingering glances and lewd comments. But now, in the privacy of her own home, Naeema wore a loose T-shirt and elastic-waisted cotton pants. Her spectacular hair, black with hints of auburn among the curls, coiled down her back in a loose braid. She still looked like the high school sophomore I'd first met, but Janice, her mother-in-law, had told me about Naeema's stature in the Islamic community.

"She's a wonderful mother, calm and wise and so patient. Other women, even those much older than Naeema, look up to her," said Janice, her eyes shining with pride in her daughter-in-law. "They're moving to Yemen in six months, and Naeema says she wants to be a midwife."

I confirmed it a week later. "Naeema, is it true that you want to be a midwife?"

A bit of her former shyness came out, but she looked right at me and said, "I'd like to very much. Middle Eastern women don't have good health care, and I'd like to help them."

"Oh, Naeema, you would be an inspirational midwife," I'd assured her, more than a little sad at the thought that I wouldn't be attending her future births.

Her labor with this fourth baby had stalled, but I didn't dare go home. "Peggy, you should take a nap," she said when I nodded off for the third time, and she made me a little nest of pillows. I curled up like a kitten in a basket and slept for nearly three hours.

When I woke up, Naeema was fixing lunch. Bonnie had arrived and sat chatting with three young women, all wearing robes in somber tones of brown, blue, or black. On the floor lay a circular tablecloth, only of course it was a floorcloth, since there was no table in the apartment. No furniture at all, actually, except for an unpainted dresser in one bedroom. They'd refused to accumulate "things," as Hameed called such nonessentials as beds and chairs, in order to simplify their lives and minimize the fuss of packing when they left for the Middle East.

"Midwives major in sleeping," I said, when I saw them smiling at me. "We can do it anywhere, anytime. Where's Hameed?"

Bonnie said, "He's at the whaddayacallit, the . . . the temple thingy."

"*Masjed*. It's just next door," murmured one of the robed women.

"You almost missed lunch," said Naeema. She set a platter of tabbouleh, a basket of pita bread, and a pitcher of ice water in the middle of the cloth, and we scooped up mouthfuls of tangy salad with pieces of the pita.

Every five or six minutes, a stillness born of peace and inward focusing came over Naeema as she paused for a contraction. When a stronger one came along, she tilted her face toward the ceiling and closed her eyes, sighing deeply. Then she had one that made her gasp, and she lowered her face and looked at me. The young women stared at her as if they were toddlers hearing Little Red Riding Hood for the first time.

"Shall I check you?" I whispered into the awed hush.

She nodded and rose straight from the floor like a flower growing toward the sun. Watching her, I wondered how she could be so pregnant and still so graceful. We went into the larger of the two bedrooms where she slipped off her cotton pants and lay on a thin futon covered with plastic and towels.

"Seven centimeters, and the bag of water's bulging," I said. "I could break it if you're tired, but it's up to you."

"No, I'm okay."

With his daughters scampering around his feet, Hameed came in the front door, turning aside for a few seconds to give the women time to cover their faces. "Hey, what's happening?" he said to Bonnie and me. He, too, had matured in the six years since we'd first met. He'd changed from a skate-boarding teenager into a hard worker and a serious student of Islam, but love still shone in his eyes whenever he looked at Naeema.

"We're waiting for the bag to break," said Bonnie. "Then the baby'll come fast."

"Naeema's never labored this long before. Why not just break it?"

My mind flashed back to Barbara, a woman I'd cared for in the hospital the previous night. "Let me answer with a story, Hameed," I said. And I told them about Barbara, a rare Kaiser patient who'd requested a midwife because she wanted a natural birth. When I met her in the evening, she was about five centimeters dilated but still not in active labor, just walking around making slow progress. Her bag of water was intact, her baby sounded perfect, and she walked the corridors with a smile on her face.

The on-call doctor made rounds at bedtime. He pointed at Barbara's name on the chalkboard and said, "What about her? She's going too slowly. I don't want to be awakened at three A.M. to do a cesarean on her when I could do it right now and not have my sleep disturbed."

When I told him she liked her slow and gentle labor, he rolled his eyes and said, "Oh, Christ, you midwives."

Just then a nurse called me into the delivery room to catch a baby. When I went back to Barbara forty minutes later, I found her in tears. While I'd been gone, the doctor had examined her, broken the bag of water, and attached a fetal monitor. He'd ordered Pitocin to speed up her contractions—and now she was writhing in pain and asking for drugs.

When I delivered her two hours later, she greeted her baby with open arms and seemed relieved her ordeal had ended. But when I later went to the recovery room to finish charting, she called me to her bedside.

"Please understand," she began. "I'm not blaming you, but that was just awful. That doctor robbed me of the birth I'd hoped for." I began to apologize for the doctor's intervention, to explain that all doctors aren't like him, but she stopped me with a hand on my arm. "I'm never coming back here to have another baby. Do you know any midwives who do home births?"

"What did you tell her?" asked Naeema.

"I gave her my phone number and told her to call me after she gets home."

"Labor's always been gentler for me with the bag intact," said Naeema, and I explained it's also gentler for the baby. Naeema wasn't exhausted, she wasn't stuck, and there were no complications at all, so it made no sense to upset Mother Nature's plan.

Another hour passed. Then the water broke while Naeema was on the toilet. With the robed women following like acolytes, Bonnie and I guided her, doubled over, to the futon in the bedroom. Hameed scrubbed his hands, knelt, and ten minutes later he delivered his first son.

"*La ilaha illa Allah,*" he whispered into the baby's ear.

By now Bonnie and I were as well trained in Muslim birth ethics as Hameed was in the mechanics of childbirth. We knew not to say a word till he'd given the traditional blessing of Islam: There is no God but God.

"A boy? A boy? Are you sure? Let me see," stammered Naeema.

"Oh, yes, we have a son at last. Praise to Allah, it's really a boy," and Hameed laid the baby on her chest. She reached out her hand to pull one fat little leg aside and then began to laugh.

Once again, I handed Hameed a Kleenex to wipe his tears and blow his nose.

Ten minutes later Naeema stood up with her baby in her arms. She walked toward the doorway where the three women sat, each with one of Naeema and

Hameed's girls on her lap, and suddenly my mind filled with images of Zelda.

Long-legged Zelda, dancing on her bed at Duke Hospital those many years ago.

I hadn't thought about that skinny black woman with her gospel tent chanting for ages. When I cared for her, she'd been about Naeema's age. Zelda's little baby would be almost forty years old by now. In those forty years, I'd changed. I had finished nursing school, married, moved to California, had three children, started an alternative birth center in Berkeley, become a midwife, and caught more than two thousand babies.

But some things hadn't changed. I still got my kicks from hanging out with women having babies. In the name of compassion and common sense, I still bent rules right and left, and I hadn't lost my appetite for drama. The rush of the unexpected, the thrill of living on the edge, the heart-stoppingly tender moments, the surprise of laughter in the midst of pain—these all charged my batteries with the energy to endure yet another sleepless night. I was no longer in charge of my own independent midwifery service, but at least I was still catching babies. And it had all started with Zelda.

"Granny Vida let me walk, yes ma'am, she let me walk and sing and dance my pains away. Everything would go much better if y'all would just lemme up," Zelda had said to me those long years ago. I'd tried my best to make her lie down, but she'd managed to get up and walk anyway. Right on top of her mattress.

Many times over the intervening years, I had conspired to protect women from the sincere but misguided intentions of the medical profession. But at nineteen, I hadn't had enough experience, power, or self-confidence to help Zelda take charge of her baby's birth.

I wish I could meet her again. I'd like to sit in a willow rocking chair on Granny Vida's porch, listening to the bees in the honeysuckle. As Zelda's grandbabies crawled around our ankles, I'd share my stories with her. Our rockers would squeak on the weathered planks, and Zelda would nod her head, saying, "Mmm-hmm, girl, mmm-hmm." She'd flash me that big grin full of crooked teeth, and then I'd feel her hand on my arm, her hand reaching across the time and space between us, and I'd grin back. I'd look off toward the hazy North Carolina hills, nodding my own head, thinking of all those babies' names inked into my blue-ruled logbook.

I went home, tired but content, and added Naeema's fourth birth to my ledger.

★   ★   ★

Two days later I returned for a postpartum home visit. After I'd checked Naeema and her son, I said, "I have something for you in my car."

"What's this?" she asked as I lugged a suitcase up the concrete steps.

"It's my going-away present, Naeema. You'll be leaving for Yemen in a few months, and you said you want to be involved in women's health over there. I'm pretty much at the end of my career, so I'm passing the torch to you."

I knelt and unfastened the clasps on the suitcase. Inside were about twenty books on midwifery, childbirth, lactation, and pediatrics. There were also two stethoscopes, a blood pressure cuff, and a set of birth instruments.

Naeema gasped, and her eyes grew misty. Then she looked around her bare apartment. On the kitchen counter stood a mayonnaise jar full of daisies and snapdragons. She snatched them up, wrapped the stems in wet paper toweling and aluminum foil, and handed them to me.

We hugged each other tightly, and suddenly I was crying. But why? Tears of parting? Or loss? Tears of nostalgia for my past or joy for her future? I couldn't have said till I looked in her eyes. Then I knew the source of my tears.

I cried with pride as I looked into the face of a midwife from the next generation of baby catchers.

Epilogue

~ The Current Situation

For several years after 1991, when I closed my private practice, certified nurse midwives were unable to obtain malpractice insurance that would allow them to be covered for home births.

Recently, insurance for home births has again become available. The American College of Nurse Midwives (ACNM) offers up to one million dollars in coverage, and premiums are generally considered affordable.

The situation with direct-entry midwives (formerly known as "lay midwives") is undergoing a rapid evolution throughout the United States. Many states now have formal programs offering midwifery education to women who have not completed nursing school. After a standardized examination is passed, the midwife is licensed and can generally obtain insurance.

What hasn't changed in the United States is the acceptance of home birth and direct-entry midwives by the ranks within organized medicine. Tremendous resistance, clearly motivated by economics, still exists on the local level to the acceptance of midwifery in general (and direct-entry midwives in particular) by many obstetricians and hospitals. Midwives who desire a private practice, and particularly those who intend to offer home births, still face greater difficulty obtaining physical backup and hospital delivery privileges.

But there is hope. What many consider the perfect combination of birth options is available in Taos, New Mexico. The Northern New Mexico Women's Health and Birth Center, begun by Elizabeth Gilmore, is staffed by certified nurse midwives, direct-entry midwives, and board certified obstetricians (a husband/wife team). Pregnant couples can select the birth attendant of their choice and may elect to deliver at home, in an out-of-hospital birthing center, or in the local hospital. Those who are supportive of mid-wives, home birth, and a woman's right to choose how, where, and by whom she will be delivered, are hopeful that this is the wave of the future.

—Peggy Vincent, RN, CNM
September 2001

Appendix I:
Pearls of Wisdom

A woman will labor more like her sisters than like her mother.

At night, in dangerous neighborhoods, walk in the middle of the street and whistle.

Carry a pillow, a blanket, and a change of clothes in your trunk.

Carry your own favorite brand of coffee or tea.

Childbirth is normal until proven otherwise.

Don't announce the sex of the baby. Let the couple discover it for themselves.

Don't wear perfume. Laboring women have a heightened sense of smell.

Fill your gas tank every Monday, Wednesday, and Friday.

First labors are long, second labors are short, but third labors are unpredictable.

For speedy dressing, skip socks and underwear, and wear wooden clogs.

If a woman wants a natural, unmedicated birth and her labor is normal, she can do it.

If you think you can predict how a woman will act in labor, you're wrong.

If you think you can predict what kind of labor a woman will have, you're wrong.

If you think you've seen it all, you're wrong.

It's better to be lucky than smart.

Keep breath mints in your purse and carry a toothbrush.

Kids do fine at births if no one forces them to be there.

Learn to nap.

Rare complications are rare. Be alert for them, but don't go looking for them.

Redheads bleed.

Restock your birth supplies as soon as you get home, no matter how tired you are.

Slow starters are often fast finishers.

Teenagers often go fast.

The minute you think you know everything you need to know, you're dangerous.

The more rigid the Birth Plan, the higher the incidence of cesarean section.

The mother of the laboring woman suffers most.

Use your car for hospital transports; forget ambulances.

Wear 100 percent cotton. Blood comes out if you soak it in cold water first.

And Murphy's Law of Midwifery: Women begin labor when it's least convenient for everyone, especially the midwife.

Appendix II:
Home Birth Supplies

Contents of my birth kits, which weighed a total of 45 lbs.:

Home Visit Bag:
> Ultrasound Doppler fetoscope and regular fetoscope
> Adult and baby stethoscopes
> Blood pressure cuff
> Baby exam bag: thermometer, tape measure, cord clamp cutter
> Erythromycin eye ointment and Vitamin K
> Nitrazine paper, Doppler gel

Blue Plastic Tackle Box:
> *Top tier:*
> > Pitocin and Methergine
> > Syringes, needles, IV intercaths, and alcohol swabs
> > Ammonia ampoules, Ketostix, and Dextrostix
> > Penlight and scrub brush
> > Spare batteries for pager, Doppler, and penlight
> *Second tier:*
> > Xylocaine and suture material
> > Cord clamps
> > Tubes for collecting cord blood
> > Infant airway and rescue blanket
> *Main compartment:*
> > Gloves (sterile and unsterile) and KY jelly
> > 4 x 4 sterile gauze packets
> > Amnihooks
> > Big mirror
> > Baby scale and flannel sling
> > Sterile instruments:
> > > 2 Mayo clamps, 2 scissors, sponge stick, needle holder, pickups

Box of Extra Supplies:
    IV setup and 2 bags of IV solution
    Blood drawing supplies
    Ambu bag
    Box of utility gloves
    Extra gloves, 4 x 4s, amnihooks, etc.

Oxygen tank. Masks for mother and baby

Supplies Provided by Home Birth Couples:

    Birth Kit ordered from Cascade Health Care Products:
        http://www.1cascade.com
    Plastic mattress protector and 2 sets of bed sheets
    Flashlight and spare batteries
    6 receiving blankets, wrapped in pairs in aluminum foil
    Pan for receiving the placenta
    Baby diapers and clothes

Appendix III:
Studies on Midwifery Safety

Butler J, Abrams B, Parker J, et al. Supportive Nurse Midwife Care is Associated with a Reduced Incidence of Cesarean Section. Am J Obstet Gynecol 1993; 168: 1407–13

Chambliss LR, Daly C, Medearis AL, et al. The Role of Selection Bias in Comparing Cesarean Birth Rates between Physician and Midwifery Management. Obstet Gynecol 1992; 80:161–65.

Davis L, Reidman G, Sapiro M, Minogue J et al. Cesarean Section Rates in Low-Risk Private Patients Managed by Certified Nurse-Midwives and Obstetricians. J Nurse Midwifery 1994; 39:91–97.

Gabay N, Wolfe S. Encouraging the Use of Nurse-Midwives: A Report for Policymakers. Public Citizen's Health Research Group, Washington DC, 1995.

Gruelich B, Paine LL, McClain C, et al. Twelve Years and More Than 30,000 Nurse Midwife Attended Births: The Los Angeles County–University of Southern California Women's Hospital Birth Center Experience. J Nurse Midwifery 1994; 39:185–96.

Harvey S, Jarrel J, Brant R, Math M, et al. A Randomized Controlled Trial of Nurse-Midwifery Care. Birth 1996; 23 (3): 128–35.

Hueston WJ, Rudy MA. A Comparison of Labor and Delivery Management between Nurse Midwives and Family Physicians. J Fam Pract 1993; 37:449–54.

Hundley VA, Cruickshank FM, Lanf GD, Glazener CMA et al. Midwife Managed Delivery Unit: A Randomized Controlled Comparison with Consultant Led Care. BMJ 1994; 309:1401–4.

Kennell J, Klaus M, McGrath S, et al. Continuous Emotional Support during Labor in a US Hospital: A Randomized Controlled Trial. JAMA 1991; 265:2197–201.

Levy B, Wilkinson F, Marine W. Reducing Neonatal Mortality Rates with Nurse-Midwives. Am J Obstet Gynecol 1971; 109:50–58.

MacDorman MF, Singh GK. Midwifery Care, Social and Medical Risk Factors, and Birth Outcomes in the USA. J Epidemiol Community Health 1998; 52:310–17.

Miller CA. Maternal and Infant Care: Comparisons between Western Europe and the United States. Int J Health Serv 1993; 23:655–64.

National Commission to Prevent Infant Mortality. Troubling Trends Persist: Short-changing America's Next Generation. Washington, DC: National Commission to Prevent Infant Mortality, March, 1992.

Paine LL, Scupholme AS, DeJoseph JF, Strobino DM. Nurse-Midwifery Care for Vulnerable Populations in the United States: The Final Report. The American College of Nurse-Midwives, Washington, DC, 1993.

Public Citizen's Health Research Group. Encouraging the Use of Nurse Midwives. Washington DC: Public Citizen's Health Research Group, 1995.

Rooks JR. Midwifery and Childbirth in America. Temple University Press, Philadelphia, 1997.

Taffel S. Midwife and Out-of-Hospital Deliveries, United States. Vital Health Stat Series 21 No. 40. Hyattsville, Maryland: National Center for Health Statistics, 1984.

Thompson JB. Safety and Effectiveness of Nurse-Midwifery Care: Research Review. In: Rooks J, Haas J (Eds). Nurse-Midwifery in America. ACNM Foundation, Washington DC, 1986.

Toward Improving the Outcome of Pregnancy: The 90's and Beyond. March of Dimes Birth Defects Foundation, 1993.

Turnbull D, Holmes A, Shields N, et al. Randomized, Controlled Trial of Efficacy of Midwife-Managed Care. Lancet 1996; 348:213–18.

Wagner M. Midwifery in the Industrialized World. Journal SOGC 1998; 20(13):1225–34.

Wagner M. Pursuing the Birth Machine: The Search for Appropriate Birth Technology. ACE Graphics, Sydney, 1994 (Available in North America at ICEA Bookcenter, tel 1-800-624-4934).

Yankou D, Petersen BA, Oakley D, et al. Philosophy of Care: A Pilot Study Comparing Certified Nurse Midwives and Physicians. J Nurse Midwifery 1993; 38:159–64.

Appendix IV:

Statistics on the Economics of Midwifery

United States Birth Statistics
Compiled by Marsden Wagner, MD, Consultant for World Health Organization
Reprinted with permission of Dr. Marsden Wagner, April 2001.

1. Percent of countries providing universal prenatal care that have lower infant mortality rates than the US: 100%
2. Percent of US births attended by midwives: 4%
3. Percent of European births attended by midwives: 75%
4. Number of European countries (Great Britain, France, Germany, Netherlands, Belgium, Denmark, Sweden, Norway, and Finland—all with over 75% of midwife-attended births) with higher perinatal mortality rates than the US: 0
5. Average cost of midwife-attended birth in the US: $1,200
6. Average cost of physician-attended birth in US: $4,200
7. Health care cost savings if midwifery care were utilized for 75% of US births: $8.5 billion/year.
8. Health care cost savings by bringing US cesarean section rate into compliance with WHO recommendations: $1.5 billion/year.
9. Health care cost savings by extending midwifery care and demedicalizing births in the US: $13–20 billion/year.

Appendix V:
Resources

National Organizations

American College of Nurse Midwives (ACNM)
818 Connecticut Ave. NW Suite 900 Washington, DC 20006
(202) 728-9860
http://www.acnm.org

Midwives Alliance of North America (MANA)
(888) 923-6262
http://www.mana.org

American College of Psychoprophylaxis in Obstetrics (ASPO)
"The Lamaze Method"
1200 19th Street, NW, Ste. 300, Washington, DC 20036–2412
(800) 368-4404 or (202) 857-1128
http://www.lamaze-childbirth.com/2000/testing_home2.html

American Academy of Husband-Coached Childbirth (AAHCC)
"The Bradley Method"
Box 5224 Sherman Oaks, CA 91413–5224
(800) 422-4784
http://www.bradleybirth.com

Books

Immaculate Deception (Suzanne Arms)—a classic
Spiritual Midwifery (Ina May Gaskin)—a classic
A Midwife's Story (Penny Armstrong)—memoir
Diary of a Midwife (Juliana Van Olfen-Fehr)—memoir
A Midwife's Tale (Laura Thatcher Ulrich)—biography
Midwives (Chris Bohjalian)—novel
The Midwife (Gay Courter)—novel

Witches, Midwives, and Nurses (Ehrenreich and English)
—sociological study
Any of Sheila Kitzinger's books

Mail-Order Products

Cascade Health Care Products (catalog of supplies for professionals
and parents)
141 Commercial N.E. Salem, OR 97301–3402
(800) 443-9942 or (503) 371-4445
http://www.1cascade.com

For aspiring midwives:

Paths to Becoming a Midwife by Jan Tritten
http://www.midwiferytoday.com/books/paths.asp

The paths to midwifery are as diverse as birthing women; this book is
unique because it doesn't insist that one path is inherently superior.
This complete book on midwifery education helps make sense of the
many options available. In this book of many voices and many
philosophies, over 125 resources, organizations, and Web links are
listed.

Appendix VI:

Sandi's Famous Caramels

2 cups white sugar
1 cup light brown sugar
1 cup light corn syrup
1 cup heavy cream
1 cup half-and-half
1 cup butter
4 teaspoons vanilla extract
1 cup chopped walnuts
Optional: chocolate for melting and dipping

You'll also need:

> a very accurate candy thermometer
> a 4-quart heavy-gauge pot
> a 9 x 9 baking pan

Combine all the ingredients except the vanilla and the nuts in a heavy-gauge 4-quart pot. (It is imperative that the pot be at least this large, because the mixture expands dramatically in volume; if it boils over, your stove will never recover.) Stir until the sugar dissolves and the butter melts.

Reduce the heat. Attach the candy thermometer to the side of the pot and cook, stirring frequently, until the thermometer reaches 240° F. Watch closely to prevent its boiling over.

After the thermometer reaches 240° F, stir constantly to avoid scorching on bottom of pan and cook until the thermometer reaches 248° F exactly. This whole process will take 35 to 60 minutes.

Remove from the heat at once and let stand 1 minute. Stir in the vanilla extract and the nuts. Quickly pour into the buttered 9 x 9-inch pan. Cool for a couple of hours.

Dip the bottom of the pan into a shallow tray of very hot water and turn the caramel slab onto a cutting board. Cut into large or small squares. Wrap individually in wax paper or dip individually into melted, highest-quality chocolate and store in the refrigerator.

Makes 2½ pounds candy, or 70 to 100 pieces, depending on size